D1447300

Laboratory Medicine:
Essentials of Anatomic and Clinical Pathology

Second Edition

John H. Dirckx, M.D.

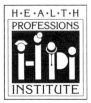

Health Professions Institute • Modesto, California • 1995

Laboratory Medicine:
Essentials of Anatomic and Clinical Pathology
by John H. Dirckx, M.D.

Second Edition

©1995 by Health Professions Institute
First edition ©1991 by Health Professions Institute

Cover: Liver showing changes of portal cirrhosis; trichrome stain. Microscopic slide courtesy of Robert W. Purvis, Sr., M.D., Modesto, Ca. Photomicrograph courtesy of Stan W. Elems, Modesto, Ca.

Published by

 Sally C. Pitman • Health Professions Institute
P.O. Box 801 • Modesto, California 95353-0801
Phone (209) 551-2112 • Fax (209) 551-0404
E-mail: hpi@hpisum.com • Web site: http://www.hpisum.com

ISBN 0-934385-61-0

Printed by
Parks Printing & Lithography • Modesto, California

Last digit is the print number: 9 8 7

For my
daughter Anne
with love

Contents

List of Tables

Page

Foreword to the Second Edition

The exhaustion of two printings of the first edition of this book has provided an opportunity to amplify and update the text. This second edition contains new material on amniotic fluid embolism, the Bethesda system for reporting cytologic findings, cytogenetic tumor markers, disseminated intravascular coagulation, fetal alcohol syndrome, placental abnormalities, TORCH infections, and Wegener's granulomatosis, as well as new entries for more than a dozen pathogenic microorganisms (Chapter 11) and a new tabulation of the effects of selected chemical poisons (Chapter 14). In addition, sections have been rewritten to reflect newer concepts of the pathology of asthma and peptic ulcer and of the role of human papillomavirus in genital cancer.

Expressions of dimensions and quantitative laboratory data have been revised to conform with current SI (Système International) guidelines. Concentrations of analytes are given in both grams (or submultiples) per unit of volume and, following in square brackets, in moles (or submultiples) per liter, thus: serum glucose, 60–115 mg/dL [3.3–6.4 mmol/L].

Again I thank the editorial staff of Health Professions Institute for their diligent and vigilant assistance. I am particularly indebted to Randy Drake for so smoothly and expeditiously incorporating the new material into this edition, and for his tactful and creative interventions. Thanks also to Sally Pitman and Ellen Drake for their proofreading skill.

Foreword to the First Edition

This survey of the principles, practice, and terminology of pathology has been designed to serve the needs of several classes of users.

For the physician and medical student it provides a concise review of essential topics in anatomic and clinical pathology with no admixture of the esoteric, the theoretical, or the trivial.

For professional and practical nurses, physician's assistants, and other healthcare workers whose training does not include formal exposure to pathology, it supplies useful background information in logical, coherent sequence.

Medical transcriptionists, medical secretaries, records clerks, insurance clerks, attorneys, and others will find this a valuable resource for tracking down the significance and bearing of pathologic terms with a minimum of effort.

In striving throughout for maximum conciseness of presentation, I have presupposed some familiarity on the part of the reader with basic medical terms and concepts. I have, however, provided an extensive coverage of histology and microscopic anatomy, without which any discussion of anatomic pathology would be largely unintelligible. An exhaustive index and a supplemental glossary enable this book to be used as a dictionary of pathology. Review questions have been included at the end of each chapter for the convenience of students.

Although most users of this book will probably find some parts of it superfluous, I venture to hope that few will feel that anything essential has been left out.

It is a pleasure to acknowledge with gratitude the valuable support and guidance of Sally Pitman, Sue Turley, and Linda Campbell of Health Professions Institute during all phases of the production of this book.

Part I

A Survey of Pathology Practice

1

The Scope and Divisions of Pathology

Pathology is the branch of medicine that studies the structural and functional changes produced in the living body by injury or disease. The application of pathologic information to medical practice occurs at several levels.

First, pathology is one of the principal basic sciences, along with anatomy, biochemistry, physiology, and pharmacology, learned during the preclinical years of medical school. Physicians' approaches to the evaluation, diagnosis, and treatment of a patient are conditioned more or less strongly by their fund of knowledge regarding the effects wrought by specific diseases on the structure and function of specific organs and tissues.

Second, in their efforts to learn the nature, cause, and extent of disease in a particular patient, and also to assess the effects of treatment, physicians may subject various tissues, fluids, or other materials removed from the patient's body to pathologic examination. Tests of blood and urine are part of any thorough diagnostic evaluation. Organs and tissues removed during surgical procedures are routinely submitted to a pathologist for gross and microscopic study. The information obtained from this study helps to confirm the preoperative diagnosis and, in cases of malignancy, to determine the extent of disease and the adequacy of surgical removal.

A third application of pathology to practical medicine occurs when an autopsy is performed to discover the cause of the patient's death and to correlate the medical history with postmortem findings. Besides providing data for official certification of the cause of death, autopsy findings may have great legal importance—for example, in a case of suspected homicide. In addition, information about the cause of death and the precise nature of the patient's disease contributes to the unending learning process of the treating physician

3

and of other health professionals who attend the autopsy as an educational experience.

Under ordinary circumstances, autopsies and pathologic examinations of tissue specimens are performed by pathologists—physicians with postdoctoral training and certification by the American Board of Pathology. The pathologist's examination of specimens is not limited to naked-eye inspection but also includes microscopic examination and perhaps chemical or other testing. For this reason, pathology is a laboratory-based specialty, and the majority of pathologists perform at least a part of their professional activities in hospitals.

The practice of pathology is divided into three principal branches. **Anatomic pathology** is concerned with the gross and microscopic changes brought about in living human tissues by disease. **Clinical pathology** refers to the laboratory examination of bodily fluids and waste products such as blood, spinal fluid, urine, and feces. **Forensic pathology** involves the application of knowledge comprised by the other two branches to certain issues in both civil and criminal law. The practice of forensic pathology is largely confined to official settings. The standard pathology residency lasts four years, the training time being variously divided between anatomic and clinical pathology. Pathologists who serve as medical examiners, coroners, or forensic consultants usually have additional training in forensic pathology.

Much of the day-by-day work in clinical pathology is done by medical technologists. These are specially trained nonphysicians who, under the supervision of a pathologist, perform routine laboratory examinations of blood, urine, and other fluids, and prepare tissue specimens for microscopic examination by a pathologist. Clinical pathology is discussed in Part V.

The bulk of this volume is concerned with anatomic pathology. Certain terms related to this field deserve clarification here. **Histology** is a division of anatomy concerned with the microscopic study of tissues. **Microscopic anatomy** applies the materials and methods of histology to specific organs and bodily structures. **Cytology** is the study of cells. **Histopathology** refers to the study of microscopic changes in tissue induced by disease or injury. **Histochemistry** is a specialized field in which chemical properties and reactions of tissues are observed microscopically. **Electron microscopy** is the study of specimens with an electron microscope, which uses a stream of electrons instead of a beam of visible light and allows much greater magnification than the light microscope used for routine laboratory work. In practice, the term **histology** is often applied to the whole range of laboratory techniques used in preparing slides of tissue specimens for microscopic study by a pathologist. **Cytology** is often used in the narrow sense of a study of cells that have been detached from a surface for microscopic study, as in a Pap smear. The pathologist's report of an autopsy or of examination of a tissue specimen is customarily dictated for subsequent transcription. This is in keeping with the usual practice of preserving permanent medical records in typewritten form. Typed records are more legible and more suitable for photocopying and microfilming than hand written records and generally take up less space. In reporting the findings, a pathologist ordinarily describes not only the abnormal features of the specimen but also identifying anatomic characteristics, gross and microscopic. This practice not only serves to document the thoroughness of his assessment, but also is necessary for a complete diagnostic appraisal of the specimen. Suppose, for example, that a surgeon submits a specimen for pathologic study which he believes to be a mesenteric lymph node but which is in fact just a mass of fat and connective tissue. If the pathologist merely states that the specimen contains no malignant cells or other signs of abnormality, without making it clear that it is not a lymph node, his report could seriously mislead the surgeon in his further management of the case.

Having described his gross and microscopic findings, the pathologist usually records a diagnosis or diagnostic impression, summarizing and coordinating those findings in the light of his specialized knowledge and experience. The diagnoses listed at the end of an autopsy report may number ten, twenty, or more. The diagnoses may be accompanied by code numbers referring to some standard system of disease nomenclature. In a case of malignancy, the pathologist's diagnosis will often include an estimate of the extent of the malignant process according to a standard grading or staging system.

Review Questions

1. Define *pathology*. Name and define its three principal branches.
2. Distinguish *histology, microscopic anatomy,* and *cytology.*
3. What information does a pathologist's report contain besides a record of abnormalities found in the specimen? Why?

2

The Gross Examination of Tissue

The purpose of this and the next three chapters is to present an overview of what anatomic pathologists do and how and why they do it. The materials examined by an anatomic pathologist fall into two major classes: specimens taken from living patients, and autopsy specimens. At autopsy it is feasible to remove vital organs such as the heart and the liver in their entirety and subject them to thorough, destructive dissection. Specimens from living patients are necessarily limited in type and volume. Such specimens are either tissues or organs removed during surgical operations or samples of material (biopsy specimens) removed from the living body for the purpose of examination.

Whereas the pathologist himself obtains and selects autopsy material for examination, specimens from the living patient are generally obtained by other physicians and submitted for study to the pathologist. Virtually all tissue specimens, regardless of how and by whom they are obtained, are subjected to certain routine procedures. As soon as possible after being removed from the body, the specimen is placed in a glass, plastic, fiberglass, or aluminum bottle, jar, or bucket containing a fluid called a **fixative**. The fixative has several purposes: to arrest the process of decomposition that begins almost at once in devitalized tissue, to kill bacteria and fungi in or on the specimen, and to begin hardening the tissue to facilitate preparation for microscopic study.

The most commonly used fixative is a 10% aqueous solution of formalin. Because formalin is made by bubbling formaldehyde gas through water, it is often called simply "formaldehyde." Formalin is inexpensive and highly suitable for most purposes. However, several other fixatives are available and may be preferred for special applications. The following list includes most of the fixatives in general use as well as certain chemicals that are included in the formulas of several fixatives.

absolute alcohol	Gendre's solution
acetic acid	glacial acetic acid
acetone	glutaraldehyde
Altmann's solution	Helly's Zenker-formalin solution
Bouin's solution	Jores's solution
buffered formalin	Kaiserling's solution
Carnoy's solution	Maximow's solution
Carson's solution	Millonig's phosphate-buffered
chlorpalladium	formalin
chromic acid	Müller's solution
Delafield's solution	neutral (buffered) formalin
Flemming's solution	osmic acid
formaldehyde	osmium tetroxide
formalin	picric acid
formalin-alcohol	potassium bichromate (or
formalin-ammonium bromide	dichromate)
formol-Müller's solution	Tellyesniczky's solution
FU−48 Zenker's solution	Zenker's solution

In performing an autopsy, the pathologist removes organs one by one and subjects them to an immediate gross examination, opening them with a knife and inspecting their internal features. In this way he can observe any abnormalities of size, shape, color, or consistency and any nodules, injury, hemorrhage, degeneration, scarring, or other significant local changes. In addition, he can select those portions of the organ most likely to be useful for microscopic study.

The pathologist's initial examination of a surgical or biopsy specimen is usually performed after the specimen has been placed in fixative. Although the fixative alters the color and consistency of the tissue to some extent, gross pathologic features can still generally be recognized. Occasionally specimens are brought directly from the operating room to the pathologist without being placed in preservative or fixative.

The pathologist performs his examination at a cutting board, which protects the top of the workbench from knife cuts and from the chemical action of fixatives. He handles the specimens with rubber gloves or with forceps, soaking up excess fluid with paper towels or other absorbent materials. He uses scalpels, razor blades, and scissors to open specimens for further examination and to trim them to the proper size for processing. One dimension, at least, of the trimmed specimen must be no more than 3–4 mm to allow penetration of processing chemicals. The trimmed pieces of tissue are placed in small flat round or oblong cassettes of perforated metal or plastic with lids of the same material, in which they will remain during the first stages of processing.

The pathologist dictates his findings during or immediately after the gross inspection and cutting of surgical specimens. This dictation typically follows a set pattern:

Identification of the Specimen

The dictation always begins with basic identifying data: the patient's name as shown on the label of the container and on the laboratory requisition accompanying the specimen, and a general indication of what material has been submitted. At every step in the handling of a specimen, care is taken to ensure that it is correctly identified. The container in which it is placed by the pathologist, surgeon, or operating room technician is labeled with the patient's name, the nature of the specimen, and often the date, the name of the person obtaining the specimen, and other information. Alternatively, a serial number or accession number may be assigned to the specimen container and the pertinent data kept in a register. If only one specimen is taken during an operation, as in an appendectomy, it may be unnecessary to identify it other than by the patient's name. When anatomically indistinguishable specimens are submitted, such as abdominal lymph nodes taken from several areas and possibly containing metastatic malignancy, they must be kept carefully separated and distinguished as to their origins.

In removing a specimen, the surgeon may cut it to a certain shape to indicate its origin or its orientation in the patient's body. Orientation may also be indicated by placement of a suture (surgical stitch) at a certain place in the specimen, such as at the uppermost point of a tumor excised from the skin. In cutting autopsy specimens from paired organs such as the lungs and the kidneys, the pathologist may indicate by the shape of the specimen which side it came from— for example, triangular for left, square for right.

After identifying the specimen, the pathologist may include clinical information (patient's medical history) in his dictation if this is available to him; often it is entered on the requisition.

Dimensions

The size of each specimen as submitted is usually determined and recorded in three planes in metric units (cm or mm). Solid organs or tumors may be weighed, if practicable, and the weight recorded in grams (g). The volume of any contained fluid (as in a cystic cavity) may be measured or (more often) estimated, and recorded in milliliters (mL) or cubic centimeters (cm³).

Gross Description

The pathologist then describes the physical features of the specimen, with particular attention to any abnormalities such as swelling, hemorrhage, scarring, or tumor. The description typically includes mention of the color, texture, and consistency of both the exterior and the cut surfaces of the specimen. Any well-defined abnormality (nodule, cyst, ulcer, perforation, scar, pigmentation) is measured as precisely as possible. Not only the exact size and location of any tumor, but also its relation to the margins of the surgical specimen, must be carefully determined to document the adequacy of removal.

Microscopic examination of certain kinds of surgical specimens is routinely omitted unless the pathologist's gross examination shows abnormalities needing further study. Surgically removed tissues that are not usually sectioned for microscopic study include hernia sacs, blood clots, varicose veins, healthy bone (e.g., a section of rib removed for access to thoracic organs), and teeth. If microscopic examination will not be done, the pathologist dictates a diagnostic impression at the conclusion of his report on gross findings.

Because the tissue specimens taken by the pathologist in the autopsy room are generally too large to be handed over directly to a histology technician for preparation of microscope slides, these specimens are subjected to further examination and selective cutting in the pathology laboratory, just as with surgical specimens. Ordinarily, however, the pathologist does not dictate a report after this second inspection and cutting of autopsy specimens, since gross findings are included in the report of the autopsy.

Review Questions

1. What are some reasons for placing tissue specimens in a fixative solution?
2. What is the most widely used fixative?
3. When the pathologist has completed the gross examination of a surgical specimen, what does he do with the tissue?
4. What are some ways by which a surgeon might indicate the origin or anatomic orientation of a specimen taken for pathologic study?
5. Name some kinds of surgical specimens that are not routinely sectioned for microscopic study.

3

The Histopathology Laboratory and the Microscopic Examination of Tissue

The preparation of microscope slides from a gross tissue specimen is a complex and exacting process consisting of many steps, some of which are performed by automatic machinery. The process actually begins when the specimen is placed in fixative. As mentioned earlier, the fixative arrests decomposition and hardens tissue. Before the tissue can be cut into transparent sections, it is necessary to make it still harder by replacing its water content with a rigid material such as paraffin or cellulose. (Bone, however, is too hard for sectioning. A specimen containing bone must be decalcified with either dilute acid, an ion exchange resin, or a chelating agent, or by electrolysis, before it can be processed. The same is true of teeth and soft-tissue specimens such as sclerotic arteries and scar tissue containing calcium.)

When the paraffin method is used, the tissue specimen is first dehydrated by immersion in a graded series of solutions of an organic solvent such as acetone, Cellosolve, ethyl alcohol, or isopropyl alcohol, which replaces the water. The dehydrated tissue is then immersed in a clearing agent such as xylene (xylol), benzene, cedarwood oil, or chloroform, which replaces the dehydrating agent and renders the tissue transparent. Certain agents (dioxane, tetrahydrofuran) can serve as both dehydrating and clearing agents. After clearing, the tissue is transferred to a bath of melted paraffin, which replaces the clearing agent and infiltrates the tissue spaces. When this infiltration is complete, a technician removes the specimen from the paraffin bath with warmed forceps and embeds it in a cube-shaped mold containing fresh melted paraffin.

When the mold has cooled, the result is a block of paraffin inside which the tissue is embedded with all its water replaced, and its empty spaces filled, by paraffin. This paraffin block is then trimmed to

Stains and Staining Methods, Mordants, Decolorizers, and Other Materials Used in Processing Histologic Sections

acetic acid
acid alcohol
acid-fast bacilli (AFB) stain
acid fuchsin
acid phosphatase
Alcian blue
alizarin
alpha-naphthol esterase
alum-carmine
ammonium silver carbonate
amyloid stain
aniline blue
auramine-rhodamine fluorescent
  stain
azocarmine
azure
basic fuchsin
Best's carmine stain
Biebrich scarlet stain
Bielschowsky's stain
Bodian stain
Brown-Brenn Gram stain
Brown-Hopp tissue Gram stain
Bullard's hematoxylin
Cajal's gold sublimate
Cajal's trichrome
carbolfuchsin
carmine
Celani's method
Congo red
cresyl fast violet
crystal violet
Dane and Herman keratin stain
Darrow red
Davenport's stain
Delafield's hematoxylin
Del Rio Hortega's method
Dieterle's silver stain

DOPA (dihydroxyphenylalanine)
  stain
Ehrlich's acid hematoxylin
elastic (elastin) stain
eosin
eosin azure
eosin-phloxine
fast blue
fast green
fast red
ferric ammonium sulfate
ferric chloride
Feulgen's method
Fite-Faraco stain
Fontana-Masson stain
Fontana's methenamine-silver stain
Foot's reticulum stain
Fouchet's reagent
fuchsin
Gallego's method
gentian orange
gentian violet
Giemsa stain
Gill's hematoxylin
Gimenez stain
gold chloride
Golgi's stain
Gomori's aldehyde fuchsin
Gomori's methenamine-silver
  (GMS)
Gram's stain
Gridley's stain
Grocott's methenamine-silver
Hale's iron stain
Harris's hematoxylin
Heidenhain's iron hematoxylin
hemalum
hematoxylin

Stains and Staining Methods, Mordants, Decolorizers, and Other Materials Used in Processing Histologic Sections

Hiss capsule stain
Holmes's silver nitrate
Holzer's method
hydrochloric acid
India ink
indigo carmine
iron hematoxylin
iron stain
Janus green B
Jenner's method
Jones's kidney stain
Kernechtrot
Kinyoun's acid-fast stain
Kleihauer-Betke stain
Langeron's iodine solution
Levine's alkaline Congo red
   method
lithium carbonate
lithium-carmine
Lorrain Smith stain
Lugol's solution
Luna modification of Bodian stain
Luxol fast blue
malachite green
Mallory-Azan stain
Mallory's iron stain
Mancini's iodine technique
Marchi's method
Masson's trichrome stain
May-Grünwald-Giemsa stain
Mayer's mucicarmine
methyl violet
methylene blue
Milligan's trichrome
mucicarmine
mucin stain
myeloperoxidase
naphthol-ASD chloroacetate
   esterase

naphthol green B
neutral red
Nissl's method
nuclear fast red
oil red O
orange G
orcein
osmic acid
osmium tetroxide
oxalic acid
Pap (Papanicolaou) stain
Pappenheim's stain
Paragon stain
Perdrau's method
periodic acid-Schiff (PAS) stain
peroxidase stain
phloxine
phosphomolybdic acid
phosphotungstic acid
phosphotungstic acid-hematoxylin
   (PTAH)
polychrome methylene blue
potassium metabisulfite
potassium permanganate
Protargol
Ramón y Cajal's stain
Ranson's pyridine silver stain
rapid mucin stain
reticulin stain
Romanowsky's stain
safranin
scarlet red
Scharlach R
Schiff's solution
Scott's solution
Seller's stain
Shorr's trichrome
silver nitrate
silver stain

Stains and Staining Methods, Mordants, Decolorizers, and Other Materials Used in Processing Histologic Sections

Snook's reticulum stain	Turnbull blue
sodium bicarbonate	Unna's stain
sodium bisulfite	uranium nitrate
sodium hydroxide	van Gieson's stain
sodium thiosulfate	Verhoeff's elastic stain
Sudan black	von Kossa's calcium stain
Sudan black B fat stain	Warthin-Starry stain
Sudan III	Wayson's stain
tetrachrome	Weigert's iron hematoxylin
thionin	Weigert-Pal method
Tilden's stain	Weil's myelin sheath stain
toluidine blue	Wilder's reticulum stain
trichrome stain	Wright's stain
Truant's auramine-rhodamine stain	Ziehl-Neelsen acid-fast stain

appropriate dimensions and cut on a microtome, a precision instrument on the order of an electric meat slicer, which makes transparent slices that are only about 5 microns (0.005 mm) thick. For technical reasons, sections are usually made by cutting across the broadest flat surface of the tissue specimen, unless the pathologist has given special instructions for an edge cut or cross section. Usually only one or two sections from each paraffin block are chosen to be made into slides. Sometimes serial sections (for example, every tenth or twentieth slice) are taken so as to provide the pathologist with a three-dimensional concept of a tissue or lesion.

Immediately after cutting, the paraffin sections are floated on a bath of warm water, which helps to smooth out wrinkles and curled edges. Each section is affixed to a separate microscope slide (a thin strip of clear glass about $1'' \times 3''$) by means of a film of albumin solution or other suitable adhesive. The slides are identified with labels bearing names or numbers matching those of the containers in which the gross specimens were submitted.

Substances other than paraffin are sometimes used to infiltrate and embed tissue for sectioning. With Carbowax, which is water-soluble, the dehydration and clearing steps can be omitted. However, obtaining satisfactory sections with Carbowax demands a high degree of technical skill. Celloidin is a suspension of a cellulose derivative in a volatile solvent. Because infiltration and embedding with celloidin do not require heat, there is less distortion of tissue than with the paraffin and Carbowax methods. However, celloidin takes much more time; as much as a month may elapse between fixation and sectioning. Commercially available embedding media besides Carbowax include Epon, Paraplast, and Parlodion.

Microscopic examination of the slide at this stage would yield little information, because all of the tissue spaces are filled with the infiltrating medium. This must be removed and replaced with water or some other suitable fluid by a reversal of the procedures used in making the block. Once the infiltrating agent has been removed and the tissue section rehydrated, the slide is immersed in one or more coloring solutions called stains. These impart a more or less intense coloration to the tissues, which greatly facilitates microscopic examination.

Seldom is only a single color applied. As will be explained further in a later chapter, different stains have affinities for different components of tissue, depending on their chemical properties. Hence it is usual to apply at least two contrasting colors. The use of standard combinations of stains enables the pathologist to recognize normal and abnormal microscopic features of tissue consistently and confidently.

In practice, staining usually involves a number of steps besides immersion of the prepared slide in a coloring agent. First a **mordant** may be applied to render the tissue chemically more receptive to staining. Many fixatives have mordant properties. After the first stain has been applied, the slide is immersed in or washed with a **decolorizer**, which removes stain from all parts of the tissue to which it has not become chemically bound. The slide is then treated with a **counterstain** of a contrasting color, which is taken up by tissues decolorized in the preceding step. A **polychrome** stain is a mixture of two or more coloring agents in one solution. With a polychrome stain, differential staining of tissue components takes place even though the tissue is exposed to all of the coloring agents simultaneously. A **metachromatic** stain is one that changes color on becoming chemically bound to certain tissues.

By far the most commonly used combination of stains for routine histopathology work is hematoxylin and eosin (H&E). Hematoxylin is a deep blue stain which imparts various shades of blue and purple to cell nuclei and other tissue components of slightly acidic nature. Eosin stains most of the other components pink to red. Many special stains and techniques are available to bring out certain features (nerve tissue, reticular fibers, lipid material, pathogenic microorganisms) that are not shown by routine stains. In submitting a tissue block to the histology technician, the pathologist may write instructions regarding the use of special stains. Some staining operations can be done by automatic machinery, but often part or all of the staining process is performed

Sample Pathology Report

TISSUE NO: DATE:
PATIENT: AGE:
SURGEON: HOSPITAL NO:
PHYSICIAN: ROOM NO:

CLINICAL DIAGNOSIS: Multiple skin lesions
PREOPERATIVE DIAGNOSIS:
POSTOPERATIVE DIAGNOSIS:
HISTORY AND OPERATIVE FINDINGS:
TISSUES: #1. Lesion, right thumb   #2. Lesion, right thigh
               #3. Lesion, left elbow   #4. Lesion, left forearm

GROSS: The specimen is submitted in four parts. Part #1, right thumb, is an ellipsoid portion of cutaneous tissue measuring $1.5 \times 1.0 \times 0.2$ cm, centrally showing sessile white papillary lesion measuring $0.3 \times 0.3 \times 0.1$ cm, sectioned and totally submitted "A."

Part #2, right thigh, is an ellipse of skin measuring $1.3 \times 0.5 \times 1.0$ cm, centrally showing an ovoid brown papillary lesion measuring $0.2 \times 0.2 \times 0.2$ cm, sectioned and totally submitted "B."

Part #3, left elbow, consists of a cutaneous ellipse measuring 1 cm on which is mounted an ovoid tan papillary lesion measuring $0.3 \times 0.2 \times 0.1$ cm, totally submitted "C."

Part #4, left forearm, consists of a cutaneous ellipse measuring $0.8 \times 0.5 \times 0.3$ cm, centrally showing a poorly defined gray area of roughened epithelium, totally submitted "D."

MICROSCOPIC: Sections of the first specimen, right thumb, show a centrally thickened epidermis with basal layer of hyperplasia, acanthosis, marked focal hyperkeratosis. Atypical changes are not evident.

Sections of the second specimen, right thigh, show sections of cutaneous tissue with centrally thickened epidermis, showing acanthosis and focal marked hyperkeratosis.

The third specimen, left elbow, shows sections of cutaneous tissue with a centrally slightly thickened epidermis showing acanthosis and rounded keratin inclusions.

The fourth specimen, left forearm, shows sections of cutaneous tissue with a slightly thickened epidermis showing slight acanthosis, basal pigmentation, rounded keratin inclusions. None of the sections show malignant change.

DIAGNOSIS: SPECIMEN #1: BENIGN SQUAMOUS PAPILLOMA.
               SPECIMEN #2: BENIGN SQUAMOUS PAPILLOMA.
               SPECIMEN #3: SEBORRHEIC KERATOSIS.
               SPECIMEN #4: SEBORRHEIC KERATOSIS.

manually. Slides are placed vertically in tall narrow glass containers called Coplin jars, which are filled with stain or other solutions.

After staining and drying, the tissue section on the slide is ordinarily protected with a cover slip, a very thin sheet of glass about ⅛" square. A film of balsam or other mounting medium is first placed over the tissue section, and the cover slip is gently dropped into place. The balsam eventually hardens around the edges, but under the cover slip it remains fluid indefinitely, preserving the section in a clear, homogeneous, refractile medium. Mounting media in common use are Apathy's medium, (Canada) balsam, Clarite, and Permount.

In most laboratories, slides are available for the pathologist's examination 24 to 72 hours after the tissue is removed from the body. Processing is speeded and simplified by the use of automated machinery that dehydrates, clears, and infiltrates tissue during the night. The preceding day's specimens are then embedded, sectioned, and stained on the following morning.

The pathologist examines or "reads" slides with a light microscope, using various magnifications as needed. The standard magnifications are scanning power (×35–50), low power (×100), and high power (×450–500). The greater the magnification, the more the detail that can be distinguished, but the smaller the zone of tissue that can be viewed without moving the slide. After reviewing the slides, the pathologist dictates his microscopic findings and then states one or more diagnoses or diagnostic impressions.

Since gross and microscopic reports are dictated on different days, they are seldom transcribed at the same session. Ordinarily the gross report is transcribed on the top half of a standard surgical pathology form. This transcription is made available to the pathologist when he examines the slides of the tissue. His dictation of microscopic findings and diagnosis is then transcribed on the bottom half of the form, and the form is returned to him for his review and signature.

Review Questions

1. Why must embedding of tissue in paraffin be preceded by dehydration and clearing?
2. What is meant by making serial sections of a specimen?
3. Define or explain: *counterstain, mordant, polychrome stain.*

4

Biopsies, Smears, Aspirations, and Frozen Sections

The term **biopsy** refers to the removal of tissue from a living patient for pathologic examination. Many factors, including the location of the tissue to be studied, the presumptive diagnosis, and the patient's general condition, influence the choice of a biopsy procedure. The following general discussion of biopsy procedures will be supplemented with more specific information in later chapters.

An **excisional biopsy** is the surgical removal of an entire tumor, lesion, or diseased organ from a living patient. The difference between the surgical removal of a tumor or abnormal tissue—which is routinely submitted to a pathologist for examination—and an excisional biopsy is merely one of viewpoint, the latter phrasing emphasizing the diagnostic intent of the procedure. Many surgical pathology specimens are, in effect, excisional biopsies. The term **incisional biopsy** refers to the surgical removal of part of a tumor, lesion, or diseased organ for pathologic study. Incisional biopsy may be preferred to complete removal of an abnormal tissue or organ for technical or cosmetic reasons, and of course total excision of a vital organ or tissue is never feasible.

In addition to these "open" biopsy procedures, a number of techniques have been devised for removing small pieces of tissue for study without making a surgical incision. These techniques are often performed by physicians who are not surgeons—sometimes even by the pathologist who will examine the specimen. A **punch biopsy** consists of the removal of a plug of skin or mucous membrane with a cylindrical punch 2–5 mm in diameter. In a **shave biopsy**, a thin layer of skin consisting mostly or entirely of epidermis is removed with a blade held approximately parallel to the surface. **Curettage** is a surgical scraping. Sometimes it is done for therapeutic reasons, as in curettage of the uterine lining for excessive menstrual bleeding. Curettage of a

17

lesion on any accessible surface may also be done to procure biopsy material. Tissue may also be snipped or snared from the lining of an internal organ or cavity with an instrument passed through an endoscope (a hollow tube with light source and optical system for the examination of internal organs such as the trachea and bronchi, the esophagus and stomach, the colon, and the bladder). **Needle biopsy** of the liver and kidney are standard procedures. A biopsy needle consists of two parts, an outer hollow cannula of large bore that is passed through the skin directly into the organ to be studied, and an inner cutting needle that slices and removes a core of tissue.

All of the biopsy procedures discussed above yield specimens of tissue that, however small and fragmentary, can be embedded and sectioned in the routine manner already described. Other standard techniques for sampling living tissue yield specimens that require special processing before they can be examined microscopically.

The term **smear** refers generically to any type of laboratory study in which material is thinly spread over the surface of a microscope slide for examination. A smear may consist of blood, sputum, feces, pus, or any other liquid or semi-solid material, and it may either be examined in its natural state or stained to show cellular details, microorganisms, parasites, or foreign material. A smear may be air-dried or it may be sprayed with or immersed in fixative before further processing or staining. Most examinations of smears pertain to clinical rather than to anatomic pathology. However, when a smear consists of cellular material removed from the body by scraping or aspiration, it is stained in much the same way as a slide made by sectioning a block of tissue, and may be examined by an anatomic pathologist.

A **Pap** (for Papanicolaou) **smear** consists of a relatively small number of cells detached from a mucous surface (most often the uterine cervix) with a wooden spatula, a suction pipette, a fine brush, or any other suitable instrument, spread on a slide, and stained to show changes in cells. **Fine-needle aspiration** is a technique used to remove cells by suction from certain structures such as the prostate, subcutaneous lymph nodes and other neck masses, and breast masses. The material obtained is smeared on a slide and stained in the same way as a Pap smear. Another way of obtaining cells for study is by **washing** a surface, such as the interior of the stomach, with saline or some other suitable fluid and collecting the washings. This method can be used to obtain cellular material from the respiratory tract and many parts of the digestive tract. Sometimes gentle brushing is used to augment the yield of cells.

Various normal and abnormal body fluids—cerebrospinal fluid, amniotic fluid, joint fluid, and pleural, pericardial, and peritoneal effusions—can be withdrawn from the body by aspiration with needle and syringe and subjected to cytologic study, as well as other examinations such as culture and chemical analysis. When it is desired to subject a clear fluid with a low cell count to cytologic study, the cells may be concentrated by centrifugation or separated by filtration.

Spinning the fluid in a centrifuge drives the cells to the bottom. The resulting sediment can either be smeared on a slide or processed as if it were a solid piece of tissue, yielding a cell block of paraffin. Alternatively, the fluid may be forced through a filter with very fine openings that trap the cells. The filter paper is then mounted on a slide and stained like a tissue section. In the Nuclepore method, fluid is forced through a filter under pressure; in the Millipore method it is drawn through by suction.

The majority of biopsies and cytologic studies are done in cases of suspected or known malignancy in order to clarify the nature and extent of disease. In examining an excisional biopsy specimen, one of the pathologist's main concerns is to determine whether all abnormal tissue has in fact been excised. Hence he pays close attention to the periphery of the specimen, and in preparing the tissue for embedding and sectioning he selects and orients the material in such a way that microscopic examination can verify whether or not all abnormal tissue is surrounded by an adequate margin of normal tissue. These findings will guide the surgeon in determining what further treatment is appropriate—chemotherapy, radiation therapy, more surgery, or simply observation.

Sometimes a surgeon needs feedback from the pathologist while an operation is actually in progress. The histologic character of a tumor may determine whether the surgeon can be content with simple excision or whether he must proceed at once with a more radical removal of tissue. When the resection of a malignancy involves extensive, mutilating surgery, the surgeon may choose to remove tissue in stages, submitting a specimen from each stage for pathologic study before deciding whether to close the incision or remove more tissue. Clearly, the routine methods of preparing specimens for histologic study cannot be used in this setting because of time limitations.

The **frozen section** technique makes it possible for a pathologist to perform a histologic examination of tissue within minutes after it is removed from the patient. This method substitutes rapid freezing of the water in the tissue for infiltration and embedding with paraffin or another artificial medium. The tissue may be frozen solid on a chilled platform called a **cryostat**, and then sectioned with a microtome in the usual way. With the **freezing microtome**, tissue is placed on a perforated stage, frozen with blasts of carbon dioxide gas, and sectioned in place with a blade that is an integral part of the instrument. Frozen sections are mounted on slides and stained rapidly. There is more distortion of tissue than with routine methods of slide preparation, and some histologic details are poorly shown, but sufficient information can be gleaned for the immediate purpose. Tissue examined by frozen section is always submitted for routine processing as well.

Review Questions

1. Define *biopsy* and distinguish several kinds of biopsy.
2. What is a smear?
3. What two methods can be used to obtain cells for study from fluids with low cell counts?
4. What is the principal advantage of the frozen section technique?

5

The Autopsy

The autopsy, necropsy, or postmortem examination (sometimes called simply a "post") is the pathologic examination par excellence. During an autopsy, every part of the body can be opened and exhaustively studied, and any organ or tissue can be removed as necessary for processing and microscopic evaluation. Fluids and other materials are readily collected for culturing, chemical testing, and other clinical pathologic studies.

The purposes of the autopsy were set forth briefly in a previous chapter. In nearly every case, the chief reason for doing an autopsy is to determine as precisely as possible the cause of death. It may already be known with a fair degree of certainty on clinical grounds that death was due, for example, to myocardial infarction or to irreversible brain damage sustained in an automobile accident. But an autopsy provides objective anatomic evidence to confirm the clinical diagnosis and to show the exact pathophysiologic mechanism of death. Sometimes two life-threatening conditions are both present at the time of death—for example, severe pneumonitis and meningitis, both due to pneumococcus. The autopsy may supply information as to which condition actually proved lethal. Occasionally the autopsy discloses an unsuspected cause of death—for example, fatal hemorrhage from a peptic ulcer in a patient under treatment for acute myocardial infarction.

An exhaustive search for the cause of death may seem like misplaced effort, since no amount of information generated by an autopsy can bring the patient back to life. But the attempt to secure full, detailed, accurate information about the cause of death is not a mere academic exercise. In every jurisdiction in the United States, a death certificate listing the cause of death must be signed by a physician and filed with the authorities before a dead body may be embalmed and buried or cremated. Although by no means are all deaths investigated by autopsy, certification of the cause of death is more likely to be accurate and complete in those that are. The validity of public health statistics compiled from data entered on death certificates depends on the caution, diligence, and thoroughness with which the certifying physicians investigated the cause of death.

In certain cases (homicide, suicide, fatal accident, death due to poison or drug overdose, and others), the law requires that an autopsy be performed by or under the auspices of a coroner or medical examiner. In addition, an autopsy may be ordered by legal authorities when a person dies during the first 24 hours after hospital admission or after surgery, or when a person with no known health problems dies suddenly. Data supplied by a medicolegal autopsy may become evidence in a criminal prosecution, a wrongful death suit, or both. Statistics on accidental death gleaned from coroners' reports have been used to support legislation concerning, for example, automobile seat belts, motorcycle helmets, drunk driving, and legal drinking age.

In a teaching hospital (one whose mission includes the training of residents, medical students, nurses, and other health professionals), the autopsy serves as a unique learning experience. Physicians at all levels of training can profit by attending autopsies. Organs and tissues removed at autopsy may be preserved and reviewed days later at a pathology conference. Microscope slides made from these tissues may be used as teaching aids for years. For the physician or physicians who were responsible for the treatment of the patient, the autopsy provides invaluable, if not always comforting, feedback on the thoroughness and accuracy of diagnostic evaluation and the appropriateness of treatment. When death occurs in the postoperative period, an autopsy may show that it resulted from surgical complications or errors of technique. Recently implanted grafts, heart valve replacements, pacemakers, and other materials or devices must be examined for signs of rejection or malfunction. When death follows the use of any experimental treatment, an autopsy is of crucial importance.

Except in those cases where an autopsy is mandated by law and performed by a coroner or medical examiner, written permission must be obtained from the next of kin before an autopsy can begin. The law makes special provision for autopsy permission when the deceased had no known family. Generally it is the responsibility of the attending physician to solicit and obtain autopsy permission. However, the pathologist must assure himself that a permission has been duly signed and witnessed before performing any examination of the body; otherwise he could be subject to legal reprisals for unauthorized mutilation of the dead. The permission form may restrict the pathologist to certain procedures only. For example, permission to open the skull may be withheld. Because microscopic examination of autopsy specimens is an integral part of the examination, the form must specify that the pathologist may remove and retain such tissues and body parts as he deems necessary.

Autopsies are performed in a hospital department set aside for this purpose. The autopsy room or morgue is usually located on a ground floor adjacent to a loading area for the convenience of undertakers, and is equipped with refrigerated lockers for the storage of bodies pending autopsy or removal. Strong illumination and adequate ventilation are essential. The autopsy is performed on a specially designed operating table provided with running water and suction equipment. Attached to the table or immediately available in the room is a cutting board for the gross examination of organs as they are removed from the body. A scale is provided for weighing organs, and graduated containers for determining the volume of fluids. The instruments used are similar to surgical instruments—scalpels, scissors, forceps, clamps, and, for cutting bone, electric saws, chisels, and hammers. In addition, a knife with a very long flat blade is used to cut sections of uniform thickness from large organs such as the spleen and kidney. Specimen containers prefilled with fixative are on hand for immediate preservation of tissues removed.

The subject of an autopsy may be called the body, the cadaver, the deceased or decedent, the patient, the remains, or the subject. The person performing the autopsy is called the prosector, the dissector, the operator, the autopsy surgeon, or simply the pathologist. He is usually assisted by a morgue attendant or diener (German *Diener* 'servant'), who looks after the autopsy facility and its equipment, moves bodies to and from the autopsy table, and helps with the actual autopsy procedure as needed.

The autopsy room is usually equipped with a pedal-activated dictating machine so that the pathologist can dictate his findings while performing the autopsy. An autopsy report or protocol so dictated will naturally follow the sequence of examination procedures as they are actually done. This sequence varies from one prosector to another and may be modified in individual cases for various reasons. In virtually all cases, however, the autopsy follows the same basic plan.

After confirming the identity of the body by means of a wrist tag, a toe tag, or both, and satisfying himself that a valid consent for the performance of the autopsy has been given in writing, the pathologist weighs the body, if equipment is available for that purpose, and determines its length from crown to heel. The entire body surface is inspected and palpated, and note is made of the color and consistency of the skin, the color and distribution of head and body hair, any deformities, swellings, or injuries (open wounds, discolorations, needle punctures), surgical or traumatic scars, and any other departure from normal and expected appearances. The presence of endotracheal tubes, intravenous lines, and catheters is noted. **Rigor mortis** refers to the stiffening of the muscles that comes on within a few hours after death and passes off after another few hours. **Livor mortis** (postmortem lividity, hypostasis) is a purplish discoloration of the skin due to engorgement of capillaries that occurs shortly after death. Lividity affects whatever parts of the body are lowermost, but does not appear in areas of the skin that have been in firm contact with a supporting surface.

The eyes and the cavities of the mouth, nose, and ears are inspected for evidence of disease, injury, or foreign material. If the eyes have been removed to provide corneal transplants, this fact is noted. The external genitalia are inspected for developmental abnormalities and signs of disease or injury. The body is turned over for inspection of the back and anus.

The thoracic and abdominal cavities are now opened. The prosector makes a Y-shaped incision through the skin and subcutaneous fat of the anterior body surface, the extremities of the Y being at the two shoulders and the pubic region. Some operators make the upper limbs of the Y above the breasts and nearly parallel to the clavicles; others cut below the breasts. Over the thorax the scalpel cuts all the way through skin and fat to the underlying breastbone and ribs. Below the level of the breastbone the operator inserts two fingers into the peritoneal cavity and lifts skin, fat, and peritoneum away from the abdominal organs so that they will not be injured as he carries the incision down to the pubes (veering around the umbilicus).

The skin is retracted from the line of the incision on each side and dissected free of the underlying tissues until wide flaps have been reflected. The thickness of the subcutaneous fat is noted and recorded. The breasts and axillary structures are examined from within and specimens are cut from any abnormal or suspicious areas. The ribs and clavicles are then cut through near their attachments to the breastbone, and the front of the bony thorax is removed in one piece.

The thoracic and abdominal organs are first inspected in their natural positions and then removed for further study. The membranous surfaces of the thoracic and abdominal cavities—pleura, pericardium, peritoneum, diaphragm, omentum—are examined for abnormalities of color or texture, adhesions, or tumors. Any blood or fluid in a body cavity is noted and if possible measured. Each organ is severed from its attachments, weighed, and opened. As the heart is removed, ligatures are placed around the stumps of the great vessels to facilitate embalming of the body by the undertaker. The intestine is removed in its entirety from just below the stomach to just above the rectum. Both solid and hollow organs are opened for inspection of internal detail. Selected features—for example, the thickness of the walls of the cardiac chambers—are measured.

Representative pieces of tissue from each organ are immediately placed in fixative. Entire organs may be preserved in large jars or buckets of fixative if they are needed for a pathology conference or "organ recital" to be held later. Blood may be withdrawn directly from the chambers of the heart for testing. Specimens may be taken for culture or other laboratory procedures, and the contents of the digestive tract may be submitted for chemical analysis. Before incising a solid organ to take material from inside for a culture, the prosector sears the surface with a hot spatula to destroy any microorganisms there, which might contaminate the culture. Any solid material removed from the body and not needed for subsequent study is placed in a large plastic bag, which is sealed at the conclusion of the autopsy and placed inside the body before it is closed.

If an examination of the brain ("head post") is to be performed, the operator makes an incision across the top of the head from ear to ear, turns flaps of scalp forward and backward, and removes the top of the skull like a cap by cutting around it with an electric saw and detaching the cap with a chisel. The brain and its membranes are observed, and any swelling, deformity, tumor, or hemorrhage is noted. The brain is cut free of its attachments and placed intact in fixative. Because brain tissue is extremely soft in its natural state, it is usually allowed to harden in fixative for several days before being cut for gross and microscopic study. If necessary, the spinal cord or specimens of bone can be removed by further manipulation of the saw and chisel. At the conclusion of the autopsy, the attendant sews the incisions shut with heavy thread or cord in a continuous or "baseball" stitch and washes the body.

Occasionally an autopsy is performed on a body that has already been embalmed. In this case, the pathologist's examination will disclose evidence of the embalmer's activities. Embalming consists of two basic procedures: replacement of the blood in the circulatory system with a preservative fluid that incidentally imparts to the skin a cosmetically acceptable hue, and introduction of a similar fluid into the thoracic and abdominal cavities through one or more punctures made with a hollow instrument. Before instilling cavitary fluid, the embalmer removes as much as possible of the contents of the digestive tract by suction through the instrument. After the instrument is withdrawn, the skin puncture site is closed with a plastic plug to prevent leakage.

Review Questions

1. List several reasons for performing an autopsy.
2. What two points must always be verified by the pathologist before an autopsy is begun, except in a forensic setting?
3. What is postmortem lividity?
4. Which major organ is sometimes removed but not opened at the time of autopsy? Why?

Part II

Normal Anatomy and Histology

6

The Cell

The essence of anatomic pathology practice is observing and interpreting changes or variations from the normal or expected appearance of tissues. Hence the pathologist must be intimately familiar with the gross and microscopic features of normal, healthy tissue, and pathology reports typically contain many references to such features. This and the next two chapters provide a concise survey of gross and microscopic anatomy, with emphasis on terminology. This material will be referred to constantly throughout the rest of the book.

For purposes of description and discussion, the human body is divided into several **systems**, each having a general biological function. For example, the function of the digestive system is to take in nutrients and dispose of associated wastes. Each system is composed of **organs**. An organ is defined as an anatomically differentiated and isolated structure with a specific function. Each of the organs that compose the digestive system—esophagus, stomach, small and large intestines, salivary glands, liver, gallbladder, pancreas—has its specific role in the overall process of digestion.

Organs are composed of **tissues**, each of which, when subjected to microscopic examination, is found to have a characteristic and more or less homogeneous composition. The stomach, for example, consists of three concentric layers, each containing a different type of tissue. The innermost layer is a lining of mucous membrane; the intermediate layer is a sheath of muscle; and the outermost layer is a coating of connective tissue.

A tissue is made up of **cells**. The cell is the smallest and simplest independent unit of living matter. Although all cells have certain features in common, many are highly specialized in structure and function. The cells of the lining of the stomach, for example, can be divided into undifferentiated columnar epithelial cells, which serve mainly as structural units or building blocks; chief cells, which produce pepsin; parietal cells, which produce hydrochloric acid; and goblet cells, which produce mucus.

This division and classification of bodily structures is not absolute. For example, the pancreas belongs to the digestive system because it produces digestive enzymes, but it also belongs to the endocrine system because it secretes insulin. Some regard the skin and even the blood as organs; others would call the skin a tissue and the blood simply a body fluid. But for practical purposes, the breakdown into systems, organs, tissues, and cells works well.

The Cell: General Features; Mitosis. The cell is both the structural and the functional unit of all living things, plant and animal. Each cell is isolated from its surroundings by an enclosing membrane. Each cell, given the proper environment and nutrients, is capable of carrying on all the vital functions proper to it, independently of other cells. Generally speaking, the function or action of a tissue is simply the aggregate of the functions or actions of its cells. The term **protoplasm** is used as a generic designation for all living material, without regard to its organization into cells or tissues.

It is convenient to start by discussing an ideal or typical cell, and then to consider how various types of cells are modified in structure for specific functions. Within each cell is a fluid called **cytoplasm**, a colloidal suspension of proteins, amino acids, carbohydrates, and electrolytes in water. The cell membrane is neither an impermeable barrier nor a biologically inert one. It allows water and substances of low molecular weight such as sodium, calcium, glucose, and amino acids to pass into and out of the cell. Only in special circumstances, however, can it be traversed by more complex substances such as enzymes and nucleoproteins. Moreover, the cell membrane actively "pumps" certain substances in and others out. This accounts for the higher concentration of potassium in a living cell than in its immediate environment, and the lower concentration of sodium.

The most conspicuous internal feature of a cell is generally its **nucleus**, a dense and roughly spherical mass of protein, DNA, and RNA, which controls such cellular functions as energy metabolism and protein synthesis. The nucleus also contains the genetic coding that determines what kind of cell this is, and that will be passed on to any daughter cells formed from it. Although all cells in the human body contain in their nuclei the genetic coding received from parental sperm and ovum, only spermatozoa and ova have the capacity to transmit this genetic material to a new individual. The **nucleolus** is a sharply defined body containing RNA that is often visible within the nucleus.

The growth of any tissue or organ comes about mainly through an increase in the number of its cells. An adult has more cells, not larger cells, than a child. In cell multiplication, one cell divides into two identical daughter cells, each of which is endowed with a full complement of genetic material, and nothing except these daughter cells remains of the parent cell. As a preliminary to cell division, the nucleus undergoes a splitting of its genetic material into two equal portions. In this process, which is called **mitosis**, the normally tangled chromatin material composing the nucleus separates into clearly distinguishable bands of DNA called **chromosomes**.

The appearance of these "mitotic figures" in many of the cells of a tissue indicates that the tissue is actively growing or developing. Most cells retain throughout life their ability to undergo mitosis and cell division when this is necessary for growth, the repair of injury, or the replacement of dead or diseased cells. Nerve cells of the central nervous system, by exception, lose their ability to reproduce even before fetal development is complete.

Other structural elements besides the nucleus can be seen in the cytoplasm of some cells. These, collectively known as organelles or organoids, include mitochondria, microsomes, the central body or centrosome, and the Golgi apparatus. Much of the ultrastructure of the cell can be seen only by electron microscopy, and is therefore not germane to routine pathology work. However, standard histologic preparations often show cytoplasmic granules that are characteristic of certain cells. In addition, the cytoplasm of some cells may contain pigment, fat globules, or minute bubbles of air or gas called vacuoles.

Cells: Variation in Structure, Function, Arrangement, and Staining Properties. While many cells are strictly limited by their genetic makeup to a single form and function, others have the capacity to undergo marked changes in type and structure to meet the evolving needs of the tissues in which they reside. Some cells are capable of traveling or migrating through tissue in response to various chemical stimuli. For example, neutrophils in great numbers can move from the blood through capillary walls and into injured or diseased tissue as part of an inflammatory response. Cells that are actively motile in a fluid medium are said to show ameboid movement—that is, movement like that of the amebas, one-celled animal organisms. In ameboid movement an extrusion of the cell called a pseudopod is first put forward, and then the rest of the cell "flows" into it.

In most tissues, cells are arranged in sheets, strands, clusters, tubules, sacs, or other characteristic patterns depending on their function. These groups of cells are held together by bands or bridges of protein between their membranes. The term **syncytium** refers to a complex of originally distinct cells that have fused to form a continuous mass of protoplasm with many nuclei but no intervening cell membranes. Cells are surrounded by or immersed in an intercellular fluid similar in composition to cytoplasm. This serves as a medium for the diffusion of nutrients, oxygen, and wastes in appropriate directions. Many tissues contain large proportions of noncellular material. For example, connective tissue consists largely of fibers formed by cells but structurally distinct from them. In some tissues, such as the outer (cornified) layers of the skin, cells that have lost their nuclei and ceased to live remain for a time as essential structural elements.

All of the cells of the body have developed from a single fertilized ovum. This development involves not only a vast increase in the number of cells but also their differentiation into many structural and functional types. As we proceed to a discussion of the various types of cells found in the human body, the reader is urged to keep in mind that cell descriptions are based primarily on the appearance of dead cells that have been chemically preserved, dehydrated, and hardened, sliced into transparent sections, and artificially colored. A histologic finding that results from the technique used to prepare a slide, rather than from any natural or pathologic process, is called an **artifact**. Vacuolation, shrinkage, and distortion of cells are often artifactual rather than pathologic in origin.

As noted earlier, most tissues do not take up chemical stains evenly. Nuclear material, which is slightly acidic, attracts basic (alkaline) stains such as hematoxylin. Cytoplasm and non-nuclear material attract acidic stains such as eosin. Many cells and tissue components are identified by and named for their staining properties: **eosinophil** 'attracting eosin,' **basophil** 'attracting basic stains,' **chromophobe** 'repelling' (literally, 'fearing') 'color,' **argentaffin** 'having an affinity for silver stains,' and so on.

Review Questions

1. Distinguish *system, organ, tissue.*
2. Describe the basic structural features of a cell.
3. What are mitotic figures?
4. What is meant by the term *artifact* with respect to a histologic section?

7

Histology: The Study of Tissues

The tissues of the body can be divided into a relatively small number of types on the basis of characteristic cells, structural organization, similarity of function, and common embryonic origin. For most purposes, a classification into five tissue types—epithelium, connective tissue, muscle, nerve, and hemolymphatic—is sufficiently specific.

Epithelium

Most of the surfaces in the body, including skin and mucous membranes, the linings of hollow and tubular organs in the digestive, respiratory, and urogenital systems, and the linings of the chest and abdominal cavities, consist of a tissue called **epithelium**. Epithelial tissue is made up almost entirely of cells, with very little intercellular material. Epithelial cells show a marked capacity for regeneration, and in some epithelial tissues, such as the lining of the digestive tract, the turnover under normal conditions is very rapid.

Epithelial cells show considerable variation in shape and arrangement, depending on whether their principal function is to contain, to conduct, or to protect. Epithelial cells are classified according to shape as **squamous** (flat, scalelike), **cuboidal**, or **columnar**. **Simple** epithelium consists of but a single layer of cells; in **stratified** epithelium there are several layers. The term **pseudostratified** is applied to certain simple columnar epithelial surfaces where variation in the positions of nuclei creates the illusion of several layers.

The free surface of an epithelial cell may show modifications of various kinds. For example, the pseudostratified columnar epithelium lining the trachea and bronchi is equipped with whiplike cilia that, by their beating motion, keep the mucus film moving upward toward the pharynx. The brush border of certain cells in the kidney, the striated border of certain cells in the intestine, and the microvilli of cells in

33

several areas are further examples of surface modifications. Underlying a zone of epithelium and separating it from deeper structures is a distinct layer of connective tissue called the **basement membrane**.

Some specialized epithelial cells have **secretory** capabilities. A secretory cell is one that produces a chemical substance whose functions are performed outside the cell. Such cells secrete mucus, digestive enzymes, and hormones. Secretory epithelium is known as glandular tissue, and any structure that is differentiated to produce a secretion may be called a **gland**.

Most glandular cells are cuboidal or columnar in shape. Some contain distinctive cytoplasmic granules representing stored secretions or their chemical precursors. A gland may consist of a single cell, such as the goblet cell, which releases its secretion of mucus directly into the interior of the trachea, stomach, or intestine. Or a group of secretory cells may be arranged in a cup- or flask-shaped **acinus** or **alveolus**. A number of these acini (alveoli) may be disposed around a single duct, which carries away their secretion, and a number of such ducts may unite to form a larger duct.

Throughout the respiratory and digestive tracts are found numerous alveolar glands whose secretions lubricate the lining surfaces. **Serous** glands produce a thin, watery secretion, while **mucous** glands produce a thicker secretion containing the protein mucin. Some gland alveoli contain cells of both serous and mucous types. Glandular structures with ducts (such as the salivary glands and the mammary glands) are called **exocrine**. Glands that release their secretions directly into the circulation (such as the thyroid and adrenal glands) are called **endocrine** or **ductless** glands, and their secretions are called **hormones**.

Certain terms and concepts regarding epithelium need clarification here. The epithelial lining found in most internal organs and ducts is known as **mucous membrane** (membrana mucosa) or simply **mucosa**. A mucous membrane may consist of squamous, cuboidal, or columnar cells. Beneath its basement membrane is a loose connective tissue layer called the **lamina propria**. Most mucous membranes are supplied with mucous glands that keep the surface lubricated. The mucosa of most of the urinary tract, however, despite its name, contains no mucous glands.

The type of epithelium that lines the pericardium, thorax, and abdomen and covers the organs they contain is called a **serous membrane** or **serosa**. Here, again, the term is misleading, for serosal surfaces do not contain serous glands. They are lubricated by a watery fluid filtered from the blood. The type of epithelium found in serosal surfaces is called **mesothelium**, and the type lining blood vessels is called **endothelium**. Both mesothelium and endothelium consist of very thin, flat, polygonal cells, but the terms refer to the location of the epithelium in each case rather than to its structural characteristics.

Connective Tissue

The term **connective tissue** includes bone, cartilage, tendons, ligaments, the dermis or true skin, subcutaneous fat, and many other supporting and investing structures. Connective tissues are, so to speak, the timbers, bricks, and mortar of the body. While varying greatly in composition, all connective tissues have certain features in common. They contain a higher proportion of noncellular material than other tissues, chiefly because bundles and networks of fibers provide more strength, cohesion, and durability than aggregations of living cells. The cells and fibers of connective tissue are embedded in a homogeneous, nonfibrous, gel-like material called **ground substance**, which is distinct from the intercellular fluid also present.

Connective-tissue cells are relatively few in type. The **fibroblast** (or **fibrocyte**) is a large flat cell with several branches or processes that extend through the surrounding tissue and may touch the processes of other fibroblasts. The function of the fibroblast is to produce fibers. In mature, healthy connective tissue, the fibroblasts are few and not especially active. In tissue that is growing or undergoing repair, fibroblasts are more numerous and more active.

Histiocytes (also called **macrophages**) are large cells of irregular shape, with small nuclei. They are at least functionally related to certain other cells found throughout the body and known generically as **phagocytes**. All of these cells have the property of surrounding and engulfing or "swallowing" foreign material, bacteria or other invading microorganisms, and degenerating or diseased tissue elements, which they then break down and remove.

Plasma cells are small, sparsely distributed cells corresponding to cells of the same name found in bone marrow and other tissues. Their function is to produce antibodies. **Mast cells** are large oval cells that produce and store complex chemical substances, including histamine and heparin, for release as needed. Certain tissues contain highly specialized **pigment cells** which produce and store the pigment responsible for the color of the skin and the iris of the eye. Bone and cartilage also contain specialized cells that will be described shortly.

Each connective-tissue fiber is actually a bundle of fibrils. Although fibrils do not branch, fibers do branch and interconnect. Connective-tissue fibers are divided on the basis of their physical characteristics into collagenous, elastic, and reticular. **Collagenous fibers** are larger in caliber and tougher than the other types. **Elastic fibers** are thinner and, as their name implies, more elastic. They show a greater tendency to form webs or lattices. **Reticular fibers** are still more delicate and still more apt to form fine networks. They have an affinity for silver stains but do not show well in routine histologic preparations. Reticular cells, found typically in association with networks of reticular fibers, are probably modified fibroblasts but may be more closely related to histiocytes.

Connective tissue can be divided on the basis of its structural organization into six distinctive types. **Loose** (or **areolar**) **connective tissue** consists of freely woven meshes of fibers with many open spaces filled by ground substance and intercellular fluid. This type of tissue is found in the subcutaneous fascia and in the stroma or structural framework of solid organs such as the liver, kidney, and pancreas. **Dense connective tissue** (also called **regular connective tissue**), which shows a more compact arrangement of fibers in sheets or cords, occurs in ligaments, tendons, and the dermis. **Reticular connective tissue**, consisting of reticular fibers and reticular cells, forms the framework of lymphoid organs (spleen and lymph nodes) and of bone marrow.

Adipose or **fatty tissue** consists mostly of specialized cells packed tightly in a sparse fibrous matrix. Each cell contains a large fat globule, which displaces the cytoplasm and pushes the nucleus against one side of the cell. Fatty tissue serves as a shock absorber and thermal insulator. It is distributed in variable amounts in the subcutaneous tissue and forms cushioning layers around certain organs such as the kidney and the eye.

Cartilage has a highly condensed but elastic ground substance that lends it both toughness and flexibility. Dense aggregations of fibers are embedded in this ground substance. Relatively rare cartilage cells or **chondrocytes** are also seen, each occupying a hollow space or **lacuna** in the cartilage. Chondrocytes have large nuclei and their cytoplasm contains fine granules and fat droplets. They are active in the formation and growth of cartilage but relatively inert in mature tissue. Regeneration of damaged cartilage occurs only to a limited extent.

Three types of cartilage are identified. **Hyaline cartilage**, by far the most abundant, contains collagenous fibers. It is found in the nose, larynx, trachea, and bronchi, and as a covering for the joint surfaces of bones. **Elastic cartilage** (also called **yellow cartilage** from its gross appearance) contains elastic fibers. It occurs in the external ear and the epiglottis. **Fibrous cartilage** (or **fibrocartilage**) features an extremely dense aggregation of collagenous fibers that make it particularly tough. It is found in the intervertebral disks.

Bone derives its unique rigidity from its calcium content. It is formed by the deposition of minute crystals of calcium salts either in a connective-tissue matrix (**intramembranous bone**, as in the cranial vault) or by replacement of hyaline cartilage (**intracartilaginous** or **enchondral** bone, as in the long bones of the extremities). The microscopic structural unit of bone is the **osteon** or **haversian system**, consisting of ten or more thin layers called **lamellae** arranged concentrically around a haversian canal. These haversian canals branch and intersect to serve as passages for blood vessels and nerves. **Osteocytes**, the characteristic cells of bone, appear in lacunae from which radiate numerous fine channels or canaliculi to accommodate the delicate processes extending from the cells. Osteoblasts are cuboidal cells with eccentric nuclei and basophilic cytoplasmic granules, which appear in developing, growing, healing, or regenerating bone. In areas where damaged or diseased bone is being broken down, multinucleated giant cells called osteoclasts are often found. These apparently arise by transformation and fusion of osteoblasts.

Muscle

The third major tissue type is **muscle**. All muscle tissue consists of bundles or sheets of long, narrow cells arranged in parallel and having the capacity to shorten under appropriate electrochemical stimulation. The collective effect of the simultaneous shortening of many thousands of muscle cells is a contraction of the muscle as a whole. Muscle tissue is divided into three distinct types.

Smooth muscle (so called by contrast with striped muscle, to be discussed shortly) consists of long, spindle-shaped cells usually found tightly packed together in sheets. Smooth muscle is also called involuntary muscle because it responds only to stimuli from the autonomic nervous system and is not under voluntary control. Smooth muscle forms part of the walls of tubular and hollow organs, including most of the structures in the respiratory, digestive, and urinary tracts, and of blood vessels other than capillaries. Smooth muscle also appears in the skin (where it is responsible for making hairs stand on end), the iris, and the spleen.

Skeletal, **striped**, or **voluntary muscle** is the type found in the large muscle masses of the trunk and extremities, which hold the body erect and serve for locomotion and other voluntary activities. Each of the voluntary muscles is made up of long cylindrical strands or fibers, which are bunched into groups called fasciculi. Muscle fibers, unlike those of connective tissue, are composed of living cells, several hundred cells sometimes combining to form a single fiber. The term **striped** refers to the fine, regular cross striations that are characteristic of skeletal-muscle fibers. This banded or striped appearance results from the arrangement in alternating layers of two proteins, actin and myosin, which are involved in muscle contraction. Changes in the bulk of a skeletal muscle due to exercise or wasting reflect changes in the size of muscle fibers, not changes in their numbers. Each muscle fiber is covered by a membrane called a **sarcolemma**. The small amount of delicate connective tissue between fibers is known as **endomysium**. **Cardiac muscle**, found only in the heart, makes up nearly the whole of that organ. In microscopic appearance it closely resembles skeletal muscle. A unique feature of cardiac muscle is the presence of **intercalated disks**, which are irregular transverse bands lying at the junctions of two cells.

Nerve

Nervous tissue is the most highly specialized type of tissue in the body, and nerve cells show the most extreme differentiation of structure. The unique property of all nerve cells is to conduct electrochemical impulses. Each nerve cell, or **neuron**, consists of a cell body (or perikaryon) with one or more processes extending from it. These processes, which function like the wires or terminals of an electrical device, are divided into two types. **Dendrites**, relatively short and extensively branching, generally conduct impulses toward the cell body, while **axons**, long and less branched, generally carry impulses away from the cell body. The axon of a spinal cord cell may be more than 50 cm long. Most neurons have relatively large nuclei with prominent nucleoli. In addition, the cytoplasm of neurons contains a coarsely granular basophilic material rich in DNA, which is called **Nissl substance**.

The nervous system is a complex network of neurons, vastly more intricate in its circuitry than any possible computer. Particularly in the central nervous system—the brain and spinal cord—neurons are densely packed together in intimate physical and electrical association. The point where the process of one neuron makes electrochemical contact with the process or body of another neuron is called a **synapse**. A nerve fiber is simply the axon of a nerve cell. Typically these fibers or axons are grouped together, in bundles of hundreds or thousands, to form the nerve tracts within the central nervous system as well as the peripheral nerves extending from it to all parts of the body. **White matter** is nerve tissue in the central nervous system that consists principally of fibers (axons), and **gray matter** is nerve tissue consisting principally of cell bodies. A **ganglion** is a mass of nerve cell bodies adjacent to a peripheral nerve.

In peripheral nerves, each axon is covered by a fine membrane, the **neurilemma** or **sheath of Schwann**, which consists of delicate Schwann cells wrapped around the axon. In addition, some axons carry a coating of fatty material called **myelin** inside the neurilemma. This myelin (or medullary) sheath shows constrictions, the nodes of Ranvier, at intervals along its course where two Schwann cells adjoin. Neurons vary greatly in the type and arrangement of their processes, depending on their function. As noted earlier, nerve cells do not normally undergo mitosis after fetal development is complete, nor can one kind of nerve cell mutate or metamorphose into another type. However, as the central nervous system matures, nerve cell processes extend, become more numerous and more complex, and establish an increasing number of connections with other neurons.

Axons within the central nervous system lack a neurilemma, but other non-nerve cells are present to serve a supporting function. These are known collectively as **neuroglia** or simply **glia**. Neuroglia is seen with difficulty in standard histologic preparations. Glial cells are classified as **astrocytes (astroglia)**, star-shaped cells with many processes, found particularly in the gray matter of the brain and spinal cord; **oligodendroglia**, smaller cells with fewer processes, found in both gray and white matter; **microglia**, very small cells resembling fibroblasts in appearance and having phagocytic functions; and **ependyma**, a columnar epithelium-like tissue lining the cavities of the brain and spinal cord.

Hemolymphatic System

The final class of bodily tissues comprises a group of cells that are found in both the circulating blood and in certain tissues and organs, particularly the bone marrow, the spleen, and the lymph nodes. These may be collectively designated **hemolymphatic** cells.

Blood consists of a fluid called **plasma** in which various cells or "formed elements" are suspended. Plasma, which is mostly water, contains electrolytes (sodium, potassium, calcium, chloride, bicarbonate), proteins (albumin, globulins), nutrients (glucose, lipids, amino acids), wastes (urea, creatinine), and dissolved gases (oxygen, carbon dioxide). Blood clots when fibrinogen (one of the globulins) is activated to form fibrin. Plasma from which the fibrin has been removed is called **serum**.

The formed elements of the blood are classified as red blood cells, white blood cells, and platelets. All of these are formed in stationary organs or tissues and released into the blood as needed. **Red blood cells** or **erythrocytes** are unique among body cells in having no nuclei throughout the entire course of their functional existence. They are formed in bone marrow by repeated divisions of large cells called erythroblasts. Through successive generations, developing erythrocytes become smaller, finally losing their nuclei just before being released into the circulation. The circulating erythrocyte is a round disc with both of its sides slightly hollowed, so that when seen on edge it has a dumbbell profile. The cytoplasm stains lightly with acidic stains. Erythrocytes are elastic and readily compressible. When found in groups they tend to form **rouleaux** (singular, **rouleau**) like stacks of coins.

The function of the erythrocyte is to carry oxygen from the capillaries of the lungs to the capillaries of the rest of the body. Each erythrocyte consists of a colloidal complex of lipid and protein material of which **hemoglobin** is the most important constituent. This iron containing substance, which is responsible for the red color of blood, forms a loose chemical union with oxygen in the lungs and releases it in the tissues. An erythrocyte survives for about 125 days after entering the circulation. Then it disintegrates and is removed from the blood, principally by phagocytes in the spleen, which conserve and recycle its iron content. Breakdown products of hemoglobin that are not recycled are responsible for the color of bile, urine, and feces.

White blood cells (leukocytes) are larger than erythrocytes and much less numerous in circulating blood, the ratio being about 600:1. Unlike erythrocytes, which perform their only function in circulating blood, leukocytes appear in the blood only when in transit from their point of production to their destination in tissues. All leukocytes have nuclei. They are divided into two major classes on the basis of their sites of production.

Leukocytes that are formed, like erythrocytes, in bone marrow are called **myeloid**, while those that are formed in lymphoid tissue are called **lymphoid**. Leukocytes of myeloid origin are further divided into granulocytes, which show conspicuous granules in their cytoplasm, and monocytes, which do not. Granulocytes are also called polymorphonuclear leukocytes because their nuclei are typically divided by shallow clefts into two to five lobes. Granulocytes are subdivided according to the staining properties of their granules into neutrophils, eosinophils, and basophils.

Neutrophils, the most numerous of all white blood cells, have granules that show approximately equal affinity for acidic and basic stains. The function of neutrophils is to engulf and digest devitalized tissue, invading microorganisms, and other foreign material. Within minutes after injury, neutrophils begin to migrate from the blood into the affected tissue. The nuclei of immature neutrophils are elongated but not lobed. Such cells are called **unsegmented neutrophils**, **stab cells**, **band cells**, or simply **bands**.

Eosinophils, normally making up no more than 5% of circulating white blood cells, have coarse granules that attract eosin and other acid dyes. Their function is unknown but their numbers increase in parasitic infestation and allergic disorders, and decrease after administration of adrenocortical steroid drugs. **Basophils** constitute 1% or less of circulating leukocytes. Their coarse granules stain with basic dyes. Their function is unknown. These three types of granulocytes (polymorphonuclear leukocytes) are formed in bone marrow by differentiation of precursor cells called **myelocytes**.

Monocytes are large cells that make up 5–8% of total circulating leukocytes. Their nuclei are large, kidney- or horseshoe-shaped, and eccentrically placed. Monocytes function as phagocytes in tissues, and are perhaps identical with histiocytes.

Lymphocytes, leucocytes of lymphoid origin, are found in lymphoid tissue (spleen, lymph nodes) and in circulating blood. Normally they make up about 25% of circulating white blood cells. Lymphocytes are slightly larger than erythrocytes and have relatively large, dark-staining nuclei. Their function is to produce antibodies.

Platelets are very small round or oval bodies found in circulating blood. They are formed in bone marrow as extrusions from the cytoplasm of giant cells with lobed nuclei called megakaryocytes. Platelets are not cells and do not have nuclei. They function in blood clotting.

Lymphoid tissue is not a separate tissue type. It consists simply of large numbers of lymphocytes in a meshwork of reticular connective tissue. Lymphocytes develop in this tissue by differentiation from reticular cells. Loose aggregations of lymphoid tissue are found in the intestinal wall and other parts of the body. More highly organized masses of lymphoid tissue occur in the spleen, thymus, lymph nodes, and tonsils.

Review Questions

1. What is the general term for the type of tissue that forms coverings and lining membranes?
2. Distinguish *serous* and *mucous* glands.
3. In what kind of structure is endothelium found?
4. What basic type of tissue contains the highest proportion of noncellular material?
5. What is the function of fibroblasts?
6. In what type of tissue are haversian systems found?
7. State two important differences between smooth and skeletal muscle.
8. What type of cell has processes called axons and dendrites?
9. What kind of sheath do some axons have in addition to a neurilemma or Schwann cell sheath?
10. Distinguish *plasma* and *serum*.
11. What are the two major groups of leukocytes?

8

Gross and Microscopic Anatomy: General Concepts

Solid and Hollow Viscera

The preceding survey of the characteristic features of various cells and tissues is intended to serve as a background for more specific details of microscopic anatomy to be given in later chapters. This chapter discusses a few basic anatomic terms and concepts.

The term **viscus** (plural, **viscera**) refers to any of the organs in the thoracic and abdominal cavities. Viscera can conveniently be classed as either solid or hollow organs, each class having its own basic structural plan. It is usual to divide the tissues composing a solid organ such as the liver or the kidney into **parenchyma**, the specialized cells that are unique to the organ and that enable it to perform its function, and **stroma**, the supporting framework of connective tissue. The stroma is also called interstitial tissue. Typically a solid organ is encased in a more or less dense **capsule** of connective tissue, from which **septa** (walls, divisions) or **trabeculae** (bands, strands) or both extend into the substance of the organ, dividing the parenchyma into small but grossly visible **lobules**. The more intimate interweaving of parenchyma and stroma is appreciable only on microscopic study.

Besides the partitioning of tissue into lobules, an organ may have several major structural divisions or lobes. The thyroid gland and the left lung have two, the right lung three, the liver four. The term **hilum** refers to a notch or cleft in the contour of an organ, where arteries, veins, ducts, or other structures enter or leave. For example, a ureter, a renal artery, and a renal vein are attached at the hilum of each kidney. The extremities of a vertically positioned organ may be referred to as **poles**—thus, the upper (or superior) pole of the kidney, the lower (or inferior) pole of the testis.

Inspection of the cut surface of certain organs, such as the kidney and the adrenal gland, reveals two grossly distinguishable zones, an outer **cortex** and an inner **medulla**. The difference in appearance between the two zones results from a different proportion between parenchyma and stroma as well as a different orientation of parenchymal elements.

The hollow interior of a tubular structure such as the aorta, the trachea, and the colon is called its **lumen**. Most hollow and tubular organs are made up of layers of different kinds of tissue. Typically there is a lining of epithelium with its basement membrane and lamina propria; then a layer of smooth muscle, often subdivided into an inner layer with fibers running circumferentially and an outer layer with fibers running longitudinally; and finally an outer coat of connective tissue. The terms **tunica** and **lamina** are used as well as English **coat** and **layer** to designate these structural divisions. In medical parlance the mucous lining of a tubular or hollow structure is often called simply the **mucosa** (for **tunica mucosa**); the muscular layer, the **muscularis** (for **tunica muscularis**); the outer layer, the **fibrosa** (for **tunica fibrosa**) in the case of an organ whose covering blends in with surrounding structures, and the **serosa** (for **tunica serosa**) in the case of an organ covered by a serous membrane.

Membranes, Blood Vessels

The peritoneum covers the entire inner surface of the abdominal cavity and all the organs it contains as one continuous serous membrane. The membranous covering of the walls of the abdominal cavity is called **parietal** peritoneum, and that of the organs is called **visceral** peritoneum. The parietal and visceral pleura respectively line the thoracic cavity and cover the lungs. The parietal and visceral pericardium respectively line the pericardium and cover the heart.

Some notion of the circulation of blood through tissues is necessary for an understanding of many basic concepts in pathology. Virtually every tissue in the body except mature cartilage and the central nervous system is filled with a meshwork of microscopic blood vessels, the capillaries, which deliver oxygen and nutrients and remove carbon dioxide and other wastes. **Arteries** carry oxygenated blood from the left ventricle of the heart to the tissues and organs of the body. The arteries keep branching repeatedly until the branches are of microscopic size. These **arterioles** branch further to become **capillaries**, whose walls are composed of a single layer of very thin epithelial cells (endothelium). Capillaries do not pass straight through tissue but branch repeatedly and join other capillaries to form a network. This arrangement of numerous connections among adjacent vessels is called an anastomosis. The flow of blood through a capillary bed is regulated by arterioles, which act as valves by virtue of the smooth-muscle fibers in their walls. For example, capillary flow in the skin is reduced by exposure to cold, increased by exposure to heat.

The joining together of many capillaries forms a **venule**, and the joining together of many venules forms a **vein**. Veins carry blood back to the heart to be reoxygenated in the lungs. Further details of the anatomy of circulation are given in Chapter 19.

A major artery is usually accompanied along its course by a vein that drains the structure supplied by the artery, and often by a nerve as well. The combination of an artery, one or more veins, and a nerve is called a **neurovascular bundle**. The vascular supply of a solid viscus usually enters at its hilum. Hollow and tubular organs in the abdominal cavity receive their blood supply through a fold of tissue that also anchors the organ to the body wall. For the small intestine this fold is called the **mesentery**. By extension, the prefix **mes(o)-** is used to name attachments of other organs: **mesoappendix**, **mesocolon**.

Sections and Directions

Certain terms in descriptive anatomy refer to imaginary cuts made through the body or through an organ in various planes. In pathology, such terms are sometimes used in this figurative sense and sometimes refer to actual cuts made through an organ or body part with a knife or microtome. A **sagittal** section divides a structure into right and left segments; a **coronal** section, into upper and lower segments; a **frontal** section, into front and rear segments. A **cross** (or **transverse**) section divides an elongated structure at right angles to its long axis (length). A **longitudinal** section divides an elongated structure parallel to its length.

The following terms are used extensively in discussing anatomic relationships:

anterior—front, toward the front of the body.

caudal—lower in the body.

cranial—higher in the body.

distal—further away from the center of the body or some other point of reference. (The thumb is distal to the wrist.)

dorsal—pertaining to or in the direction of the back.

inferior—lower, downward.

lateral—further away from the midline of the body. (The lungs are lateral to the heart.)

medial—nearer to the midline of the body. (The nipple is medial to the axilla.)

posterior—rear, toward the back.

proximal—nearer to the center of the body or some other point of reference. (The wrist is proximal to the thumb.)

superior—upper, upward.
ventral—pertaining to or in the direction of the front surface of the body.

Review Questions

1. Distinguish *parenchyma* and *stroma*.
2. Distinguish *cortex* and *medulla*.
3. What English words are roughly synonymous with Latin *tunica* and *lamina*?
4. What is the difference between visceral and parietal peritoneum?
5. What structures are typically found in a neurovascular bundle?

Part III

General Pathology

9

Pathologic Change and Pathologic Diagnosis

Diagnostic Focus of Pathology

Pathology is a diagnostic science. Although the pathologist's findings and conclusions may strongly influence the course of treatment chosen for a patient, the pathologist himself does not prescribe medicine or perform surgery. His chief concern is to supply diagnostic information to the treating physician. Moreover, he makes no attempt to assess symptoms such as pain, itching, or nausea, but rather confines his attention to those features of disease that can be objectively observed and perhaps even measured.

This emphasis by the pathologist on objective interpretation is reflected in a dual signification for many everyday diagnostic terms. For example, the clinician diagnoses pneumonitis (inflammation of the lung) on the basis of clinical symptoms—fever, chills, cough productive of purulent sputum, and chest pain—and of physical findings such as characteristic sounds heard through a stethoscope. The pathologist diagnoses pneumonitis only when he has seen gross and microscopic evidence of inflammation in lung tissue—something no one is likely to do as long as the patient is alive.

History of Pathology

The historical roots of pathology lie in the dim past when man first speculated about the causes of disease. Primitive peoples with little insight into the workings of nature are apt to attribute disease to evil spirits, divine vengeance, or witchcraft. Our remote ancestors entertained such beliefs, and members of some undeveloped cultures entertain them today.

The Greek physician Hippocrates (460–377 BC) is honored as the father of medicine because he argued that disease is a purely natural phenomenon, subject to rational explanation and amenable to rational treatment. The doctrines of Hippocrates, as modified and augmented by Galen (AD 129–199), dominated Western medical thought until the beginning of the modern scientific era. According to Hippocratic medicine, health depends on a proper balance of four bodily "humors" (blood, phlegm, yellow bile, and black bile), and disease results when there is an excess of one or more of these with respect to the others. This abortive attempt to formulate reasons for the changes that take place when a person gets sick became the basis for a system of therapeutics that relied heavily on phlebotomy (bloodletting) and the administration of violent emetics and cathartics to rid the body of excessive or "peccant" humors.

Developments in anatomy, chemistry, and particularly microscopy during the eighteenth century led to a revolution in pathologic thinking. The old Hippocratic-Galenic theories were rejected in favor of a rigorously scientific pathology based on correlation of symptoms and physical findings with gross and microscopic changes detected on postmortem examination. The pioneer of this new anatomic pathology was an Italian physician and anatomist, Giovanni Battista Morgagni (1682–1771), whose epoch-making work, *The Seats and Causes of Disease,* was published in 1761. The German pathologist Rudolf Virchow (1821–1902) carried the science further by explaining disease in terms of changes in the behavior and interrelations of cells. His *Cellular Pathology* was published in 1858.

It was also during the nineteenth century that the French chemist Louis Pasteur (1822–1895) and the German physician Robert Koch (1843–1910) demonstrated conclusively that some diseases are caused by microorganisms that multiply in the body, produce toxic wastes capable of interfering with normal functions, and induce similar disease on being transmitted to healthy persons.

One of Virchow's most memorable contributions to modern pathologic thinking was his statement, "Disease is life under altered conditions." Although even today we find it hard not to think of a disease as a "thing" that someone "has," disease is merely an abstraction—a state, quality, or condition somehow different from that indefinable state, quality, or condition we call "health." The major premise of pathology is that specific causes of disease are consistently associated with specific changes in bodily structure and function. Often a further premise must be that the specimen of blood, urine, or tissue submitted to pathologic study is representative of what remains in the patient's body.

Changes in form and structure are the province of the anatomic pathologist, while changes in function or activity, as observed or measured through laboratory study of blood, urine, and other body fluids, are the province of the clinical pathologist. The distinction is far from absolute, for each branch of pathology constantly makes use of the data and conclusions of the other. In each branch, a thorough familiarity with what is normal—that is, an appreciation of the full range of variations in form or function that are compatible with health—must precede any attempt to identify abnormality.

The Diagnostic Process

In performing a gross examination of a tissue specimen, the anatomic pathologist looks for departures from expected color, size, shape, surface texture, internal consistency, and homogeneity, as well as for any tumors, cysts, hemorrhage, exudate, tissue death, scarring, or abnormal deposition of materials such as fat or calcium. In examining microscopic sections of tissue he observes the type, size, shape, number, and distribution of cells present, the configuration and staining properties of their nuclei, cytoplasmic granules, vacuoles, or deposits, the type and distribution of intercellular material such as connective-tissue fibers, extravasated blood, fibrinous or other exudates, and any variations from expected tissue architecture.

Arriving at a pathologic diagnosis is not simply a question of recognizing certain patterns that are characteristic of certain diseases. This visual recognition is only the starting point for an analysis of all available data leading to a diagnostic formulation that includes, when possible, the cause of the disorder in this particular patient, its chronology and degree or extent, and its relation to other abnormal conditions, past and present. In examining tissue from a living patient, the pathologist regards the specimen not as a static product of past events but rather as a momentary glimpse of a dynamic process that is still going on.

The diagnosis may be purely local, referring only to the specimen submitted—for example, a basal cell carcinoma of the cheek, completely excised and contained in its entirety in the surgical specimen submitted. On the other hand, assessment of a small piece of tissue may enable the pathologist to diagnose a widespread or systemic condition. For example, certain findings in a lymph node may indicate a malignant process affecting the entire lymphatic system, and certain changes in the kidney may point to a diagnosis of diabetes. More than once, an astute pathologist has diagnosed measles before the rash appeared by finding Warthin-Finkeldey giant cells in an appendectomy specimen.

General pathology is concerned with the investigation and description of classes or patterns of abnormal changes in tissues, regardless of the specific organ or region in which the tissue is located. These patterns of change, which are relatively few in number, will be discussed in the next six chapters.

Review Questions

1. What scientific advances during the 18th and 19th centuries profoundly altered the scope and viewpoint of pathology?
2. What is meant by saying that disease is life under altered conditions?
3. What kinds of change in the gross and microscopic features of a tissue specimen are taken into account by the pathologist in arriving at a diagnosis?
4. What other kinds of information does the pathologist consider?

10

Disorders of Development, Growth, and Nutrition

Disorders of Development

Developmental (or **congenital**) **disorders** are those that are built into the body during fetal development. They may arise from abnormalities already present in the fertilized ovum (hereditary or genetic disorders, such as mongolism and muscular dystrophy), or they may be caused by adverse environmental factors during fetal development (such as fetal alcohol syndrome due to maternal alcoholism, and congenital blindness due to maternal rubella). A developmental disorder may affect only one organ or tissue—indeed, it may be microscopic—or, on the other hand, it may produce striking deformities and lethal or life-threatening dysfunctions affecting the whole body. Abnormal formation of a tissue or organ is called **dysplasia**. (The term is also applied to acquired malformations or changes in cells.) **Hypoplasia** refers to underdevelopment of a structure, **aplasia** to extreme underdevelopment, and **agenesis** to complete failure of formation (congenital absence).

Many genetic disorders exist only at the cellular or biochemical level. These have been called **inborn errors of metabolism.** For example, hemophilia is a hereditary inability to form coagulation factor VIII, a plasma protein needed for normal blood clotting. Sickle cell anemia is a genetically transmitted disorder in which an abnormal hemoglobin (hemoglobin S) is synthesized instead of the normal kind, with the result that erythrocytes are malformed and unduly fragile. Diabetes mellitus is a group of diseases in which the endocrine tissue of the pancreas (the islets of Langerhans) fails to produce adequate insulin for normal carbohydrate use by cells. Even though an inborn error of metabolism may be molecular in nature and difficult or impossible for the anatomic pathologist to detect, it can have wide-

Inborn Errors of Protein Metabolism

Disease	Chemical Defect	Clinical Features	Pathologic Features
Hemophilia A	Failure to form coagulation factor VIII.	Excessive bleeding, hematomas, hemarthrosis, anemia.	
Hemophilia B (Christmas disease)	Failure to form coagulation factor IX.	Excessive bleeding, hematomas, hemarthrosis, anemia.	
Congenital agammaglobulinemia (Bruton's disease)	Failure to form immunoglobulins.	Heightened susceptibility to certain bacterial and viral infections.	Absence of plasma cells, absence of germinal centers in lymphoid tissue.
Sickle cell anemia, sickle cell trait	Formation of abnormal hemoglobin S.	Hemolytic anemia, jaundice, bone and abdominal pain, cardiomegaly, cholelithiasis.	Sickle-shaped erythrocytes, erythroid hyperplasia of marrow, widespread hemosiderosis, thrombosis, infarction.
Thalassemia, thalassemia minor	Defective synthesis of hemoglobin.	Anemia, hepatosplenomegaly, weakness, dyspnea, osteoporosis.	Extramedullary hematopoiesis in liver and spleen.

Inborn Errors of Amino Acid Metabolism

Disease	Chemical Defect	Clinical Features	Pathologic Features
Phenylketonuria (PKU)	Failure to convert phenylalanine to tyrosine.	Mental retardation, seizures, reduced skin pigment.	Incomplete myelination of nerve fibers in brain and spinal cord.
Alkaptonuria	Deficiency of homogentisic acid oxidase.	Dark urine, articular chondritis.	Blue-black pigmentation (ochronosis) of cartilage, tendons, arterial intima.
Albinism	Defect in melanin synthesis.	Absence of pigment from skin, hair, eyes, premature wrinkling of skin, keratoses.	Absence of melanocytes.
Cystinuria	Various abnormalities in metabolism of cystine.	Cystine calculi in urinary tract, obstructive uropathy.	Absence of descending loop of Henle from renal tubules.
Hartnup disease	Impaired transport of mono-amino-monocarboxylic acids.	Photodermatitis, ataxia, tremors, psychiatric disorders.	Erythroid hyperplasia of marrow.
Glucose-6-phosphate dehydrogenase deficiency	Deficiency of glucose-6-phosphate dehydrogenase.	Hemolytic anemia after exposure to primaquine, sulfonamides, nitrofurans, fava beans.	
Maple syrup urine disease (ketoaciduria)	Block in decarboxylation of branched-chain alpha-ketoacids.	Odor of maple syrup in urine, mental retardation, seizures, coma.	

Inborn Errors of Carbohydrate Metabolism

Disease	Chemical Defect	Clinical Features	Pathologic Features
Hurler's syndrome (gargoylism)	Excessive production of mucopolysaccharides.	Short stature, coarse features, skeletal deformities, corneal opacities, hepatosplenomegaly.	Irregular enchondral ossification, distention of fibroblasts and macrophages by mucoid material, mucopolysaccharides in intima of arteries.
Marfan's syndrome (arachnodactyly)	Abnormal formation of connective tissue.	Long, slender habitus, skeletal malformations, subluxation of lens, cataract, cardiomegaly, dissecting aneurysm of aorta.	Medial necrosis of large arteries, cardiac valvular abnormalities, cardiac hypertrophy.
Osteogenesis imperfecta	Abnormal formation of connective tissue.	Blue ocular scleras, fractures of bone after slight trauma, deafness due to otosclerosis.	Thin bone cortex, enlarged haversian canals and canaliculi, spindle-shaped fibroblasts replacing osteoblasts.
von Gierke's disease	Deficiency of glucose-6-phosphatase.	Hepatomegaly, cachexia, hypoglycemia, acidosis.	Glycogen vacuoles in cytoplasm and nuclei of hepatocytes and in renal tubule cells.
Pompe's disease	Deficiency of alpha-glucosidase.	Growth retardation, macroglossia, cardiomegaly, neurologic abnormalities.	Massive deposits of glycogen in skeletal, cardiac, and smooth muscle.
Galactosemia	Deficiency of galactose-1-phosphate uridyl transferase.	Mental retardation, hepatosplenomegaly, cataracts.	Fatty infiltration and cirrhosis of liver.

Inborn Errors of Lipid Metabolism

Disease	Chemical Defect	Clinical Features	Pathologic Features
Tay-Sachs disease (amaurotic familial idiocy)	Deficiency of hexosaminidase A.	Mental retardation, blindness, spasticity, seizures.	Cerebral atrophy, foam cells (macrophages) containing ganglioside.
Gaucher's disease	Deficiency of glucocerebrosidase.	Mental retardation, hepatosplenomegaly, purpura, erosion of bones.	Demyelination of nerve fibers in central nervous system, gliosis, deposits of kerasin in lungs, kidneys, thyroid, adrenals.
Niemann-Pick disease	Deficiency of sphingomyelinase.	Mental retardation, hepatosplenomegaly.	Accumulation of sphingomyelin in liver, spleen; demyelination and gliosis in central nervous system.
Krabbe's disease	Deficiency of galactosylceramidase.	Mental retardation, muscle rigidity, seizures.	Absence of myelin, multinucleate globoid cells, sclerosis of brain.
Fabry's disease (angiokeratoma corporis diffusum)	Deficiency of ceramide trihexosidase.	Telangiectases, corneal opacities, edema, renal failure.	Deposition of globotriaosylceramide in arterial intima and media, myocardium, kidney.

Inborn Errors of Pigment Metabolism

Disease	Chemical Defect	Clinical Features	Pathologic Features
Crigler-Najjar syndrome	Deficiency of glucuronyl transferase.	Jaundice, spasticity.	Bile pigment in basal ganglia (kernicterus), inspissated bile in hepatic canaliculi.
Dubin-Johnson syndrome	Impaired excretion of conjugated bilirubin.	Jaundice, hepatomegaly.	Green, blue, or black liver.
Congenital porphyria	Formation of excessive porphyrin in marrow.	Pink urine, photodermatitis, anemia, splenomegaly.	Redness of bone.

Inborn Errors of Mineral Metabolism

Disease	Chemical Defect	Clinical Features	Pathologic Features
Hemochromatosis (bronze diabetes)	Increased absorption of iron.	Bronze pigmentation of skin, diabetes mellitus, hepatomegaly, hypogonadism, polyarthritis.	Hemosiderin in hepatocytes, Kupffer cells, spleen, pancreas; portal cirrhosis, fibrosis; hepatocellular carcinoma.
Wilson's disease (hepatolenticular degeneration)	Excessive absorption and impaired excretion of copper.	Kayser-Fleischer ring in cornea, splenomegaly, jaundice, spasticity.	Shrinkage and cavitation of basal ganglia, hepatic cirrhosis.
Hypophosphatasia	Deficiency of alkaline phosphatase.	Skeletal defects, bone pain, hypercalcemia, nephrocalcinosis.	Inadequate calcification of osseous matrix.

spread and devastating effects on health. All three of the examples given above are life-threatening diseases.

Numerous inherited metabolic errors have been identified, and no doubt many more exist. The accompanying table of some of the better known ones may be taken as a representative sampling.

During the third week following conception, the embryo differentiates into three primitive layers of cells. Each of these **germ layers** will give rise to a specific group of tissues and organs as development proceeds. The **ectoderm**, or outer layer, forms the epidermis, the nervous system including the specialized sensory structures of the eye and ear, and the enamel of the teeth. The **mesoderm**, or middle layer, forms connective tissue (including cartilage and bone), muscle (all types), the circulatory and genitourinary systems, and the spleen. The **endoderm**, or inner layer, forms the epithelial linings of the respiratory, digestive, and excretory systems, the liver, and the pancreas. Some congenital disorders affect derivatives of only one of these germ layers. Thus an ectodermal dysplasia may result in abnormalities of the skin, the eyes, and the central nervous system.

Further embryonic development involves a complex series of divisions, foldings, and fusions as the basic plan of the body is laid down and the organs begin to form. Any disturbance during this critical period can result in faulty development or in complete fusion. Examples of such disorders are an abnormal communication between two heart chambers, incomplete closure of the spinal column (spina bifida), and cleft palate. Flaws of development may result in zones of essentially normal tissue forming in the wrong places, or in abnormal proportions or combinations of normal tissue. Tissue that appears at an abnormal site is said to be **ectopic** or **heterotopic**. For example, implants of thyroid tissue may appear in the ovary. An abnormal combination of tissues in their normal location is called a **hamartoma**.

Disturbances of fetal development can result from maternal malnutrition or infection or from intrauterine exposure to drugs, chemical poisons, or ionizing radiation. Harmful influences acting early in pregnancy, particularly during the first trimester, typically cause spontaneous abortion or severe fetal malformation (failure of organs or limbs to develop; cardiac and neural anomalies). Once the major organ systems are formed, adverse influences on the fetus can cause defects in tissue differentiation, low birth weight, premature birth, or stillbirth.

A **teratogen** is any substance or condition that can induce congenital malformations. Recognized teratogens include drugs (thalidomide, anticancer agents, hormones), chemicals (lead, ethyl alcohol), and maternal infections that spread to the fetus. Tetracycline antibiotics administered during pregnancy can cause discoloration and

Nutritional Deficiency Syndromes

Nutrient	Clinical Disorder	Pathologic Findings
Vitamin A (retinol, dehydroretinol)	Night blindness, xeroderma, follicular hyperkeratosis.	Atrophy and proliferation of basal cells; squamous metaplasia of epithelium in respiratory and digestive tracts, bladder, uterus.
Vitamin B$_1$ (thiamine)	Beriberi: polyneuritis, tachycardia, edema. Wernicke's, Korsakoff's encephalopathies.	Degeneration of myelin sheaths of peripheral nerves; fragmentation of axons; neuronal degeneration and gliosis in central nervous system; hydropic degeneration of myocardial fibers.
Niacin (nicotinic acid)	Pellagra: dermatitis, glossitis, diarrhea, paresthesias, spasticity, dementia.	Mucosal inflammation and ulceration, atrophy of gastric mucosa, fatty change, and necrosis of liver.
Vitamin B$_6$ (pyridoxine)	Glossitis, polyneuritis, seizures.	
Vitamin B$_{12}$ (cobalamin)	Pernicious anemia: megaloblastic anemia, weakness, weight loss, glossitis. Combined system disease: anesthesia, paresthesias.	Megaloblastic bone marrow, hypersegmented neutrophils, granulocytopenia; patchy degeneration of posterior and lateral columns of spinal cord.
Vitamin C (ascorbic acid)	Scurvy: hyperkeratosis of skin; swollen, bleeding gums; weakness, myalgia, impaired wound healing.	Proliferation of fibroblasts, disorganization of connective tissue, ill-formed capillaries.

Nutritional Deficiency Syndromes (continued)

Nutrient	Clinical Disorder	Pathologic Findings
Vitamin D (calciferol)	Rickets (infants): skeletal deformity, bowing of long bones, hypertrophy of epiphyses. Osteomalacia (adults): softening, deformities, fractures of bones.	Overgrowth of poorly mineralized osteoid, proliferation of fibroblasts, enlarged marrow cavities.
Vitamin K (phytonadione, menaquinone, menadione)	Hemorrhages, petechiae.	
Protein	Kwashiorkor: muscle wasting, hepatosplenomegaly, abdominal distention, abnormalities of hair, skin, and nails, delayed wound healing.	Fatty infiltration of liver, hepatic necrosis, atrophy of pancreatic acini.
Iron	Iron-deficiency anemia: pallor, fatigue, dyspnea, cardiomegaly, edema, glossitis.	Hypochromic microcytic anemia, hyperplastic marrow with reduced stainable iron.
Iodine	Cretinism (infants): mental retardation, macroglossia, skeletal defects. Myxedema (adults): mental impairment, coarsening of skin and hair, hypogonadism. Endemic goiter.	Deposition of mucoid material in subcutaneous tissue, muscle; hydropic degeneration of myocardial fibers. Thyroid gland enlarged, vascular; papillary hyperplasia of follicles.
Fluoride	Increased incidence of dental caries.	

hypoplasia of dental enamel. Intrauterine exposure of a female fetus to the estrogen diethylstilbestrol has resulted in deformities of the genital tract and increased risk of clear cell adenocarcinoma of the cervix or vagina. Fetal alcohol syndrome, which occurs in at least one-half of infants born to women who abuse alcohol chronically during pregnancy, includes mental and growth retardation, spinal defects, cardiac valvular and septal defects, and pixielike facial features (broad flat nose, hypoplastic upper lip, and short palpebral fissures).

The risk of teratogenesis is particularly high with four maternal infections: toxoplasmosis, rubella, cytomegalovirus disease, and herpes simplex, represented by the acronym TORCH. All of these can cause malformations of the brain and the eye. In addition, rubella, which unlike the other TORCH infections does the most damage when contracted during the first trimester, causes malformations of the ear and the heart.

Disorders of Growth and Nutrition

Growth refers generally to an increase in the number of cells rather than to differentiation of cells or increase in cell size. Even when not due to hereditary factors, disorders of growth can begin early in fetal development if the maternal environment is deficient in essential nutrients. Low birth weight is a common feature of many prenatal nutritional syndromes. But most **nutritional disorders** begin after birth. Good health requires a regular intake of water, proteins, carbohydrates, fats, vitamins, and minerals. Dietary deficiencies of any of these during infancy and childhood may result in stunting of growth or in abnormalities of development. For example, inadequate vitamin D intake can lead to rickets, in which bones are improperly formed. Deficient intake of iron at any age can lead to anemia, a shortage of erythrocytes in the circulation. Even when dietary intake is adequate, the absorption of certain nutrients can be blocked by congenital or acquired abnormalities of the digestive system. Such blockages are the basis for several **malabsorption** syndromes. In sprue, for example, the absorption of fat in the small intestine is deficient, so that dietary fat passes out of the body in the stools (steatorrhea).

A general deficiency of all nutrients results in **cachexia** (inanition, starvation), manifested by depletion of fat stores, wasting of muscles, and widespread deterioration of cellular functions. In our culture, overnutrition or exogenous **obesity** is a more frequently encountered threat to health than inanition. In obesity the amount of adipose tissue in the body, particularly in the subcutaneous fat layer, is increased. Obesity is associated with a higher incidence of many diseases, including hypertension, diabetes, coronary artery disease, degenerative joint disease, and some malignancies. The mortality rate in morbid obesity (twice the ideal weight or greater) is ten times that of the nonobese population.

Hormonal factors play a vital role in nutrition and growth. Abnormal increase or decrease of hormone levels due to disease of endocrine glands can induce local or generalized disturbances of growth and development. Growth hormone from the pituitary gland regulates increase in body length and other developmental changes during childhood and adolescence. Deficiency of growth hormone during childhood results in dwarfism. Deficiency of thyroid hormone in childhood causes a nutritional and metabolic retardation known as cretinism. Adrenal disease causing a decline in cortisol levels (Addison's disease) is associated with muscle wasting. The effects of hormone deficiencies are discussed further in Chapter 25.

Hypertrophy and hyperplasia refer to excessive growth or development of a tissue or organ. **Hyperplasia** is an increase in the number of cells or other structural elements, **hypertrophy** an increase in the size of cells or fibers. In practice this distinction is often ignored. Overdevelopment may be hormonally induced. An excessive amount of growth hormone in childhood leads to gigantism, or abnormally increased stature. If growth hormone levels rise only after closure of the growth centers in the long bones, the result is a deforming enlargement of the hands, feet, and face called acromegaly. Overdevelopment can also be genetically induced, as in excessive growth of the long bones in arachnodactyly. Increased local circulation, as in arteriovenous fistula, can cause enlargement of an extremity. Compensatory, adaptive, or reactive hyperplasia occurs when part of an organ (e.g., liver or thyroid) is lost and the remaining part enlarges to compensate for the loss. An organ may hypertrophy to meet increased demands placed on it, as when the muscular wall of the left ventricle thickens to compensate for a leaky mitral valve. **Dystrophy** refers to abnormal (not necessarily deficient) development as a result of inappropriate nutrition. (The term is also applied to congenital or acquired disorders not directly resulting from nutritional causes.) The abnormal transformation of one fully differentiated tissue type into another—for example, the transformation of columnar epithelium into squamous epithelium—is known as **metaplasia**.

Review Questions

1. Distinguish *hypoplasia, aplasia,* and *agenesis.*
2. List some inborn errors of metabolism and describe their effects on health and well-being.
3. What are the three germ layers?
4. Strictly speaking, how does *hypertrophy* differ from *hyperplasia*?

11

Inflammation, Allergy, and Infection

Inflammation

Inflammation is the most basic of all abnormal responses of living tissue. Not only is it the most commonly encountered of these responses, but it frequently occurs along with, or as a consequence of, other patterns of response. **Inflammation** is a general term for the reaction of living tissue to injury or irritation. The gross features of inflammation—redness, heat, swelling, and pain—have been recognized for many centuries. The biochemical and histologic correlates of these phenomena are still under study today. Although, in certain diseases, inflammation occurs in many organs and tissues throughout the body, the pathology of inflammation is best understood as a local event or series of events.

A wide variety of injuries and irritations can elicit an inflammatory response from living tissue—a response that is always strikingly similar, with only minor variations depending on the nature of the stimulus. Causes of inflammation can be divided into two broad categories: pathogenic (disease-causing) microorganisms, and physical or chemical injury. The latter category includes cutting, crushing, burning, freezing, electrical shock, radiation, various types of foreign body, and irritation or poisoning by chemical agents. In addition, certain processes originating inside the body—tissue death due to circulatory impairment, the formation and spread of a malignant tumor, the production of abnormal antibodies that attack normal tissue—can set off an inflammatory response.

For convenience, inflammation is usually thought of as involving two distinct processes: an acute response to injury or irritation, in which the body seeks to contain or limit the damage; and a repair phase in which destroyed tissue is regenerated or replaced by scar tissue. Actually these processes overlap, one grading imperceptibly into the other.

The **acute phase** of inflammation consists of a response on the part of capillaries and certain cells to chemical substances released by damaged tissue. The **capillaries** in a zone of inflamed tissue dilate. Although many of the channels in a capillary bed are normally shut down, they all tend to open as part of an inflammatory reaction. In fact, if inflammation persists for more than a few hours, endothelial buds begin to form from capillaries and give rise to new capillaries. At the same time, capillary walls thicken, so that the net effect is congestion or engorgement of tissues with blood rather than an increased flow of blood through the tissues. This increased amount of blood in the tissues, or **hyperemia**, accounts for the familiar observation of redness and heat in an inflamed part, and is the basis for the word *inflammation*. As a result of vascular engorgement, plasma leaks from capillaries and venules into the tissue spaces producing swelling or **edema**.

Of more obvious benefit is the **cellular** component of the inflammatory response. Substances released by damaged tissue attract certain types of cells into the area of injury, a process called **chemotaxis**. Phagocytic cells assemble with remarkable speed, engulfing, breaking down, and removing dead tissue, foreign material, or invading microorganisms. The principal phagocytes are the **histiocytes** (macrophages) of connective tissue and the neutrophils and monocytes of the circulating blood. Histiocytes migrate into the battle zone from surrounding tissue. Leukocytes, particularly **neutrophils**, arrive via the circulation and emerge through capillary walls by a process called diapedesis. In the presence of large fragments of foreign material, many histiocytes may join together to form a syncytium or **multinucleate giant cell** to deal with the invader more efficiently.

Variable numbers of mast cells, plasma cells, eosinophils, and other cells of blood and tissue may also participate in the cellular response, depending on the inciting cause. **Lymphocytes**, whose function is to produce antibodies, appear in increasing numbers as the inflammatory response continues, and in chronic inflammation they are usually the principal cell found. Plasma cells and eosinophils are also more likely to appear in chronic inflammation.

The pathologist refers to a collection of unusual numbers of cells in tissue as an **infiltrate**. An infiltrate of neutrophils and histiocytes will generally be interpreted as a sign of acute inflammation; a lymphocytic infiltrate ("small round cell infiltrate" or "mononuclear cell infiltrate") suggests a more chronic process. The term **exudate** is used in a somewhat general way for any abnormal collection of fluid formed by release of plasma from the circulation into the tissues. A serous exudate is low in protein; a fibrinous exudate is rich in protein, including fibrin. Generally an exudate tends to localize injurious material and limit its spread. An exudate may form on and cling to an epithelial surface; it may accumulate in a body cavity; or it may simply filter into and distend the intercellular spaces of tissue, producing local swelling (edema). When an exudate contains a large amount of dead tissue along with large numbers of neutrophils, it is called **pus**, and its formation is known as suppuration. In severe inflammation, damaged capillaries may allow red blood cells to leak into tissue spaces. This local **hemorrhage** is not part of the inflammatory reaction but rather becomes part of the problem: the extravasated erythrocytes must now be engulfed and broken down by macrophages along with other degenerated tissue elements.

The **repair phase** of inflammation may begin even before the acute phase has reached its peak. Repair of damaged tissue takes place in two distinct ways. Some tissues are able to replace lost or destroyed cells through **regeneration**—an increase in the number of cells by mitosis and division of existing cells (reactive hyperplasia). The liver and epithelial tissues in general have a high potential for regeneration. Peripheral nerves and skeletal muscle have some; cardiac muscle, cartilage, and fat have little; and nerves in the central nervous system have none. When cells cannot be replaced by regeneration, the body does the next best thing and produces a patch of scar tissue.

Wound repair begins with proliferation of capillaries along the wound edges. Loops of newly formed capillaries form minute but grossly visible red granules on the surface of this healing tissue, hence the term **granulation tissue**. Meanwhile, a fibrin-rich exudate forms in any open spaces. Fibroblasts migrate into this medium from surrounding tissue and produce collagenous fibers, bridging the wound or tissue defect with a zone of scar. This process is known as **fibrosis**. The composition of scar tissue is essentially the same whether it is formed in burned skin, cardiac muscle devitalized by blockage of a coronary artery, or a lung segment ravaged by tuberculosis. The formation of scar tissue in an exudate, a blood clot (thrombus), or a mass of necrotic (dead) tissue is known as **organization**. Sometimes fibrosis results in the "walling off" of a mass of foreign material that cannot be broken down (e.g., a bullet) or of a cavity in tissue left by injury or sloughing.

Once the scar is formed, the capillaries within it are gradually obliterated. With the passage of time, scar tissue tends to shrink and become more dense. Mature scar tissue has no circulation, no feeling, no ability to contract, no sweat glands or hair follicles; it is just fibrous tissue. Generally this is better than nothing, but when fibrosis is excessive it can become a liability. Scar tissue can produce deformity, obstruct normal passages, and compress nerves, causing pain or paralysis. Scar tissue that forms in an area of exudate between two serous surfaces can result in adhesions—such as between the lung and the chest wall, or between adjacent loops of intestine. Fibrosis is a lasting marker of past inflammation. The degree of fibrosis is generally in proportion to the severity and extent of the original injury and the duration of the inflammatory response. A smoldering inflammatory reaction that is kept going by chronic infection or retained foreign material may result in the formation of **granulomas**—microscopic or grossly evident nodules of excessive fibrous reaction.

Allergy

Allergy or **anaphylaxis** is a condition of induced hypersensitivity to certain foreign substances (allergens), such as inhaled pollens or swallowed foods or medicines. After an initial exposure to these substances, certain persons form complex proteins called antibodies. On subsequent exposure, a reaction occurs between the allergen and the antibody, culminating in a release of histamine from mast cells. The local effect of histamine release is capillary dilatation and edema. In the skin this can take the form of hives (**urticaria**) or other types of eruption. In the respiratory tract, allergy can cause congestion of mucous membranes, excessive production of mucous and serous secretions, and bronchiolar spasm and edema (**asthma**). Serum sickness is a syndrome of fever, urticaria, and joint inflammation due to allergy to foreign protein, such as in serum or antivenin of animal origin. Severe anaphylaxis can cause widespread vascular collapse, shock, and death (**anaphylactic shock**). Many allergic reactions are transitory, leaving no visible change in tissue specimens. Severe or chronic allergy can cause inflammatory changes, in which eosinophils are conspicuous.

In a number of diseases (rheumatoid arthritis, lupus erythematosus, periarteritis nodosa), the basic abnormality appears to be formation of an antibody that reacts with the body's own tissues to induce local inflammation and destruction. These **autoimmune** disorders are also called **collagen diseases** because they attack principally connective tissue. (See table, pp. 69–71.)

Infection

Infection means the proliferation of microscopic organisms within the living body, to the detriment of that body. Infectious diseases are also called contagious, communicable, or transmissible diseases because, with few exceptions, they can be transmitted in one way

Autoimmune (Collagen) Diseases

Disease	Clinical Features	Pathologic Features
Arteritis— Systemic necrotizing vasculitis (periarteritis nodosa, polyarteritis nodosa)	Variable: fatigue, abdominal pain, skin eruption, fever, arthritis, subcutaneous nodules, nephritis, central nervous system symptoms.	Nodular lesions of arteries throughout body; mucoid degeneration and necrosis of media, inflammation of all layers, replacement by fibrinous material, aneurysm, infarction, fibrosis.
Granulomatous vasculitis (temporal arteritis, giant cell arteritis)	Headache, painful swelling of temporal artery, visual impairment. Associated polymyalgia rheumatica: weakness, myalgia, fever, weight loss.	Chronic granulomatous inflammation of cranial arteries beginning in internal elastic membrane, spreading to media and adventitia.
Takayasu's disease (pulseless disease, aortic arch syndrome)	Fever, fatigue, arthralgia, absence or weakness of peripheral pulses, syncope, congestive heart failure.	Inflammation, thrombosis, obliteration of branches of aortic arch.
Goodpasture's syndrome (pneumorenal syndrome)	Dyspnea, hemorrhagic pneumonitis, nephritis, renal failure.	Intra-alveolar hemorrhage, nodular thickening of alveolar septa, hyaline change in renal glomeruli, proliferative glomerulitis.
Hashimoto's disease (lymphocytic thyroiditis)	Goiter, dysphagia, fever, myxedema.	Massive infiltration of lymphoid tissue with germinal centers replacing thyroid follicles, depletion of colloid, interstitial fibrosis.
Idiopathic thrombocytopenic purpura (ITP)	Petechiae, purpura, mucosal hemorrhage.	Thrombocytopenia, increased megakaryocytes with smooth borders in marrow.

Autoimmune (Collagen) Diseases *(continued)*

Disease	Clinical Features	Pathologic Features
Lupus erythematosus (LE)— Discoid lupus erythematosus	Scaly erythematous patches, especially of face and scalp.	Hyperkeratosis; hyperemia, telangiectasia, lymphocytic infiltration of dermis.
Systemic (disseminated) lupus erythematosus (SLE)	Malar rash, photosensitivity, arthralgia, weight loss, fever, pleuritis, pericarditis, nephritis.	Hemolytic anemia, leukopenia, lupus erythematosus cells and antinuclear antibodies in blood, widespread swelling of collagen with fibrinoid change, inflammation and sclerosis of small vessels, endothelial proliferation of glomeruli, Libman-Sacks verrucous endocarditis.
Polymyositis-dermatomyositis— Primary idiopathic polymyositis	Widespread muscle pain and weakness, wasting, weight loss, splenomegaly, dysphagia, diplopia.	Antinuclear antibodies in blood, hyaline degeneration of skeletal muscle fibers, loss of striations, interstitial fibrosis, lymphocytic infiltrates; 15–20% have malignancies of lungs, ovary, breast, stomach.
Dermatomyositis	Widespread muscle pain and weakness, wasting, weight loss, splenomegaly, dysphagia, diplopia; lilac rash of forehead, eyelids, cheeks, knuckles; telangiectases.	As above.

Autoimmune (Collagen) Diseases *(continued)*

Disease	Clinical Features	Pathologic Features
Progressive systemic sclerosis—Scleroderma	Raynaud's phenomenon, edema and hardening of skin beginning on extremities, arthritis.	Antinuclear antibodies in blood, perivascular infiltrates of inflammatory cells in dermis, fibrosis in skeletal and cardiac muscle, endothelial proliferation.
CRST syndrome	Calcinosis cutis, Raynaud's phenomenon, sclerodactyly, telangiectases.	As above.
CREST syndrome	Calcinosis cutis, Raynaud's phenomenon, sclerodactyly, telangiectases, esophageal dysfunction.	As above.
Rheumatic fever	Tachycardia, cardiac murmurs, migratory polyarthritis, subcutaneous nodules, erythema marginatum, chorea.	Aschoff bodies (fibrinoid degeneration and granulomatous inflammation) of cardiac valves, myocardium, fibrinous pericarditis, synovitis.
Rheumatoid arthritis	Joint pain, swelling, stiffness, deformity, fever, weight loss, subcutaneous nodules, splenomegaly.	Rheumatoid factors and antinuclear antibodies in blood, villous hypertrophy of synovial membranes, granulomatous pannus invading cartilage, ankylosis.
Sjögren's syndrome (keratoconjunctivitis sicca)	Dryness of mouth and eyes, painful swelling of parotid glands, hoarseness, cough, dysphagia.	Atrophy of parenchyma of lacrimal and salivary glands, interstitial fibrosis.
Wegener's granulomatosis	Fever, weakness, weight loss, ulcerative rhinitis, cough, dyspnea, renal failure.	Anticytoplasmic antibodies in blood, necrotizing vasculitis, granuloma formation, segmental necrotizing glomerulonephritis.

or another from one person to another. It is customary and convenient to discuss infection along with inflammation because in most infectious diseases there is a marked inflammatory response, which accounts for the most striking and characteristic signs and symptoms. The clinical picture and pathologic findings in an infectious disease depend chiefly on the biological properties of the infecting organisms, but also on the route by which they enter the body, their number and virulence, and such host factors as general health and the possession of protective antibodies. Some microorganisms that a normal body can harbor without ill effects are capable of invading tissues and causing disease when host defenses are impaired by nutritional deficiency, disturbances of the immune system, or preexisting infection with another organism. Infectious agents that lie in wait for a breakdown in host defenses are called **opportunistic**.

Many infections are purely local, as in the case of a dental abscess or a fungal infection of the feet. Others are systemic, spreading through the body by the blood or lymphatic channels and producing widespread, perhaps fatal, disease. Regional spread can also occur, as in the familiar example of a head cold that evolves into a chest cold. Not every infection is due to a single species of organism in pure strain; mixed infections are common in certain parts of the body and in debilitated patients.

In response to some infections, the body can produce antibodies that are capable of inactivating invading microorganisms and bringing the infection to an end. In some cases, protective antibodies continue to be formed throughout life (as, for example, after measles and chickenpox). In other diseases (the common cold, staphylococcal abscess), any antibodies formed either are not protective or do not continue to be formed after recovery.

Bacterial Infection

A detailed discussion of medical microbiology is beyond the scope of this book. For our purposes it will be sufficient to divide pathogenic organisms into four classes—bacteria and rickettsiae, fungi, viruses, and parasites—and to make a few remarks about each class. **Bacteria** are one-celled organisms capable of multiplying rapidly by cell division. By no means are all bacteria harmful, and some are even beneficial, including those that live in the normal human colon. Pathogenic bacteria vary greatly in structure, growth characteristics, and ability to harm a human host, and they cause a correspondingly broad range of diseases, including boils, streptococcal pharyngitis, some kinds of pneumonia and meningitis, most urinary tract infections, tetanus, cholera, typhoid fever, tuberculosis, syphilis, and gonorrhea.

Bacteria are classified on the basis of shape, staining properties, cultural characteristics, and other variables. **Cocci** are round, **bacilli** rod-shaped. **Staphylococci** are cocci which form in grape-cluster shapes. **Streptococci** are cocci that occur as pairs or chains. **Spirochetes** are spiral-shaped bacteria.

Bacteria can be seen in sections of infected tissue, particularly after the application of the types of staining techniques that are used to examine smears of pus or exudate. Two types of staining for bacteria deserve mention here. The **Gram stain** has been a standard technique for many decades. Crystal violet is first applied, along with a mordant containing iodine. Certain bacteria, called gram-positive, take up this stain and resist decolorization with alcohol. Other organisms, called gram-negative, do not retain the stain after washing with alcohol. These are counterstained red with safranin in the final step of the technique. The **acid-fast stain** is used to detect Mycobacteria, including the organisms that cause tuberculosis and leprosy. In this technique a carbolfuchsin stain is applied and the specimen is then washed in acidified alcohol. Only Mycobacteria take up the red stain and retain it after acid decolorization—hence, "acid-fast." Acid-fast organisms cannot be satisfactorily stained by the Gram method.

Pathogenic bacteria do much of their harm by producing waste products called **toxins**. Toxins vary widely in their capacity to damage tissue and to break down normal defenses against the growth and spread of bacteria. Some toxins work locally, such as the streptococcal toxins that break down bridges between cells and allow the bacteria to infiltrate tissue more readily. Others have remote or systemic effects, such as toxins produced by tetanus organisms, which can induce generalized convulsions and paralysis. The presence of toxins (not necessarily of bacterial origin) in the circulation is known as **toxemia**.

Pathogenic bacteria multiply generally in intercellular fluid, occasionally in cavities and tissue spaces such as the urinary bladder, the pericardium, or a joint space. A suppurative infection which remains localized—"walled off" by tissue reaction—is called an **abscess**. This type of infection is commonly caused by staphylococci and some other organisms. Infection that spreads readily through tissue spaces, causing diffuse swelling, such as that induced by some streptococci, is called **cellulitis**. **Septicemia** is the invasion of the blood stream by significant numbers of virulent organisms from a focal infection. This may result not only in severe systemic symptoms—fever, chills, and circulatory collapse—but also in the formation of secondary abscesses remote from the original focus.

Only a few types of bacteria are capable of invading cells. Rickettsiae are very small bacilli that reproduce inside host cells and cause a variety of diseases, including typhus and Rocky Mountain spotted fever, most of them characterized by fever and rash. Chlamydias, which cause ocular and genital infections, are also intracellular bacteria. None of these intracellular organisms can be detected in routine histologic preparations. Indeed, the diagnosis of infectious disease generally requires cultures, serologic testing, and special staining procedures that pertain to clinical rather than to anatomic pathology.

Fungi, Viruses, and Parasites

Fungi are less important than bacteria as causes of human disease. Most of the pathogenic fungi cause only superficial infections of skin and mucous membranes, hair, and nails (such as athlete's foot and ringworm of the skin), but a few are capable of systemic spread to produce severe, even life-threatening disease of the lungs, central nervous system, or other tissues. Two forms of fungi are recognized. A **yeast** is a unicellular organism that reproduces by budding. A **mold** consists of multicellular, filamentous masses (mycelia) of branching tubules called hyphae, which reproduce by various means. A few fungi can exist in either form, but most occur in only one form.

Several types of fungi may be present on normal skin and in other areas of the body, and only invade tissue when there is some impairment of local or general defenses. In fact, all fungi possess only slight invasive abilities. Typically a fungus elicits only a mild inflammatory reaction, but often a very chronic one. Fungi cannot be identified in tissue sections without special staining procedures.

Unlike bacteria and fungi, **viruses** are not living organisms. A virus is a very small segment of genetic material (DNA or RNA) encased in a protective protein shell. Upon entering a living cell, the virus assumes control of that cell's function and reproduction. The normal operations of the cell are suspended and it becomes a factory for the synthesis of more virus. Finally the cell disintegrates, releasing hundreds of new virus particles, which can then invade other cells. Viral infection typically elicits an acute, self-limited inflammatory response, without suppuration or fibrotic reaction. Viruses show a predilection for skin and mucous membranes, and even those that cause systemic disease often produce eruptions of papules or vesicles (as in measles and chickenpox).

Viruses cause many important diseases, including the common cold, influenza, measles, mumps, chickenpox, warts, herpes simplex, hepatitis, poliomyelitis, AIDS, and rabies. Virus particles are much too small to be seen by light microscopy—as many as 100 000 of them may be present within a single cell—but cells infected with virus show characteristic changes that may enable the pathologist not only to recognize that infection is present but even to identify the specific virus involved. Among these changes may be mentioned cytoplasmic and intranuclear inclusion bodies and the formation of multinucleate giant cells.

Parasites are a heterogenous group of organisms that spend part or all of their life cycles on or in the human body, causing varying degrees of disease by depriving the host of nutrients, invading or disrupting tissues, and eliciting allergic and inflammatory reactions. Some parasites, such as the protozoans that cause malaria and amebic dysentery, are microscopic; others, such as liver flukes and intestinal worms, are not. Parasites are more of a health problem in the tropics than in the temperate zone, but a few (pinworms, Trichomonas) are found in all latitudes, and any of them can appear in returned travelers. Many parasites, or their cysts or eggs, can readily be identified in tissue sections.

Clinical and pathologic features of the principal bacteria, fungal, viral, and parasitic diseases are summarized in the tables on the following pages.

Review Questions

1. List various causes of inflammation.
2. What is responsible for the redness and heat in inflamed tissue?
3. What is phagocytosis?
4. What is granulation tissue?
5. Distinguish beneficial from harmful types of antibody formation.
6. Name some autoimmune or collagen diseases.
7. What is the standard staining method in bacteriology?
8. Distinguish *abscess* from *cellulitis*.
9. In what important ways do viruses differ from bacteria and fungi?
10. What are some ways in which a parasite may affect the health of the host?

Infections Due to Gram-Positive Bacteria

Organism	Disease	Clinical Features	Pathologic Features
Staphylococcus aureus	Pyoderma and soft tissue infections: folliculitis, abscess, furuncle, carbuncle, impetigo.	Pain, swelling, hyperemia, suppuration, fever, chills.	Inflammatory cell infiltrates, focal necrosis, fibrosis.
	Visceral infections: pneumonitis, lung abscess, osteomyelitis, septicemia, endocarditis, meningitis, brain abscess.		
	Toxic shock syndrome.	Fever, erythroderma, mucosal hyperemia, gastroenteritis, jaundice, renal failure, vascular collapse.	
	Scalded skin syndrome (Ritter's disease).	Erythema, bullae, exfoliation.	
	Food poisoning.	Transitory gastroenteritis.	
Streptococcus pyogenes	Cellulitis, erysipelas, impetigo.	Erythema, edema, septicemia.	Inflammatory cell infiltrates, focal necrosis, fibrosis.
	Pharyngitis ("strep throat"), otitis media, pneumonia.		

Infections Due to Gram-Positive Bacteria (continued)

Organism	Disease	Clinical Features	Pathologic Features
Streptococcus pyogenes (cont.)	Toxic shock syndrome.	Fever, erythroderma, hepatic and renal failure, shock, necrotizing fasciitis.	Thrombocytopenia, inflammatory cell infiltrates, focal or widespread necrosis, fibrosis.
	Scarlatina (scarlet fever).	Fever, erythema, circumoral pallor, strawberry tongue, septicemia.	Dermal edema, lymphoid hyperplasia, mononuclear infiltrates in heart, liver, kidneys.
	Acute rheumatic fever.	Tachycardia, fever, cardiac murmurs, arthritis, subcutaneous nodules, erythema marginatum, chorea.	Aschoff bodies (fibrinoid degeneration and granulomatous inflammation) of cardiac valves, myocardium; pericarditis, synovitis.
	Acute glomerulonephritis.	Headache, edema, tachycardia, hypertension.	Renal edema, punctate hemorrhages, exudative inflammation of glomeruli, fibrinoid necrosis, capillary thrombosis.
Streptococcus agalactiae	Streptococcal disease of the newborn.	Septicemia, pneumonitis, meningitis.	
Streptococcus pneumoniae (pneumococcus)	Lobar pneumonia.	Chills, fever, dyspnea, cough, rusty sputum, pleuritic pain.	Edema, lobar consolidation, fibrinous exudate, extravasation of erythrocytes, hepatization, fibrosis.
	Acute sinusitis, otitis media, meningitis.		

Infections Due to Gram-Positive Bacteria *(continued)*

Organism	Disease	Clinical Features	Pathologic Features
Enterococcus	Infective endocarditis.	Fever, cardiac murmur, spleno-megaly, septic emboli, hyper-trophic osteoarthropathy.	Vegetations on valve margins containing fibrin, bacteria, necrotic debris.
Bacillus anthracis	Anthrax.	Cutaneous: necrotic ulcer at site of inoculation; lymphadenitis, fever, septicemia, meningitis.	Focal inflammation, hemorrhage, necrosis; organisms in blood vessels, lymph nodes.
		Pulmonary (woolsorter's disease): dyspnea, hemoptysis, septicemia.	Hemorrhagic necrosis of alveolar septa.
Clostridium tetani	Tetanus.	Muscle rigidity and spasm in jaw, abdomen, back; fever, headache, seizures.	
Clostridium botulinum	Botulism (due to ingestion of toxin in spoiled food).	Headache, nausea, weakness, diplopia, dryness of mouth, mydriasis, respiratory paralysis.	Thrombosis of small cerebral vessels, ganglion cell degenera-tion, hyperemia of viscera, brain.
Clostridium perfringens (C. welchii)	Gas gangrene.	Cellulitis, purulent discharge, crepitation.	Bubbles of gas in subcutaneous tissue and muscle, edema, necro-sis of muscle.

Infections Due to Gram-Positive Bacteria (continued)

Organism	Disease	Clinical Features	Pathologic Features
Clostridium difficile	Pseudomembranous enterocolitis.	Copious watery diarrhea, toxemia, hemorrhage, perforation of bowel, circulatory collapse.	Mushroom caps of mucus-like pseudomembrane, edema, inflammatory cell infiltrates, mucosal necrosis.
Listeria monocytogenes	Listeriosis.	Meningoencephalitis, lymphadenitis, septicemia, endocarditis, abscesses, papular eruption.	Abscesses of spleen, adrenals, lungs, digestive tract, brain and meninges.
Erysipelothrix rhusiopathiae	Erysipeloid.	Reddish-blue localized eruption at site of inoculation, fever, arthritis, septicemia.	
Corynebacterium diphtheriae	Diphtheria.	Pharyngitis with edema, membrane formation, respiratory obstruction, myocarditis, polyneuritis.	Edema, hyperemia, necrosis of epithelium, adherent membrane of necrotic tissue, fatty degeneration of heart, cloudy swelling of kidneys.
Corynebacterium minutissimum	Erythrasma.	Intensely red macules, usually in groin; little or no inflammation.	Organisms in stratum corneum or skin scrapings.

Infections Due to Gram-Negative Bacteria

Organism	Disease	Clinical Features	Pathologic Features
Neisseria meningitidis (meningococcus)	Meningococcal meningitis.	Headache, purpura, nuchal rigidity, seizures, delirium, shock.	Edema, punctate hemorrhages of meninges, purulent subarachnoid exudate, adrenal hemorrhage (Waterhouse-Friderichsen syndrome).
Neisseria gonorrhoeae (gonococcus)	Gonorrhea.	Male: dysuria, urethral discharge. Female: dysuria, salpingitis, pelvic inflammatory disease, infertility.	Mucosal inflammation and necrosis, fibrosis. Organisms in neutrophils.
	Ophthalmia neonatorum.	Conjunctivitis, corneal ulceration, panophthalmitis, blindness.	Focal inflammation, necrosis, fibrosis.
Bordetella pertussis	Whooping cough (pertussis).	Coryza, conjunctivitis, paroxysmal cough.	Hyperplasia of peribronchial lymphoid tissue; necrotizing inflammation of respiratory epithelium; bronchopneumonia.
Pasteurella multocida	Animal bite infections.	Pain, swelling, hyperemia, suppuration.	Focal inflammation and necrosis.
Francisella tularensis	Tularemia.	Ulcer or conjunctivitis, regional or generalized lymphadenitis, pneumonitis.	Neutrophilic infiltrates, granulomas with epithelioid giant cells in liver, spleen, lungs, kidneys.

Infections Due to Gram-Negative Bacteria (continued)

Organism	Disease	Clinical Features	Pathologic Features
Brucella abortus, B. melitensis, B. suis	Brucellosis (undulant fever).	Intermittent fever, malaise, fatigue, muscle and bone pain, lymphadenitis, splenomegaly.	Monocellular epithelioid cells, giant cells, lymphocytes in liver, spleen, lymph nodes, bone marrow.
Afipia felis	Cat-scratch disease.	Papule or pustule at inoculation site, malaise, fever, regional lymphadenitis, rash, pharyngitis, pneumonitis.	Local inflammation, lymphoid hyperplasia, stellate granulomas.
Yersinia pestis	Plague (bubonic, septicemic, pneumonic).	Lymphadenitis, purpura, hemorrhagic pneumonitis, septicemia, meningitis.	Lymphoid hyperplasia of lymph nodes, spleen; focal necrosis, acute hemorrhagic nephritis.
Yersinia enterocolitica	Enterocolitis.	Diarrhea, bloody stools, fever, abdominal pain, arthritis, erythema nodosum.	Inflammation, necrosis, hemorrhage of intestinal mucosa, mesenteric lymphadenitis.
Salmonella typhi	Typhoid fever.	Lethargy, headache, cough, diarrhea, rose spots, bradycardia, splenomegaly.	Leukopenia, mononuclear cell proliferation in lymph nodes and spleen; necrosis and ulceration of Peyer's patches.

Infections Due to Gram-Negative Bacteria *(continued)*

Organism	Disease	Clinical Features	Pathologic Features
Salmonella (various species)	Salmonellosis.	Enterocolitis.	
	Osteomyelitis.	Bone pain, inflammation of soft tissues.	Infarction, necrosis, sclerosis of bone.
	Salmonella food poisoning.	Chills, fever, abdominal cramps, vomiting, diarrhea.	
Shigella dysenteriae, S. boydii, S. flexneri, S. sonnei	Bacillary dysentery.	Abdominal pain, bloody diarrhea, fever, dehydration, toxemia, seizures.	Focal inflammation and necrosis of intestinal mucosa.
Vibrio cholerae	Asiatic cholera.	Copious rice-water diarrhea, dehydration, acidosis, shock.	Necrosis of gastrointestinal epithelium, inflammatory cell infiltrates of lamina propria; lymphoid hyperplasia of ileum.
Spirillum minus	Sodoku (spirillary rat-bite fever).	Local inflammation at bite, regional lymphadenitis, splenomegaly, purplish rash.	Local inflammation; degenerative changes in liver and kidneys.
Campylobacter fetus (C. jejuni)	Enterocolitis.	Abdominal pain, fever, bloody diarrhea, arthritis.	Mucosal ulceration, necrosis, hemorrhage.

Infections Due to Gram-Negative Bacteria (continued)

Organism	Disease	Clinical Features	Pathologic Features
Klebsiella pneumoniae	Friedländer's pneumonia.	Fever, chest pain, cough, hemoptysis.	Lobar consolidation, fibrinous pleuritis, alveolar necrosis, inflammatory cells, organisms in tissue and exudate.
Moraxella catarrhalis	Pharyngitis, sinusitis, otitis media, bronchitis.		
Haemophilus influenzae	Sinusitis, otitis media, meningitis.		
Haemophilus ducreyi	Chancroid.	Genital papule becoming ulcer, suppurative inguinal lymphadenitis	Epithelial necrosis, perivasculitis, thrombosis, fibrosis.
Gardnerella vaginalis	Bacterial vaginosis.	Foul discharge.	
Calymmatobacterium granulomatis	Granuloma inguinale.	Genital ulcer with exuberant granulation tissue, purulent exudate.	Acute and chronic inflammatory cell infiltrates, Donovan bodies in monocytes.
Bartonella bacilliformis	Oroya fever.	Fever, anemia, hepatosplenomegaly, lymphadenitis.	Endothelial proliferation in capillaries, lymphoid hyperplasia in spleen and lymph nodes, hepatic degeneration.
	Verruga peruana.	Red cutaneous and mucosal granulomas, bone pain.	

Infections Due to Gram-Negative Bacteria (continued)

Organism	Disease	Clinical Features	Pathologic Features
Pseudomonas mallei	Glanders.	Ulcer at site of inoculation, lymphadenitis, septicemia, pneumonitis.	Focal necrosis, abscesses, thrombosis, fibrosis.
Escherichia coli (invasive or toxigenic)	Diarrheal disease.	Nausea, abdominal cramps, diarrhea.	
	Hemorrhagic colitis.	Nausea, abdominal cramps, bloody diarrhea.	Hyperemia and ulceration of colonic mucosa.
	Hemolytic-uremic syndrome.	Fever, diarrhea, acute renal failure.	Anemia, thrombocytopenia, endothelial hyaline thrombi of glomeruli, renal cortical necrosis.
Escherichia coli, Proteus vulgaris, P. mirabilis	Cystitis, pyelonephritis, peritonitis, septicemia.		
Pseudomonas aeruginosa	Wound and burn infections.	Blue-green pus.	
	Ecthyma gangrenosum.	Cutaneous or mucosal nodule with central necrosis and surrounding erythema.	Organisms in venules, thrombosis, minimal neutrophilic reaction, necrosis.
	Cystitis, meningitis, otitis externa.		

Infections Due to Gram-Negative Bacteria *(continued)*

Organism	Disease	Clinical Features	Pathologic Features
Helicobacter pylori	Gastritis, peptic ulceration of stomach and duodenum.	Dyspepsia, pyrosis, gastrointestinal hemorrhage, perforation, obstruction.	Local or diffuse inflammation, atrophy, ulceration, fibrosis of gastrointestinal mucosa.
Capnocytophaga canimorsus	Dog-bite infections.	Cellulitis, septicemia, meningitis, endocarditis.	
Eikenella corrodens	Opportunistic infections.	Fever, lymphadenitis, endocarditis, stomatitis, pleuritis.	
Bacteroides fragilis	Abdominal abscess, peritonitis, septicemia.		

Infections Due to Miscellaneous Bacteria

Organism	Disease	Clinical Features	Pathologic Features
Mycobacterium tuberculosis	Tuberculosis.	Granulomatous pneumonitis, fever, cachexia, hemorrhage from lungs, lymphadenitis, pleuritis, meningitis.	Neutrophilic exudates, fibrinous exudate, epithelioid cells, giant cells, caseous necrosis, fibrosis, calcification.
Mycobacterium avium-intracellulare (*M. avium* complex)	Tuberculosis, particularly in AIDS.	As above.	As above.
Mycobacterium leprae	Leprosy (Hansen's disease).	Lepromatous: generalized cutaneous macules and nodules; deforming infiltrations of face and extremities; anesthesia.	Proliferation of dermal histiocytes containing bacilli (lepra cells), histiocytes in neurons.
		Tuberculoid: focal granulomatous nodules of skin, anesthesia.	Epithelioid cells, lymphocytes, Langhans giant cells, cellular infiltrates in dermal nerves.
Mycobacterium marinum	Fish tank (swimming pool) granuloma.	Solitary or several cutaneous papules, nodules, abscesses, or ulcers, regional lymphadenitis.	Granuloma formation, caseous necrosis.
Mycoplasma pneumoniae	Primary atypical pneumonia (mycoplasmal pneumonia).	Headache, fever, cough, substernal pain.	Hemorrhagic consolidation of lung, mucopurulent exudate in alveoli.
Chlamydia pneumoniae	Pneumonia, bronchitis.	Fever, cough, chest pain, wheezing, induction or exacerbation of asthma.	

Infections Due to Miscellaneous Bacteria (continued)

Organism	Disease	Clinical Features	Pathologic Features
Chlamydia trachomatis, types A to C	Trachoma.	Conjunctivitis with ulcers, granulomas, scarring of cornea, blindness.	Papillary hypertrophy of conjunctiva, follicles, pannus, fibrosis of cornea, lymphocytic infiltrates.
C. trachomatis, type L	Lymphogranuloma venereum.	Ulcer, lymphadenitis, proctitis, rectal stricture.	Acute inflammation, fibrosis.
C. trachomatis, types D to K Ureaplasma urealyticum	Nongonococcal urethritis, cervicitis, salpingitis.	Urethral discharge, dysuria, mucopurulent cervical exudate, pelvic pain, fever; perihepatitis (Fitz-Hugh-Curtis syndrome), infertility, inclusion conjunctivitis (inclusion blennorrhea).	Edema, inflammatory cell infiltrates, mucosal necrosis, suppuration.
Legionella pneumophila	Legionellosis (legionnaires' disease, Pontiac fever).	Fever, chills, chest pain, hemoptysis, diarrhea.	Patchy pneumonitis, inflammatory cell infiltrates, alveolar septal necrosis, hemorrhage, consolidation, cavitation.
Streptobacillus moniliformis	Haverhill fever.	Chills, headache, myalgia, arthritis.	Inflammatory changes in liver, kidneys, myocardium; microinfarcts of spleen.
	Streptobacillary rat-bite fever.	Inflammation at bite, macular rash, arthritis.	

Infections Due to Spirochetes

Organism	Disease	Clinical Features	Pathologic Features
Treponema pallidum	Syphilis.	Primary: painless indurated ulcer (chancre) at site of inoculation, regional lymphadenitis, fibrosis.	Acute and chronic inflammatory cell infiltrates, mucocutaneous inflammation and necrosis, obliterative endarteritis, thrombosis, necrosis, fibroplasia.
		Secondary: maculopapular rash, mucous patches, alopecia, lymphadenopathy, gummata.	
		Latent (tertiary): cardiovascular, central nervous system damage.	
		Congenital: deafness, Hutchinson's teeth, interstitial keratitis, frontal bossing, saber shins.	
Treponema pertenue	Yaws (frambesia).	Widespread papular granulomas or ulcers of skin and mucous membranes.	Epithelial hyperplasia, hyperkeratosis, granulomas, gummata, necrosis.
Borrelia recurrentis	Relapsing fever.	Recurrent high fever with headache, delirium, hepatosplenomegaly, jaundice, gastrointestinal bleeding.	Organisms in spleen and brain; gastrointestinal mucosal hemorrhages.

Infections Due to Spirochetes *(continued)*

Organism	Disease	Clinical Features	Pathologic Features
Borrelia burgdorferi	Lyme disease.	Erythema chronicum migrans, fever, arthritis, myalgia, aseptic meningitis, neuritis, myocarditis.	Lymphoid hyperplasia, perivascular mononuclear cell infiltrates, obliterative vasculitis, neuronal degeneration; spirochetes in dermis, lymph nodes, synovium, liver, spleen, CNS.
Leptospira icterohemorrhagiae	Weil's disease (leptospirosis).	Headache, myalgia, vomiting, diarrhea, hepatomegaly, jaundice, oliguria, petechiae, epistaxis, pneumonitis, myocarditis, gastrointestinal hemorrhage.	Hemorrhages in skin, muscle, gastrointestinal mucosa; hepatic inflammation and necrosis; interstitial nephritis.

Infections Due to Rickettsias

Organism	Disease	Clinical Features	Pathologic Features
Rickettsia rickettsii	Rocky Mountain spotted fever.	Severe headache, myalgia, petechiae, periorbital edema, bronchopneumonia, arterial thrombosis.	Vasculitis, destruction of endothelium of small vessels, thrombosis, mononuclear infiltrates in muscle, heart, brain, lungs.
Rickettsia prowazekii	Epidemic typhus (including Brill-Zinsser disease).	Headache, myalgia, macular or petechial rash, circulatory collapse, coma.	Vasculitis in heart, lungs, brain; interstitial myocarditis.
Rickettsia mooseri	Endemic typhus.	Headache, myalgia, maculopapular rash, splenomegaly, lymphadenitis, cough.	Endothelial swelling and proliferation, vascular necrosis, thrombosis.
Rickettsia tsutsugamushi	Scrub typhus.	Eschar at site of mite bite, headache, cough, lymphadenitis, splenomegaly.	Vasculitis, perivascular mononuclear infiltrates.
Rickettsia akari, R. conorii	African tick-borne fever (fièvre boutonneuse).	Buttonlike necrotic lesion at inoculation site, chills, myalgia, lymphadenitis, maculopapular rash.	Endothelial swelling, perivascular infiltrates.
Coxiella burnetii	Q fever.	Headache, myalgia, cough, hemoptysis, chest pain, hepatosplenomegaly, jaundice.	Interstitial pneumonitis, granulomatous hepatitis.

Infections Due to Rickettsias (continued)

Organism	Disease	Clinical Features	Pathologic Features
Ehrlichia canis, E. chaffeensis	Ehrlichiosis.	Fever, headache, myalgia, diarrhea, lymphadenitis, hepatosplenomegaly.	Neutropenia, lymphopenia, thrombocytopenia, anemia; organisms in lymph nodes, spleen, kidney, liver, bone marrow; cytoplasmic inclusions (morulae) in peripheral neutrophils.
Rochalimaea henselae	Cat-scratch disease.	Lymphadenitis.	Necrotizing inflammation of lymph nodes.
	Bacillary angiomatosis (especially in AIDS).	Vascular cutaneous and hepatic tumors.	Cutaneous angiomata, focal hepatocellular necrosis with hemorrhagic cysts.

Systemic Fungal Infections

Organism	Disease	Clinical Features	Pathologic Features
Coccidioides immitis	Coccidioidomycosis (San Joaquin Valley fever).	Cough, weakness, arthralgia, lymphadenitis, meningitis.	Bronchiolar and alveolar inflammation, focal abscesses, necrosis, giant cells, cavitation.
Histoplasma capsulatum	Histoplasmosis.	Cough, chest pain, hemoptysis, myalgia, splenomegaly, hepatomegaly, lymphadenitis, gastrointestinal ulcers, meningitis.	Epithelioid granulomas, caseation, cavitation, calcification, mucosal ulceration.
Blastomyces dermatitidis	North American blastomycosis.	Cough, chest pain, cachexia, papular dermatitis (Gilchrist's disease), osteomyelitis, involvement of central nervous system and urinary tract.	Dermal microabscesses, miliary granulomas of lungs, caseation, fibrosis.
Paracoccidioides brasiliensis	South American blastomycosis.	Oral and nasal ulcers, abdominal pain, diarrhea, lymphadenopathy, involvement of liver and spleen.	Suppuration, abscess formation, granulomas, fibrosis, caseation, small round cell infiltrates.
Candida albicans	Candidosis (moniliasis, thrush).	Cutaneous and mucosal edema and hyperemia, mucosal patches, esophagitis, pneumonitis, pyelonephritis, endocarditis.	Hyphae in tissues, granuloma formation.

Systemic Fungal Infections *(continued)*

Organism	Disease	Clinical Features	Pathologic Features
Cryptococcus neoformans	Cryptococcosis (torulosis, European blastomycosis).	Cough, weight loss, acneiform pustules, granulomatous ulcers and nodules.	Granulomas, macrophages, giant cells.
Aspergillus niger	Aspergillosis.	Cough, hemoptysis, dyspnea, fever, arthralgia.	Hyphae and fibrin in bronchi, suppuration, granuloma formation.
Mucor	Mucormycosis (zygomycosis).	Purulent sinusitis, otitis, pneumonitis.	Inflammation, suppuration, necrosis, arteritis, thrombosis.
Rhizopus	Zygomycosis.	Purulent sinusitis, otitis, pneumonitis.	Inflammation, suppuration, necrosis, arteritis, thrombosis.
Actinomyces israelii	Actinomycosis.	Induration and swelling of jaw, sinus tract formation, pus containing "sulfur granules," sweats, cachexia, cough, hemoptysis.	Granulomas surrounded by neutrophils, abscesses, sinuses, fibrosis.
Nocardia asteroides	Nocardiosis.	Chest pain, cough, dyspnea, weakness, weight loss, spread to brain, liver, kidney.	Suppurative pneumonitis, lung abscess.
Torulopsis glabrata	Opportunistic infections in immunodeficiency.	Cholecystitis, endocarditis, pneumonitis, esophagitis, pyelonephritis.	

Superficial Fungal Infections

Organism	Disease	Clinical Features	Pathologic Features
Trichophyton, Microsporum, Epidermophyton floccosum	Tinea capitis.	Scaly macules of scalp, hair loss.	Inflammation about follicles.
	Tinea corporis, cruris.	Scaly round macules, central clearing.	Hyphae in stratum corneum or scrapings.
(All three cause the first four conditions in the second column.)	Tinea unguium.	Deformity, crumbling, separation of nail.	Hyphae in nail.
	Tinea pedis.	Dermatitis, scaling, fissuring, maceration.	Inflammation, hyphae in stratum corneum or scrapings.
Pityrosporum orbiculare (Malassezia furfur)	Tinea versicolor.	Scaly macules of upper trunk, darker than untanned skin, lighter than tanned skin.	Hyphae in stratum corneum or scrapings.
Piedraia hortai	Piedra.	Stony hard black nodules on beard or scalp hairs.	Green or brown hyphae in stratum corneum or scrapings.
Phaeoanellomyces werneckii (Cladosporium werneckii)	Tinea nigra.	Scaly black macules.	Lymphatic vessels thickened, granulomas with central necrosis.
Sporothrix schenckii (Sporotrichum schenckii)	Sporotrichosis.	Cutaneous pustules, mucosal ulcers, lymphangitis, lymphadenitis.	Dermal microabscesses containing fungi, fibrosis, epidermal hyperplasia and hyperkeratosis.
Phialophora pedrosoi	Chromomycosis.	Warty gray papule or nodule, lymphedema, ulceration.	

Infections Due to DNA Viruses

Virus	Disease	Clinical Features	Pathologic Features
Orthopoxvirus	Smallpox (variola).	Fever, pustular eruption, hemorrhage, septicemia.	Acanthosis, epidermal inclusions (Guarnieri bodies), ballooning degeneration, mononuclear infiltrates, dermal necrosis.
Parapoxvirus	Orf.	Papule, vesicle, eschar at site of inoculation, lymphadenitis.	Proliferation, ballooning and reticular degeneration of epidermis.
	Molluscum contagiosum.	Pearly umbilicated papules.	Large dyskeratotic cells with inclusions (Lipschütz bodies).
Herpesvirus, type 1	Herpes labialis (facial herpes simplex).	Cluster of painful vesicles becoming ulcers, regional lymphadenitis.	Ballooning degeneration of stratum spinosum, intranuclear inclusion bodies, dermal congestion and inflammatory cells.
type 2	Herpes progenitalis (genital herpes).	As above.	As above.
type 3	Varicella (chickenpox).	Vesicular, pustular exanthem and enanthem, fever, encephalitis, pneumonitis.	Ballooning degeneration, inclusion bodies.
	Herpes zoster (shingles).	Vesicular eruption, neuritic pain in one dermatome.	As above.

Infections Due to DNA Viruses *(continued)*

Virus	Disease	Clinical Features	Pathologic Features
Herpesvirus *(cont.)* type 4 (Epstein-Barr virus)	Infectious mononucleosis. Burkitt's lymphoma. Nasopharyngeal carcinoma.	Fever, pharyngitis, lymphadenitis, splenomegaly, prostration, jaundice. Rapidly growing malignant tumor of jaw.	Atypical lymphocytes, lymphoid hyperplasia, mucosal ulceration.
type 5 (cyto-megalovirus)	Cytomegalovirus disease.	Fever, weakness, lymphadenitis, splenomegaly. Congenital: jaundice, purpura, mental retardation, pneumonitis, chorioretinitis.	Mononucleosis, foci of cyto-megalic cells in liver, lungs, kidneys, pancreas, lymphoid tissue.
Adenovirus	Common cold, exudative pharyngitis, pneumonitis.	Fever, rhinitis, cough, malaise, myalgia, dysphagia, lymphadenitis	Epithelial edema, hyperemia, necrosis, lymphoid hyperplasia.
types 8, 19	Epidemic keratoconjunctivitis.	Pain in eye, lacrimation, photophobia, conjunctival injection, corneal opacities, lymphadenitis.	As above.
types 3, 7	Pharyngoconjunctival fever.	Fever, pharyngitis, conjunctivitis.	As above.
types 11, 21	Acute hemorrhagic cystitis.	Dysuria, hematuria.	As above.
Human papilloma-virus (HPV)	Verruca vulgaris (wart).	Rough, irregular cutaneous papule.	Hyperkeratosis, acanthosis, vacuoles in stratum granulosum, mononuclear infiltrates.
types 6,11	Condyloma acuminatum.	As above.	As above.

Infections Due to DNA Viruses (continued)

Virus	Disease	Clinical Features	Pathologic Features
Human papilloma-virus (cont.) types 33, 35, 39, 40, 43, 45, 51–56, 58	Condyloma acuminatum; dys-plasia of genital skin, mucosa.	As above.	As above; low grade dysplasias, carcinoma.
types 16, 18	Flat genital warts; dysplasia or cancer of cervix, penis.		As above; dysplasias, invasive carcinoma.
Parvovirus B–19	Erythema infectiosum ("fifth disease") (children).	"Slapped cheek" erythema, generalized reticular to maculo-papular rash.	
	Aplastic anemia syndrome.	Fever, headache, rash, arthritis.	Aplastic anemia, thrombocyto-penia, neutropenia, erythroid hypoplasia and giant proerythro-blasts in marrow.

Infections Due to RNA Viruses

Virus	Disease	Clinical Features	Pathologic Features
Poliovirus	Poliomyelitis.	Headache, meningeal irritation, muscular weakness, residual flaccid paralysis.	Chromatolysis, neuronophagia of anterior horn cells of spinal cord, perivascular lymphocytic infiltrates, myocarditis.
Coxsackievirus A, types 2, 4, 5, 6, 8, 10	Herpangina.	Vesicular pharyngitis, lymphadenitis, fever.	
type 16 & others	Hand, foot, and mouth disease.	Papulovesicular eruption, oral ulcers.	
various types	Aseptic meningitis.	Fever, headache, vomiting, stiff neck.	Pleocytosis of cerebrospinal fluid.
Coxsackievirus B	Epidemic pleurodynia (Bornholm disease). Myocarditis, pericarditis, endocarditis. Aseptic meningitis.	Severe pain in chest or abdomen, fever, headache.	
Echovirus	Aseptic meningitis. Diarrheal disease.		
type 16	Boston exanthem.	Fever, headache, exanthem.	
Rhinovirus Coronavirus	Common cold.	Fever, rhinitis, malaise, myalgia, cough, pharyngitis.	Epithelial edema, hyperemia, necrosis.

Infections Due to RNA Viruses *(continued)*

Virus	Disease	Clinical Features	Pathologic Features
Hepatitis A	Infectious hepatitis.	Anorexia, jaundice, fever, malaise, abdominal pain.	Degeneration and necrosis of hepatocytes, inflammatory cell infiltrates of sinusoids and portal areas.
Hepatitis E	Hepatitis E.	As above.	As above.
Hepatitis B	Serum hepatitis.	Vomiting, abdominal pain, fever, jaundice, rash, arthritis.	Edema, degeneration, necrosis of hepatocytes, perilobular inflammatory cell infiltrates, portal cirrhosis, hepatocellular carcinoma.
Hepatitis C	Transfusion hepatitis.	As above.	As above.
Hepatitis D	Coinfection with hepatitis B.	As above.	As above.
Flavivirus	Yellow fever.	Fever, headache, hemoptysis, black vomit, jaundice.	Midzonal hepatic necrosis, acidophilic Councilman bodies, fatty change, renal tubular degeneration, splenic congestion, focal hemorrhages of gastrointestinal tract, lungs, brain.
	Dengue (breakbone fever).	Fever, chills, severe bone and joint pain, rash.	Endothelial swelling, perivascular mononuclear infiltrates.

Infections Due to RNA Viruses (continued)

Virus	Disease	Clinical Features	Pathologic Features
Flavivirus (cont.)	Encephalitis (Japanese B, St. Louis).	Fever, headache, meningeal irritation, stupor, coma, seizures, paralysis.	Neuronal degeneration and necrosis in brain and spinal cord, perivascular mononuclear infiltrates, encephalomalacia, gliosis.
Alphavirus	Encephalitis (Venezuela, Eastern, and Western equine).	As above.	As above.
Bunyavirus	California encephalitis.	As above.	As above.
Hantavirus	Korean hemorrhagic fever.	Fever, purpura, renal failure, shock.	Thrombocytopenia, vasculitis.
	Hantavirus pulmonary syndrome.	Fever, myalgia, vomiting, cough, respiratory distress.	Thrombocytopenia, hypoalbuminemia, lactic acidosis, pulmonary septal and alveolar edema, pleural effusion.
Rubivirus	Rubella.	Lymphadenitis, maculopapular rash, arthritis. Congenital: cataracts, deafness, cardiac anomalies.	Leukopenia, lymphoid hyperplasia.
Rotavirus	Infantile gastroenteritis.	Diarrhea, abdominal pain, fever, dehydration.	Inflammation and necrosis of small intestinal mucosa.

Infections Due to RNA Viruses (continued)

Virus	Disease	Clinical Features	Pathologic Features
Orthomyxovirus	Influenza.	Fever, chills, malaise, myalgia, cough, headache, pneumonitis, myocarditis, pericarditis, Reye's syndrome, Guillain-Barré syndrome.	Tracheobronchial mucosal inflammation and necrosis, interstitial pneumonitis.
Paramyxovirus	Mumps.	Fever, painful swelling of parotid glands, orchitis, meningoencephalitis, pancreatitis.	Edema of parotid glands, inflammation, lymphocytic infiltrates, necrosis of ductal epithelium.
	Respiratory syncytial disease.	Fever, cough, dyspnea, cyanosis.	Bronchopneumonia, bronchiolitis, multinucleate giant cells with cytoplasmic inclusions.
Morbillivirus	Measles (rubeola).	Coryza, conjunctivitis, cough, maculopapular exanthem, oral enanthem (Koplik's spots), encephalomyelitis.	Mononuclear and neutrophilic exudates, lymphoid hyperplasia, Warthin-Finkeldey giant cells in lymphoid tissue and skin.
Rhabdovirus	Rabies.	Headache, anorexia, spasm, encephalitis.	Cerebral congestion and edema, perivascular mononuclear infiltrates, neuronal degeneration, Negri bodies in neurons, demyelination.

Infections Due to RNA Viruses *(continued)*

Virus	Disease	Clinical Features	Pathologic Features
Rhabdovirus *(cont.)*	Marburg disease, Ebola disease.	Fever, myalgia, headache, pharyngitis, gastroenteritis, rash, hemorrhages, hepatic and renal failure.	Necrosis of liver, pancreas, kidney.
Arenavirus	Lymphocytic choriomeningitis.	Flulike illness, meningitis, headache, nausea, lethargy.	Leukopenia, lymphocytic infiltrates of meninges.
	Lassa fever.	Fever, oral ulcers, myalgia, petechiae, pneumonitis.	Mucosal necrosis, myocardial and renal tubular degeneration.
Orbivirus	Colorado tick fever.	Fever, chills, headache, vomiting, rash.	
Retrovirus	Acquired immune deficiency syndrome (AIDS).	Fever, lymphadenitis, weight loss, and susceptibility to Kaposi sarcoma, *Pneumocystis carinii* pneumonia, cryptosporidiosis, esophageal candidiasis, and other opportunistic infections.	Lymphopenia, pathology of specific disease.

Infections Due to Unidentified or Unclassified Viruses

Disease	Clinical Features	Pathologic Features
Norwalk disease.	Vomiting, diarrhea, fever.	
Roseola infantum (exanthema subitum).	Fever, maculopapular rash.	
Kawasaki disease (mucocutaneous lymph node syndrome).	Fever, cervical and oropharyngeal injection, strawberry tongue, edema and erythema of extremities, exanthem, periungual desquamation, myocardial infarction.	Lymphoid hyperplasia, coronary arteritis, pericardial effusion.

Diseases Due to Protozoan Parasites

Organism	Disease	Clinical Features	Pathologic Features
Entamoeba histolytica	Amebic dysentery.	Colic, bloody diarrhea, tenesmus, nausea, weight loss, intestinal perforation, hepatic abscess.	Flask-shaped ulcers of colonic mucosa, coagulation necrosis, neutrophils, amebas in tissues, granuloma (ameboma) formation, necrotic "anchovy paste" material in hepatic abscess.
Giardia lamblia	Giardiasis.	Colic, diarrhea, weakness, weight loss, and malabsorption of fats, carbohydrates, vitamins A and B_{12}.	Mucosal inflammation, cholangitis, cholecystitis.
Trichomonas vaginalis	Trichomonal vaginitis, urethritis.	Female: vulvovaginitis, cervicitis, discharge. Male: urethritis, prostatitis.	Mucosal inflammation.
Cryptosporidium	Cryptosporidiosis.	Watery diarrhea, dehydration, malabsorption.	Organisms in small intestinal mucosa, superficial inflammation.
Isospora belli	Coccidiosis.	Fever, malaise, diarrhea.	Organisms in small intestinal mucosa, superficial inflammation.
Leishmania donovani	Kala-azar (visceral leishmaniasis).	Fever, lymphadenitis, hepatosplenomegaly, wasting.	Lymphoid hyperplasia, organisms in macrophages of spleen, liver, lymph nodes, bone marrow.

Diseases Due to Protozoan Parasites *(continued)*

Organism	Disease	Clinical Features	Pathologic Features
Leishmania tropica	Oriental sore (cutaneous leishmaniasis).	Papules, granulomatous ulcers, scarring.	Proliferation of amastigotes (Leishman-Donovan bodies) in dermal cells, epidermal ulceration, tuberculoid lesions.
Leishmania brasiliensis	Espundia (uta, chiclero ulcer, mucocutaneous leishmaniasis).	Polypoid granulomas, destructive ulcers of skin and mucous membranes, hepatosplenomegaly, subcutaneous nodules.	Proliferation of amastigotes (Leishman-Donovan bodies) in dermis, submucosa, subcutaneous tissues, necrosis, tuberculoid lesions.
Trypanosoma cruzi	Chagas' disease (American trypanosomiasis).	Edema and discoloration about orbit at site of inoculation (Romaña's sign), fever, hepatosplenomegaly, cardiac failure.	Invasion of liver, spleen, lymph nodes, skeletal and cardiac muscle, central nervous system, gastrointestinal tract by organisms; focal and diffuse inflammation, degeneration.
Trypanosoma rhodesiense, T. gambiense	African sleeping sickness.	Headache, anorexia, weakness, lethargy, posterior cervical lymphadenitis (Winterbottom's sign).	Inflammation of blood vessels and lymphatic channels and sinuses; diffuse meningoencephalitis, lymphoid hyperplasia, meningeal petechiae, gliosis, myocarditis.

Diseases Due to Protozoan Parasites *(continued)*

Organism	Disease	Clinical Features	Pathologic Features
Plasmodium vivax	Benign tertian malaria.	Regularly recurring fever and chills, anemia, splenomegaly, jaundice, hemoglobinuria (black-water fever).	Parasites filling sinuses of spleen and liver and inside erythrocytes and Kupffer cells; capillary thrombosis, renal tubular degeneration.
P. falciparum	Malignant tertian malaria.	As above.	As above.
P. malariae	Quartan malaria.	As above.	As above.
P. ovale	Ovale malaria.	As above.	As above.
Toxoplasma gondii	Toxoplasmosis.	Congenital: hydrocephalus, chorioretinitis, hepatosplenomegaly, pneumonitis. Acquired: Fever, lymphadenitis, hepatosplenomegaly, myocarditis.	Sinusoidal hyperplasia of lymphoid tissue, large epithelioid histiocytes with foamy cytoplasm.
Pneumocystis carinii	Interstitial plasma cell pneumonitis.	Dyspnea, tachypnea, cyanosis.	Lungs firm, rubbery; epithelial hyperplasia, foamy eosinophilic material in alveoli, cysts.
Babesia microti	Babesiosis.	Fever, chills, malaise, spleno-megaly, hemolytic anemia, renal failure.	Lymphoid hyperplasia, renal tubular degeneration.
Babesia bigemina	Texas fever.	As above.	As above.

Infections Due to Trematodes (Flukes)

Organism	Disease	Clinical Features	Pathologic Features
Fasciola hepatica	Fascioliasis.	Diarrhea, cachexia, arthritis, urticaria, jaundice, cholangitis, hepatic abscess.	Hyperplasia of bile duct epithelium, periductal inflammation and fibrosis, focal hepatic necrosis.
Clonorchis sinensis	Clonorchiasis.	Vomiting, diarrhea, jaundice, hepatomegaly, cachexia.	As above.
Fasciolopsis buski	Fasciolopsiasis.	Diarrhea, weakness, peripheral edema.	Mucosal necrosis and abscess formation in small intestine.
Paragonimus westermanni	Paragonimiasis.	Hemoptysis, diarrhea.	Organisms, cysts in lung, brain; pneumonitis.
Schistosoma mansoni	Bilharziasis.	Pruritus, hepatosplenomegaly, diarrhea, cachexia, hepatic failure, rectal polyps.	Colonic mucosal edema, inflammation, necrosis; organisms in venules of colon, rectum, liver; hepatic cirrhosis.
Schistosoma japonicum	Schistosomiasis japonicum.	Dermatitis, cough, diarrhea, hepatosplenomegaly, ascites.	Small intestinal mucosal inflammation, necrosis, polyps; eggs in intestinal venules; hepatic cirrhosis
Schistosoma haematobium	Schistosomiasis haematobium.	Dysuria, hematuria, obstructive uropathy.	Hyperplasia, inflammation, necrosis of bladder mucosa.
Schistosoma sp.	Swimmers' itch.	Pruritus, macules, pustules.	Cercariae of avian schistosomes in skin; local inflammation.

Infections Due to Intestinal Worms

Organism	Disease	Clinical Features	Pathologic Features
Taenia solium, T. saginata, Hymenolepis nana, Dibothriocephalus latus	Tapeworm infestation.	Abdominal pain, diarrhea, anemia, malabsorption.	Eosinophilia, tapeworm segments and ova in stools.
Ancylostoma duodenale, Necator americanus	Hookworm disease.	Pruritus at site of skin invasion (ground itch), headache, diarrhea, cough, anemia, nutritional deficiency.	Edema, inflammation, necrosis of small bowel mucosa, fatty infiltration of liver, erythroid hyperplasia of bone marrow.
Ascaris lumbricoides	Ascariasis.	Colic, nausea, vomiting, cachexia, intestinal obstruction.	Acute and chronic inflammation, eosinophils in gastrointestinal mucosa and lung.
Strongyloides stercoralis	Strongyloidiasis.	Diarrhea, abdominal pain, urticaria, weight loss, invasion of lungs, central nervous system.	Hyperemia, edema, necrosis of small bowel mucosa, parasites in crypts of Lieberkühn, focal pneumonitis, intra-alveolar hemorrhage.
Trichuris trichiura	Trichuriasis (whipworm).	Nausea, vomiting, diarrhea, rectal prolapse.	Worms in mucosa of cecum and appendix, focal ulceration and hemorrhage.

Infections Due to Intestinal Worms (continued)

Organism	Disease	Clinical Features	Pathologic Features
Enterobius vermicularis	Enterobiasis (pinworm, seatworm).	Anal pruritus.	Worms in rectum, cecum, appendix; shallow mucosal ulcers.
Anisakis marina	Anisakiasis (eosinophilic granuloma).	Colic, nausea, vomiting, fever.	Larvae in mucosa of stomach and small intestine, edema, granuloma formation.

Diseases Due to Tissue Worms

Organism	Disease	Clinical Features	Pathologic Features
Taenia solium, T. saginata	Cysticercosis.	Subcutaneous nodules, seizures, iritis.	Acute and chronic inflammation, eosinophils, fibroplasia, calcification of cysts.
Echinococcus granulosus	Echinococcosis.	Local swelling, bone pain, pathologic fractures, focal symptoms.	Unilocular cysts of liver, lung, bone, brain; inflammatory cells, eosinophils, fibrosis, calcification, pressure necrosis.
Trichinella spiralis	Trichinosis.	Fever, periorbital edema, muscle pain, weakness, myocarditis, meningoencephalitis.	Cysts and focal inflammation in skeletal muscle, loss of cross striations, basophilic degeneration; calcification of cysts.

Diseases Due to Tissue Worms *(continued)*

Organism	Disease	Clinical Features	Pathologic Features
Toxocara canis	Visceral larva migrans.	Abdominal pain, weight loss, cough, arthritis.	Eosinophilic granulomas of liver, lungs, kidneys, skeletal and cardiac muscle; giant cells surrounding larvae.
Ancylostoma brasiliense	Cutaneous larva migrans.	Pruritus, papular eruption, burrows.	Larvae in epidermis, eosinophilic infiltrate.
Dracunculus medinensis	Dracontiasis (Guinea worm).	Subcutaneous worm; pruritus, vomiting, diarrhea.	Worm in subcutaneous or connective tissues, body cavities.
Onchocerca volvulus	Onchocerciasis.	Pruritus, myalgia, lymphadenitis, lymphedema.	Microfilariae in subcutaneous tissue, skin, eye; inflammation, eosinophils, fibroplasia, abscess formation.
Loa loa	Loiasis (Calabar swelling).	Subcutaneous nodules, burrows; worm under skin, conjunctiva.	Microfilariae in blood; subcutaneous inflammation.
Wuchereria bancrofti	Filariasis (elephantiasis).	Headache, weakness, vomiting, myalgia, lymphadenitis, severe chronic lymphedema.	Microfilariae in blood, granulomas of lymphatic system, obliterative lymphangitis, lymphoid hyperplasia, fibroplasia.

Diseases Due to Arthropods

Organism	Disease	Clinical Features	Pathologic Features
Sarcoptes scabiei	Scabies.	Pruritic papules, burrows, secondary infection.	Mites in cutaneous burrows or skin scrapings, focal inflammation.
Phthirus pubis	Phthiriasis.	Pubic itching, lice and nits on pubic hairs, bluish macules.	
Pediculus capitis	Pediculosis capitis.	Pruritus, papules, lice and nits on scalp hairs.	
Pediculus corporis	Pediculosis corporis.	Pruritus, papules, lice and nits on body hairs.	

12

Disorders of Circulation

Hyperemia, Edema

The critical importance of a normal circulation for the health and functioning of all bodily tissues is emphasized by the variety and severity of disorders that can result when this circulation is altered or impaired.

As noted in the preceding chapter, inflammation is accompanied by hyperemia (increased blood in tissues, due to engorgement of capillaries) and edema (tissue swelling due to leakage of plasma from the circulation into intercellular spaces). Hyperemia or edema or both can occur in various other conditions as well.

Hyperemia (congestion) may be either active or passive. **Active hyperemia** occurs when the flow of blood into an area is increased by widespread dilatation of arterioles. Besides being part of an inflammatory reaction, this arteriolar dilatation can result from increased environmental temperature, emotional stimuli (blushing), or local or systemic disease or poisoning that impairs vascular tone. In active hyperemia, tissues are redder than normal because of their increased content of oxygenated blood.

Passive hyperemia is caused by a slowing or stoppage of the venous outflow of blood from an organ or tissue. Such a slowing of venous return of blood to the heart can be caused by anything that obstructs or compresses a major vein, including a blood clot, a tumor, scar tissue, or a pregnant uterus. Local impairment of venous drainage induces a condition called **stasis**, in which blood stagnates in a capillary bed. A more generalized slowing of venous return occurs in congestive heart failure. When the pumping action of the heart is reduced by valvular disease, coronary artery disease, or any other cause, it fails to empty itself completely with each contraction. As a consequence, back-pressure builds up in the veins, and the tissues become

112

congested. When the left ventricle fails, congestion occurs in the lungs; with right ventricular failure, the entire systemic circulation becomes congested. In longstanding heart failure, many organs develop changes known collectively as **chronic passive congestion**. Unlike active hyperemia, passive congestion results in a decrease of oxygen supply to tissues and a buildup of waste products. Passively congested tissues and organs become cyanotic (blue) because of their increased content of nonoxygenated blood. Capillaries must dilate to accommodate the increased volume of blood. Edema results from both the rise in capillary pressure and increased permeability of capillaries and venules. Red blood cells as well as plasma may leak into intercellular spaces. In time, edema fluid may be replaced by fibrosis. All of these changes tend to impair the function of an organ such as the liver or the lung more or less severely, and once fibrosis occurs the impairment may be irreversible.

Edema (also known as hydrops or dropsy) may be local or generalized, depending on its cause. **Lymphedema** is an increase in tissue fluid due to local obstruction of lymphatic channels by a tumor, scarring, or chronic inflammation in lymph nodes. **Angioneurotic edema** is a local allergic response resulting from a sudden change in vascular tone and permeability. A variety of other conditions can produce increases in capillary permeability of a more widespread distribution. These include severe systemic infections, asphyxia, and intoxication with various chemicals. **Osmotic edema** results from retention of sodium in cardiac, renal, hepatic, or endocrine disease or from a decrease in the concentration of albumin in plasma. The osmotic effect of a normal level of albumin is to hold the water content of the blood in the circulation despite the pressure within the system. A decline in the production of albumin (as from starvation or liver disease) or loss of albumin from a diseased kidney (nephrotic syndrome) results in leakage of plasma water into tissue spaces.

An edematous solid organ appears swollen, with a tense, glistening capsule. Its cut surface bulges and exudes fluid. **Ascites** is the presence of edema fluid in the abdominal (peritoneal) cavity; pericardial and pleural effusions are called, respectively, **hydropericardium** and **hydrothorax**. Edema that is most prominent in the lower extremities is called **dependent**. **Anasarca** is a generalized edema of the whole body.

Ischemia, Thrombosis, Embolism

Ischemia is a reduction in the supply of blood to a tissue or organ. It can result from obstruction of a single major artery by a clot or external compression, or from generalized narrowing of arterioles by vascular disease. An organ or tissue that is suddenly and completely deprived of its blood supply cannot long survive the lack of oxygen and essential nutrients and the accumulation of harmful waste products. However, tissues vary greatly in their ability to tolerate ischemia, and the more slowly it develops, the less devastating its effects. Many tissues are able to compensate for ischemia of gradual onset by developing a **collateral circulation**, consisting of newly formed arterioles and capillary beds. Ischemic tissue is abnormally pale and may become edematous because of increased capillary permeability. Prolonged ischemia may result in atrophy (reduction in size), fibrosis, and permanent loss of function. Severe acute interruption of blood supply to any tissue may culminate in infarction (necrosis, death of tissue). Atrophy and necrosis are discussed in Chapter 13.

Blood coagulates when the soluble plasma protein called fibrinogen is converted to fibrin, an insoluble gel that forms strands in which blood cells become enmeshed. The formation of fibrin depends on the presence of calcium and certain other plasma or tissue components. Several alternative series of biochemical reactions, some of them involving platelets, can lead to clotting of blood. A clot that forms within the circulatory system is called a thrombus, and the process of its formation is called **thrombosis**. This can result from local disease or injury of a vessel wall, circulatory stasis, or an increase in the coagulability of the blood. A thrombus may completely obstruct the vessel in which it forms. If this is an artery, thrombosis will result in ischemia or infarction of the tissue supplied by the artery; if a vein, in passive congestion of the tissue or organ drained by the vein. Meanwhile, the thrombus undergoes a gradual process known as **organization**. Capillary buds and inflammatory cells enter it from the vessel wall and eventually break it down, leaving behind a mass of fibrous tissue. **Canalization** (recanalization)—the opening of a new passage through the obstructed vessel—may occur in time. Thrombosis is particularly common in the veins of the pelvis and lower extremity. A thrombus can also develop on the interior wall of a cardiac chamber (**mural thrombus**) under certain conditions.

Because blood in some parts of the circulatory system normally clots after death, it is important for the pathologist to distinguish between thrombi and **postmortem clots**. A thrombus is adherent to the vessel wall, tough, and friable; a postmortem clot is soft, homogeneous, and easily separated from the wall of the vessel in which it forms. Depending on their color, postmortem clots may be called either currant jelly clots or chicken fat clots.

Anything other than fluid blood moving through the circulatory system is called an embolus, and the process of its formation or release into the circulation is called **embolism** or embolization. A thrombus detached from its site of formation is by far the most common kind of embolus, and **thromboembolic disease** is an important cause of disability and death. A thrombus from a systemic vein passes through the right atrium and right ventricle to lodge in a branch of the pulmonary artery (**pulmonary embolism**). This can result in fatal circulatory collapse—a common cause of death in elderly and debilitated persons and those suddenly immobilized by injury or surgery. If the patient survives the embolic episode, he may develop a **pulmonary infarction**—a zone of tissue death in the affected lung. A mural thrombus from the left atrium or left ventricle can pass through the aorta to block a major artery, producing ischemia or infarction of an organ or an extremity. The release of many thrombotic fragments into the circulation is called a "shower" of emboli. **Septic emboli** are fragments of an infected thrombus which, upon being released into the circulation, can not only obstruct small vessels but carry infection to sites remote from the original focus.

Materials other than thrombi can enter the circulation and cause embolic phenomena. **Air embolism** occurs when a substantial volume of air is introduced into a vein as a result of injury, misadventure during certain surgical procedures, or in a deliberate attempt to cause death. Air that reaches the right ventricle interrupts blood flow through the heart. **Fat embolism** results when fat from injured adipose tissue or marrow from a fractured bone enters the circulation. Extensive fat embolism may lead to a syndrome of respiratory failure, neurologic dysfunction, and petechial rash occurring 1–3 days after long-bone fracture. **Amniotic fluid embolism** due to entrance of amniotic fluid into the maternal circulation before or during labor usually causes respiratory distress and circulatory collapse (possibly anaphylactic) and may be accompanied by disseminated intravascular coagulation. The mortality rate is high. At autopsy the pulmonary vessels are stuffed with epithelial cells, hair, and amorphous debris of fetal origin. Drugs and other materials injected for recreational purposes can also act as emboli.

Hemorrhage, Shock

The escape of whole blood from the circulation is called **hemorrhage**. Generally this results from direct injury to one or more vessels, but it can also occur when the wall of a vessel is weakened by disease such as arteriosclerosis or inflammation. **Ecchymosis** is the release of blood into the skin after injury. **Purpura** refers to widespread zones of skin hemorrhage due to generalized vascular disease, deficiency of platelets, or circulating toxins. A **hematoma** is a collection of extravasated blood in tissue.

Shock is an acute, life-threatening state of hypotension (subnormal blood pressure) with inadequate blood flow through vital organs. In shock there is a disparity between the volume of the circulatory system and the volume of blood it contains. A reduction in blood volume is known as hypovolemia. The sudden loss of a large amount of blood from the circulation triggers various compensatory mechanisms, including an increase in the force and rate of the heartbeat, a shift of fluid from intercellular spaces into the circulation, and a shutting down of less important capillary beds such as those in the skin and the digestive system. These compensatory mechanisms account for some of the more conspicuous features of **hemorrhagic (hypovolemic) shock**, such as pallor and coldness of the skin and increased pulse rate. After the rapid loss of about 40% of total blood volume, adequate perfusion of vital organs cannot be maintained by compensatory mechanisms, and death occurs. Hypovolemic shock can also occur when a large volume of plasma is lost from the circulation, as in dehydration and severe burns. Shock can occur in a person with normal blood volume if the arteries undergo widespread dilatation. This happens in severe septicemia (**septic shock**) and in various chemical intoxications.

Review Questions

1. Distinguish active from passive hyperemia.
2. Define or explain: *ascites, embolism, ischemia, shock, thrombosis.*

13

Atrophy, Degeneration, and Necrosis

This chapter discusses a diverse group of tissue disorders, in each of which microscopic changes reflect metabolic or nutritional derangements at the cellular level. In most of these disorders, gross changes and functional impairment are evident as well.

Atrophy

Atrophy is a decrease in the bulk of a tissue or structure that was formerly of normal size and development. Generally it results from the reduction or withdrawal of some essential substance. Hence atrophy may be caused by impairment of blood supply, deficiency in the intake or absorption of nutrients, or failure of hormone stimulation. Atrophy implies both a grossly evident decrease in the size of a structure and a reduction in the number of cells composing it. Microscopic examination usually shows a change not only in the absolute number of cells but in their proportion and arrangement.

Many cells, especially those of cardiac muscle, acquire yellow or brown pigment granules (lipofuscin) on undergoing atrophy. This coloration is evident on gross inspection of tissue. Secretory epithelium, such as that of the liver and kidney, is particularly susceptible to reduction in cell number and disturbance of cellular organization. Connective tissue is less subject to atrophy and in fact the fibrous and fatty stromal elements of an atrophic organ may increase, offsetting in some degree the gross reduction in its bulk. Skeletal muscle atrophy involves a reduction in cell size. Some kinds of atrophy may be considered normal. The thymus gland usually undergoes atrophy during infancy, the tonsils after puberty. Atrophy of the ovaries and breasts normally follows menopause.

Cachexia (wasting) or general atrophy as a consequence of starvation was mentioned in Chapter 10. Cachexia can also result from any severe systemic disease (chronic infection, widespread malignancy) that impairs general metabolism. Fat and muscle are the tissues that are most conspicuously reduced in cachexia. **Senile atrophy** refers to a group of irreversible chemical changes that take place with aging. Certain tissue elements—elastic fibers, bone, and nerve cells—are particularly subject to senile atrophy, though the type and degree of change vary greatly from person to person. Some features of senile atrophy are probably due to impairment of circulation by vascular disease, itself often a form of senile change.

Many forms of atrophy are purely local. Chronic ischemia from any cause can lead to atrophy of the affected organ or tissues. **Pressure atrophy** results when a tissue is subject to constant or intermittent pressure, as from a swelling, tumor, or deformity in an adjacent structure. The basis of pressure atrophy is generally a disturbance of the blood and the lymphatic circulation. Obstruction of a duct, such as the ureter or the hepatic duct, can result in such a buildup of pressure within the organ normally drained by that duct that atrophy ensues.

Disuse atrophy results when a part is subjected to prolonged inactivity or immobilization. Muscle and bone are especially vulnerable to this kind of atrophy. **Neurotrophic atrophy** affects skeletal muscle whose nerve supply has been interrupted by injury or disease. **Endocrine atrophy** is a reduction in parenchymal elements, with decline in function, of a tissue or organ whose normal hormonal stimulation has been lost. For example, the thyroid and adrenal glands undergo atrophy when the pituitary gland (the source of thyroid stimulating hormone and adrenocorticotropic hormone) is destroyed by disease or surgically removed.

Degeneration

Degeneration is a broad term referring to a heterogeneous group of disorders characterized by changes in tissue chemistry. In most of these disorders, microscopic examination reveals swelling of cells and accumulation or deposition in their cytoplasm of substances not normally seen there. Abnormal deposits of material may also occur in intercellular spaces. Special staining may be required to show or to identify abnormal materials in and among cells. Degenerations are classified according to which of these materials are present.

Degenerative changes involving alteration of tissue proteins are among the most common. Abnormal deposits of protein are identified in microscopic sections by their eosinophilic staining properties, that is, their attraction for eosin and other acidic stains. **Albuminous degeneration** (also called parenchymatous degeneration and cloudy swelling) is a common and often reversible change seen in certain organs (particularly the heart, liver, and kidneys) as a result of various systemic conditions—high or prolonged fever, toxemia, or starvation. Affected organs are grossly enlarged, with tenseness of their capsules or covering membranes. Their cut surfaces bulge and appear gray and cloudy or opalescent. On microscopic examination, parenchymal cells are swollen and their cytoplasm appears cloudy or granular. **Hydropic degeneration** presents a similar appearance grossly and has similar causes, but on microscopic examination cells are found to be more markedly distended and their cytoplasm shows vacuoles rather than granules.

Hyaline degeneration includes several unrelated disorders in which tissue elements are changed into or replaced by hyaline (glassy, refractile, transparent) eosinophilic material. Hyaline change can take place in any tissue subjected to chronic inflammation, and it may accompany or follow scarring, atrophy, or senile degeneration. **Zenker's waxy degeneration** is a kind of hyaline change seen in skeletal muscle.

Amyloid is a hyaline protein material that can be distinguished from similar substances by staining with Congo red or by application of iodine. Immunoperoxidase staining using antibodies to various amyloid proteins provides more specific identification. In primary amyloidosis, which is of unknown cause, deposits of amyloid appear chiefly in cardiac and skeletal muscle. Secondary amyloidosis, occurring as a sequel or complication of chronic infection (especially tuberculosis) involves primarily the spleen, kidneys, liver, and adrenals. Amyloid deposits are particularly likely to occur in blood vessel walls. Severe amyloidosis can impair organ function.

Mucinous degeneration refers to any tissue disorder accompanied by abnormal accumulation or deposition of mucin, the protein component of mucus. Excessive mucin can be found in tumors formed from mucus-producing glands, or in glands whose ducts have been obstructed. Mucin is slightly acid and hence attracts basic dyes. **Mucoid** is a similar substance produced by connective tissue and found in increased amounts in myxedema (resulting from deficiency of thyroid hormone) and in myxoma (a type of connective tissue tumor). **Fibrinoid**, a breakdown product of diseased collagen, may be seen in various degenerative processes affecting connective tissue, particularly autoimmune disorders.

Degenerative changes involving abnormal deposition of adipose or lipid material (fat) are also common. Routine techniques of tissue preparation remove fat, leaving empty spaces in the sections. Treatment of tissue with osmic acid before dehydration, clearing, and infiltration fixes the fat and colors it black. Sudan III and other stains are useful for showing adipose material, especially in frozen sections. **Fatty infiltration** is an increase in the fat content of connective-tissue (stromal) components of various organs, which occurs in obesity and other disturbances of lipid metabolism. When severe, it can impair the function of the affected organ by compressing or displacing parenchymal cells. In contrast, **fatty degeneration** refers to the appearance of fat inside parenchymal cells, such as those of the heart, liver, and kidneys, which have sustained metabolic damage as a result of anemia, toxemia, chronic infection, certain chemical intoxications, and other severe systemic disorders. Fatty changes in the liver commonly occur in chronic alcoholism and in both obesity and undernutrition. An organ affected by fatty degeneration has a yellowish color, a greasy or buttery texture, and a flabby consistency, and may be slightly swollen. Fat deposits may appear in grossly evident patches or streaks, producing a "tigroid" appearance.

Cholesterol is a lipoid (fatlike) material normally present in blood and tissues. Deposits of cholesterol can occur in certain tissues, particularly blood vessels, when circulating levels are elevated as a result of diabetes, hypothyroidism, kidney disease, or hereditary disturbance of cholesterol metabolism. Atherosclerosis, a deposition of cholesterol in the lining of arteries accompanied by fibrosis, is a major cause of stroke and heart attack. Cholesterol is a normal component of bile and may form deposits in the wall of the gallbladder, especially when the gallbladder is chronically inflamed. In addition, cholesterol is an important constituent of gallstones.

Several other normal substances may appear in abnormal amounts or locations in tissue as a reflection or accompaniment of biochemical dysfunction. Deposition of **calcium** in tissues other than bones and teeth is abnormal, except that the pineal gland normally shows some calcification after age 20. Calcium appears in microscopic sections as irregular masses of basophilic (blue) material. **Dystrophic calcification** is a deposition of calcium in chronically inflamed, fibrotic, or degenerating tissue, as in tendinitis, osteoarthritis, pulmonary tuberculosis, and in aging blood vessels with or without cholesterol deposits. **Metastatic calcification** is deposition of calcium in normal tissues as a result of an excessive level of calcium in the blood. The lungs, kidneys, and blood vessels are most susceptible; **calculi** (stones) may also form within the urinary tract. **Ossification** implies not only pathologic calcification but formation of bone tissue with haversian systems.

Glycogen is a starchlike carbohydrate that serves as a storage form of glucose, the principal sugar used by the body in energy metabolism. Glycogen is synthesized in the liver and stored in liver and skeletal muscle cells, to whose cytoplasm it normally imparts a finely granular appearance. Abnormal deposition of glycogen in cells occurs in diabetes and in hereditary abnormalities of glycogen storage. Special stains may be used to show glycogen.

Salts of **uric acid**, a normal breakdown product of certain foods, accumulate in the blood and tissues in gout and other metabolic disorders. Formation of urate crystals in joints causes the pain and swelling of acute gouty arthritis. Nodular urate deposits in subcutaneous tissue are called **tophi**. Urates may also contribute to the formation of urinary calculi.

Hemosiderin is an iron-containing breakdown product of hemoglobin. Normally, small amounts of hemosiderin are present in macrophages of the liver and spleen and in other cells. Excessive hemosiderin deposits (**hemosiderosis**) may be found in macrophages and other cells in any condition in which many red cells are broken down (hemolysis), in chronic passive congestion, and after local hemorrhage into tissues. In **hemochromatosis**, large amounts of iron and hemosiderin are deposited in the skin and cardiac muscle and in parenchymal cells of the liver and pancreas, as a result of a disturbance of iron metabolism.

Bilirubin, the pigment of bile, is formed by the further degradation of hemoglobin in the liver. Disease of the liver or obstruction of its ducts can cause a rise in the level of bilirubin in the blood. When this rise is sufficient to impart a yellow or green color to tissues, the condition is known as **jaundice**. **Porphyrins** (coproporphyrin and uroporphyrin), additional breakdown products of hemoglobin, may accumulate in tissue and impart a pink to purple color to urine, teeth, bones, and even the skin in persons with various metabolic and hematologic disorders (porphyrias).

Melanin, the normal pigment of the skin and of the iris, may be increased in certain abnormal conditions. Sun exposure, pregnancy, and adrenocortical deficiency (Addison's disease) cause bronzing of the skin due to increase of melanin. Melanin is responsible for the tan, brown, or black color of pigmented lesions such as freckles, moles, and malignant melanoma. Melanin pigmentation may occur at sites of chronic inflammation or trauma in the skin and in the cartilage and urine (ochronosis) of persons with alkaptonuria, an uncommon inborn error of metabolism. Deposits of foreign material, such as injected inks (tattoos) and absorbed heavy metals (lead, silver), can also cause pigmentation in skin and other tissues.

Necrosis

Necrosis refers to a group of physical and chemical changes in a cell, tissue, or organ that reflect total and permanent cessation of all biological processes and functions—in a word, death. Severe trauma, chemical poisoning, severe or chronic inflammation or degeneration, and any interruption in the supply of oxygen and nutrients may lead to necrosis. On gross examination, necrotic tissue appears white, gray, or yellow, and opaque. On microscopic examination, necrotic cells have more intensely eosinophilic cytoplasm than living ones and their nuclei may show shrinkage and distortion (pyknosis), fragmentation (karyorrhexis), or dissolution (karyolysis). As time passes, cell membranes rupture and architectural details of tissue are lost.

Various types of necrosis are described on the basis of associated physical changes. In **coagulation necrosis**, the usual pattern, plasma proteins gel and solidify, whereas in **liquefaction necrosis** (characteristic of the central nervous system) the dead tissue becomes fluid. **Caseous necrosis**, seen in tuberculosis, involves the conversion of tissue into microscopic masses of homogeneous, cheesy material. A zone of necrotic tissue typically acts as an irritant and elicits an inflammatory reaction in adjacent tissue. It may also show zones of hemorrhage. **Fat necrosis**, a local necrosis of adipose tissue, may result from trauma or ischemia. It is also seen in pancreatic disease, in which local release of fat-digesting enzymes may convert fatty tissue to whitish, opaque, nodular material, which is subject to calcification.

Gangrene is an extensive local necrosis, usually in an extremity, due to circulatory impairment. Dry gangrene is a purely ischemic disorder; wet gangrene implies secondary infection of a necrotic limb.

Infarction is localized necrosis of a zone of tissue due to obstruction of an artery or, occasionally, a vein. In some tissues, such as the kidney, infarction produces a pale, bloodless zone of necrosis (anemic infarct). In others, such as the lung and cardiac muscle, necrosis is preceded or accompanied by considerable hemorrhage from damaged vessels (hemorrhagic infarct). Typically an infarct assumes a wedge shape with the narrow end pointing toward the obstructed vessel.

Putrefaction or decay refers to the decomposition of the body as a whole after death. It is due in part to the action of bacteria normally resident in the intestine. Another element in the decomposition of the dead body is autolysis, or breakdown of cells and tissues by the action of their own chemical components. This is particularly conspicuous in the stomach; gastric juice begins to digest the stomach lining within minutes after death. Gases generated in a putrefying body (cadaverine, putrescine, and others) have an oppressive, nauseating odor. They may cause marked swelling of soft tissues and may distend or even rupture the bowel and other body cavities and spaces. Blood and tissue fluids in which gases of putrefaction are dissolved have a foamy or frothy appearance.

Review Questions

1. Mention some types of atrophy that are normal or expected.
2. What is the common feature of all types of hyaline degeneration?
3. Distinguish *fatty degeneration* from *fatty infiltration*.
4. What substance is deposited in the walls of atherosclerotic blood vessels?
5. What substance breaks down into hemosiderin and bilirubin?
6. What is the name of the pigment normally found in the skin and the iris?
7. Define or explain: *infarction, necrosis, putrefaction.*

14

Physical and Chemical Injury

Physical Trauma

Physical injury and chemical poisoning are important causes of tissue damage, disease, and death. **Physical trauma**, broadly conceived, includes any damage to tissues caused by exposure to excessive kinetic, thermal, electrical, or radiant energy. Friction, stretching, compression, cutting, tearing, or crushing of tissue by physical force causes damage in proportion to the amount of force applied and the type and volume of tissue exposed to it. Disruption of capillaries or larger vessels with focal or diffuse hemorrhage is a feature of most physical trauma. Rigid tissues such as bone, cartilage, and teeth are subject to cracking or shattering (fracture). In soft tissues, distortion of normal architecture occurs at gross and microscopic levels, with tearing or bursting of cell membranes, separation of connective tissue fibers, loss of cellular organization, collapse or disruption of ducts, passages, and other tissue spaces with escape of secretions or contained fluids and gases, and general fragmentation of tissue. In cutting and puncturing wounds due to sharp objects, injury may be largely limited to separation of tissues without extensive damage beyond the margins of the wound.

An inflammatory response begins promptly in any injured tissue whose blood supply has not been critically impaired, as described in Chapter 11. Destroyed or devitalized tissue undergoes necrosis and is removed by macrophages or by sloughing, while surrounding tissues supply endothelial buds and fibroblasts for regeneration and repair. Infection is a common consequence of trauma, especially when bacteria from the skin, the bowel, or the respiratory tract are introduced into areas of hemorrhage, exudate, degeneration, or necrosis. Fibrotic scarring as a late result of extensive injury may cause severe deformity and dysfunction.

Damage due to excessive **heat** is usually confined to the skin. Depending on the amount of heat and the duration of exposure, a burn can induce a spectrum of injury ranging from hyperemia and edema to coagulation and carbonization (charring) of protoplasm. Vesication (blistering) occurs when there is an effusion of fluid under the epidermis. **Chilling** of tissue causes a general retardation of biochemical reactions and a reduction of blood flow through capillary beds, and may lead to edema, vesication, and denaturation of protein.

Electrical shock results from a flow of electrical current through tissues. This may generate enough heat to produce local burns. An electrical current can also interfere with the physiology of nerve and muscle cells, causing failure of respiration, fatal disturbance of cardiac rhythm, or both.

Radiant energy of various wavelengths can damage tissue. **Ionizing radiation** (x-rays, gamma rays) can not only alter the chemistry of cytoplasm and intercellular fluid but also block cell mitosis and induce aberrant cell division and tumor formation. Cells in mitosis are much more vulnerable to the effects of ionizing radiation than other cells. **Sunlight** and **ultraviolet radiation** from other sources can produce acute burns not unlike thermal burns. Prolonged exposure to lower doses of solar irradiation causes tanning (increase in pigment cells), accelerates degeneration and atrophy of both dermis and epidermis, and may promote malignant change.

Chemical Poisons

The variety of ways in which **chemical poisons** can do harm is almost as broad as the variety of poisons. Chemical poisons in gas, liquid, or solid form can exert their effects on contact with skin and mucous membranes or by being swallowed, inhaled, or injected. Strong mineral acids (sulfuric acid, nitric acid) have an immediate and undiscriminating corrosive action on all tissues. Heavy metals (lead, mercury, arsenic) interfere with the metabolism of any cells to whose cytoplasm they penetrate. Organic solvents (benzene, carbon tetrachloride) have a predilection for nerve tissue because of its high content of fatty material. Carbon monoxide competes with oxygen for binding sites on hemoglobin molecules in red blood cells. Some substances block mitosis in certain types of cells. Benzene, for example, can interfere with formation of red blood cells. Drugs and certain plant poisons may exert a highly specific action on one type of tissue— for example, the conduction system of the heart—or may interfere with one specific type of biochemical reaction—for example, the synthesis of essential clotting factors. Establishing a diagnosis of chemical poisoning usually depends on identification of the poison by chemical analysis of blood, tissue, secretions, or waste products. The accompanying table summarizes information on the toxic effects, chiefly systemic, of selected chemical poisons.

Review Questions

1. List several types of physical trauma.
2. Name various ways in which chemical poisons affect body structure and function.

Effects of Chemical Poisons

Poison	Clinical Features	Pathologic Features
Arsenic Acute	Vomiting, diarrhea, abdominal cramps, skeletal muscle cramps, oliguria, shock.	Gastrointestinal ulceration, hyperemia and petechial hemorrhage of viscera, serous effusions, focal hepatic necrosis, renal tubular necrosis.
Chronic	Cutaneous pigmentation, peripheral neuropathy.	Hyperkeratosis, myelin degeneration of peripheral nerves, hepatic cirrhosis.
Benzene	Tachypnea, cardiac arrhythmias, visual blurring, seizures, coma.	Aplastic anemia due to marrow suppression, hemosiderosis, and centrilobular necrosis of liver.
Carbon monoxide	Flushing or cyanosis of skin, CNS depression, paralysis, seizures, shock, neurologic sequelae.	Cerebral edema and petechiae, neuronal degeneration, degeneration of liver, kidney, myocardium; carboxyhemoglobin in blood.
Cyanide	Cyanosis, respiratory depression, shock.	Visceral edema, gastrointestinal mucosal hemorrhage, fatty degeneration of liver.
Fluoride Acute	Vomiting, muscle twitching, tetany.	Pneumonitis, pulmonary edema, necrotizing gastritis.
Chronic	Dental mottling.	Osteosclerosis.

Effects of Chemical Poisons *(continued)*

Poison	Clinical Features	Pathologic Features
Lead		
Acute	Abdominal cramps, vomiting.	Gastrointestinal inflammation.
Chronic	Muscle cramps, abdominal cramps, seizures, peripheral neuropathy, anemia.	Cerebral edema, neuronal degeneration, myelin degeneration of peripheral nerves, anemia, basophilic stippling of erythrocytes, porphyrins in blood and urine.
Mercury		
Acute	Sialorrhea, abdominal pain, vomiting, bloody diarrhea, oliguria, shock.	Coagulation necrosis of gastric and colonic mucosa; degeneration and necrosis of proximal convoluted tubules.
Chronic	Tremors, hyperreflexia.	Cerebral cortical neuronal degeneration.
Methyl alcohol	Headache, visual impairment, nausea, vomiting, dyspnea, cyanosis, abdominal pain.	Cerebral edema, meningeal petechiae, neuronal necrosis of retina, pleural hemorrhage, degeneration of liver and kidney, metabolic acidosis.
Mushroom (*Amanita*)	Vomiting, diarrhea, hepatomegaly, oliguria, jaundice, seizures.	Hepatic necrosis, metabolic acidosis.
Nitrogen oxides	Cough, dyspnea, chills (silo filler's disease).	Pulmonary edema, obliterative bronchiolitis.
Petroleum distillates	Vomiting, cough, bronchopneumonia, seizures.	Pneumonitis, cerebral edema, myelitis, marrow depression.

Effects of Chemical Poisons *(continued)*

Poison	Clinical Features	Pathologic Features
Phenol	Dyspnea, cough, headache, weakness, nausea, dark urine.	Pulmonary edema, hepatic and renal degeneration, cerebral edema, necrosis of bladder epithelium.
Phosphorus Acute	CNS depression, seizures, respiratory arrest, garlic odor on breath.	Fatty degeneration of kidney, heart, brain; peripheral hepatic necrosis.
Chronic	Jaundice, renal failure.	Osteomalacia, necrotizing and suppurative osteomyelitis of maxilla and mandible ("phossy jaw"), hepatic cirrhosis.
Snake venom (pit viper)	Local pain, hypesthesia, nausea, dyspnea, cyanosis, fever, shock.	Hemolysis, neuronal degeneration, local necrosis.
Thallium	Ataxia, lethargy, seizures, dyspnea, fever, abdominal and limb pain, hair loss.	Inflammation of gastrointestinal mucosa, fatty degeneration of liver and kidney, pneumonitis, vacuolar degeneration of adrenal and thyroid glands.

15

Neoplasia

Neoplasia may be defined as an erratic, uncontrolled growth of cells that serves no useful or beneficial purpose. The product of neoplasia may be called a growth, tumor, or neoplasm. Various explanations have been offered for the occurrence of neoplasia, but none of these fits all cases. Among causes that seem to explain certain types of neoplasms may be mentioned an aberrant repair process after chronic inflammation; alteration of cell genetics by chemical poisons, ionizing radiation, or viral infection; hormonal stimulation; depression of cellular immunity; and hereditary factors. Neoplastic cells arise from normal cells by abnormal mitosis and generally bear some resemblance to their cells of origin. However, their genetic coding is permanently deranged, and this is often reflected in irregularity of structure (atypia). Moreover, neoplastic tissue generally fails in some measure to duplicate the internal organization and architecture of normal tissue. For example, glandular structures may be ill-formed or nonfunctioning, and the expected proportions and relations between parenchyma and stroma may not be preserved. Neoplasia is sometimes difficult to distinguish histologically from chronic inflammation.

A neoplasm that is capable of causing death by extending into or spreading to normal tissue and destroying it is called cancerous or malignant; one that does not do so is called benign. It is noteworthy that a histologically benign tumor can cause death by compressing some vital structure or eroding a major blood vessel, and on the other hand, a slowly growing malignancy may not prove lethal if a more rapidly progressive fatal condition supervenes. Some tumors are inherently malignant from their earliest origins, while others begin as benign tumors and undergo malignant degeneration. Most benign tumors, however, remain benign.

As mentioned in previous chapters, much of the day-by-day practice of pathology is concerned with the identification of malignancies and the determination of their extent and expected future behavior. Several features are more characteristic of malignant neoplasms than of benign ones. First, a malignant tumor is more likely to display **anaplasia**—the presence of primitive cells, or more undifferentiated cells than are normally present in the affected tissue. Second, a malignant tumor typically enlarges by infiltration and invasion of surrounding tissues, whereas a benign tumor expands while remaining sharply localized and readily distinguishable from surrounding normal tissue. Often a benign tumor has a definite capsule. Third, a malignant tumor tends to grow faster than a benign one. Fourth, a malignant tumor is capable of **metastasis**—establishing secondary foci of malignant cells at sites remote from the primary tumor. Metastasis can be lymphatic, through lymph channels; hematogenous, through the blood circulation; or by direct implantation, as in the peritoneal cavity and central nervous system, where seeding of a fluid medium with malignant cells can result in development of metastatic tumors over the surface bathed by that fluid (drop metastases). Each type of tumor has its preferred sites for metastasis. In general, tumors of epithelial origin (carcinomas) tend to metastasize by lymphatic channels, tumors of connective tissue origin (sarcomas) by the blood stream. Metastasis to a vital organ such as the brain, the lung, or the liver is a common mechanism of death in malignant disease. The presence of widespread metastases (carcinomatosis) is often associated with cachexia, toxic manifestations, and increased susceptibility to infection.

Malignant cells display a number of distinctive morphologic features. They tend to vary more in size (anisocytosis) and shape (pleomorphism) than normal cells, and to form irregular clusters instead of showing the polarity of normal cell aggregations. The nuclei of malignant cells tend to be larger than the nuclei of nonmalignant cells in proportion to their cytoplasm (high nuclear/cytoplasmic ratio) and to vary more in size, shape, and structure. These nuclei also tend to stain more darkly (hyperchromasia) and to show prominent nuclear membranes and one or more large, acidophilic nucleoli. Mitotic figures are more frequent in malignant tissue, and are often multipolar or otherwise anomalous. The cytoplasm of malignant cells often contains vacuoles. Giant-cell formation is characteristic of some malignancies.

A neoplasm is called hormone-dependent when its development results in part from stimulation by a normal or abnormal level of hormone in the circulation. For example, cancer of the prostate depends on testicular androgen, and does not develop in men who have been castrated. Conversely, both benign and malignant tumors arising from glandular tissue can produce excessive levels of hormone that cause remote or systemic effects (functioning tumors). Hormonelike substances produced by tumors arising from nonglandular cells may also induce remote effects (paraneoplastic syndromes).

Because the proliferation of neoplastic tissue is not subject to normal controls, it often outstrips the available blood supply. Many tumors, especially malignant ones, contain areas of degeneration, necrosis, and hemorrhage. Cysts formed within a tumor may be lined with secretory epithelium and contain serous, mucinous, or other secretion, or they may simply be clefts or spaces formed by degeneration of tissue and filled with necrotic debris. Calcium deposits may develop in degenerating tumor tissue. In a scirrhous tumor, exuberant production of connective tissue fibers (desmoplasia) yields a dense, woody or stony consistency. Some malignancies, particularly rapidly growing ones, elicit intense inflammatory reaction in surrounding tissues. A malignant tumor developing on a surface, such as skin or mucous membrane, may evolve in one of three patterns: as a thickened plaque, infiltrating laterally; as a polypoid or fungating mass growing away from the surface; or as an ulcer formed by undermining and destruction of surface epithelium.

The **grade** of a malignant neoplasm is a quantitative estimate of its malignant potential, generally based on the percentage of anaplastic (undifferentiated) cells it contains. Grading correlates generally with the expected future behavior of a tumor, a high-grade malignancy being more prone to invade and metastasize than a low-grade one. The following widely used grading system is called the Broders index:

Grade 1: one-fourth undifferentiated cells
Grade 2: one-half undifferentiated cells
Grade 3: three-fourths undifferentiated cells
Grade 4: all cells undifferentiated

Staging of a malignancy is a formulation of its current extent, an attempt to describe its behavior up to the present. A tumor that remains confined to its tissue of origin is said to exist **in situ** (carcinoma in situ). A system of staging used for many tumors is the TNM (tumor-node-metastasis) classification. In each class, a number represents the degree of spread, 0 meaning "none" or "undetectable." Thus, T2, N1, M0 would indicate a locally invasive tumor with involvement of regional lymph nodes but no distant metastases. Elaborate TNM codes have been worked out for several types of tumor.

Both grading and staging of tumors are important in prognosis, in choice of therapy, and in statistical recording (tumor registry).

Nomenclature of the Commoner Neoplasms

Origin	Benign Neoplasms	Malignant Neoplasms
Epithelium		
surface epithelium	papilloma	epidermoid carcinoma
secretory epithelium	adenoma	adenocarcinoma
endothelium, lymph vessel	lymphangioma	lymphangioendothelioma
endothelium, blood vessel	hemangioma	hemangioendothelioma
Connective Tissue		
adult fibrous tissue	fibroma	fibrosarcoma
fat	lipoma	liposarcoma
cartilage	chondroma	chondrosarcoma
bone	osteoma	osteogenic sarcoma
embryonic fibrous tissue	myxoma	myxosarcoma
notochord	chordoma	chordoma
nerve sheath	neurofibroma	neurogenic sarcoma
Muscle		
skeletal muscle	rhabdomyoma	rhabdomyosarcoma
smooth muscle	leiomyoma	leiomyosarcoma
Nerve		
neuron	neuroma	neuroma
Hemolymphatic Tissue		
bone marrow		myeloma
lymphoid tissue		lymphoma

Review Questions

1. List four major differences between benign and malignant neoplasms.
2. Distinguish between grading and staging of malignant neoplasms.
3. Define or explain: *anaplasia, desmoplasia, hyperchromasia, pleomorphism.*

Part IV

Special Pathology

16

The Skin

Gross and Microscopic Anatomy

The skin or integument covers the entire external surface of the body. Skin normally varies in texture, thickness, pigmentation, and distribution of sweat glands and hair follicles from one part of the body to another, and from one person to another on the basis of age, sex, race, and other constitutional factors. At the orifices of the respiratory, digestive, and genitourinary systems, skin shows a transition to mucous membrane. Histologically the skin consists of two layers of essentially different tissue, an outer epithelial layer or epidermis and an inner layer of connective tissue called the dermis, corium, or true skin.

The **epidermis** contains but two kinds of cell, the keratinocyte and the melanocyte. **Keratinocytes** are by far the more numerous. The epidermis is divided into four zones or strata on the basis of various stages in the development of keratinocytes. The **stratum germinativum** or basal cell layer, the deepest zone, consists of cylindrical or polygonal cells with deeply staining nuclei. These are sometimes known as prickle cells because of their conspicuous, thornlike intercellular bridges. By their continued duplication, the cells of the stratum germinativum maintain a steady supply of new epidermal cells. Some authorities divide the basal cell layer into a deeper stratum germinativum and a more superficial stratum spinosum.

Melanocytes or melanoblasts, which produce the pigment melanin, are distributed through the stratum germinativum in varying numbers. By embryonic origin they are neural rather than epithelial cells. Melanocytes are more plentiful in certain areas of the body surface, such as the genitals and the nipples. They have long, branching, tubular processes that extend among the keratinocytes in the more superficial layers of the epidermis, and through which they inject pigment into these keratinocytes. In routine histologic preparations, melanocytes may not show their pigment. When a section of skin is treated with DOPA (dihydroxyphenylalanine, which is essential for natural melanin synthesis), only melanocytes darken.

The basement membrane on which the stratum germinativum rests is not flat but corrugated. Elevations of the dermis called **dermal papillae** extend upward into the epidermis, and projections of epidermis called **rete pegs** extend downward into the dermis. This mechanical interlocking of the two layers greatly enhances the cohesion and tensile strength of the integument.

The **stratum granulosum** lies just above the stratum germinativum and consists of two to five layers of flattened polygonal cells with prominent cytoplasmic granules composed of keratohyalin. These are cells that were formed in the stratum germinativum and are now moving outward. Some of them already show nuclear disintegration. The **stratum lucidum** is a layer of further flattened cells, without nuclei. The outermost layer or **stratum corneum** consists of dead, scalelike cells composed largely of keratin. All of these zones can be distinguished in thick skin such as that of the palms and soles. In thin skin only the stratum germinativum and stratum corneum may be clearly evident.

The **dermis** is a thin but tough layer of connective tissue containing collagenous, elastic, and reticular fibers in varying proportions. In the deeper **reticular layer** the fibers are more densely woven and are disposed roughly parallel to the skin surface. The **papillary layer** consists of numerous club- or fingerlike dermal papillae, which extend upward between the rete pegs of the epidermis. Some of these papillae contain capillary loops, while others contain sensory nerve endings (Meissner's corpuscles). The dermis is richly supplied with blood vessels, lymphatic vessels, and sensory nerves. It contains the usual connective tissue cells, including a few fat cells, and scattered smooth muscle fibers. Dermal chromatophores similar to melanocytes are occasionally found in the dermis. Beneath the dermis is a layer of loose connective tissue containing variable amounts of fat and called the superficial fascia, panniculus adiposus, pannus, tela subcutanea, fibrofatty layer, or hypodermis.

Nails are plates of keratin material that develop in a fashion similar to the stratum corneum of the epidermis from a region of specialized tissue called the nail matrix. **Hairs** are formed in hair follicles, tubular structures lying at the junction of the epidermis and the dermis and incorporating tissue from both. The hair itself consists of epithelial cells that lose their nuclei as the hair grows out. In the scalp and other areas of the body, each hair follicle has an arrector pili muscle attached to it, a small bundle of smooth-muscle cells responsible for the erection of hairs.

Sebaceous or **oil glands** are usually found in association with hair follicles, the combination of one of each being referred to as a pilosebaceous unit. These simple alveolar glands produce an oily secretion called sebum, which serves to protect the skin and retard water loss from it. Lying in the dermis, the sebaceous gland empties its secretion by a short duct directly into the hair follicle. The funnel-shaped portion of the hair follicle between the sebaceous gland duct and the skin surface is called the infundibulum. Sebaceous glands are more plentiful in some parts of the body surface (e.g., the face and axillae) than in others. They appear independent of any hair follicles in the skin of the lips and the external genitalia. **Sweat** or **sudoriferous glands** are coiled, tubular arrangements of secretory cells located in the dermis or subcutaneous tissue. Each sweat gland communicates with the skin surface by a straight duct that passes perpendicularly up through the epidermis to end at a pore.

Pathologic Study of the Skin

Human skin is subject to a broad variety of trophic, inflammatory, and degenerative disorders, some of them having little clinical importance, and many of them of unknown origin. For the majority of these conditions, dermatologists and other physicians can establish a working diagnosis and a plan of treatment after reviewing the patient's history and conducting a gross examination of the lesion or lesions.

The practicing pathologist's principal concern with skin is in the evaluation of relatively small biopsy specimens removed to aid in the diagnosis of local or general skin diseases whose nature cannot be determined by other means. The pathologist is also frequently called upon to examine excised neoplasms of the skin, not only for histologic diagnosis but to assess the adequacy of removal. Skin may be included in various other types of surgical specimens, such as excised scars and fistulous tracts, devitalized tissue debrided from wounds or ischemic zones, amputated extremities, and mastectomy specimens.

A punch biopsy consists of a plug of skin 3–4 mm in diameter removed with a cylindrical punch under local anesthesia. The punch is rotated slightly as it advances through epidermis and dermis into the subcutaneous fat. In a shave biopsy, a scalpel or razor blade is moved along parallel to the skin surface with a slight sawing motion so as to remove a thin layer consisting mostly of epidermis. For malignant neoplasms, total excision is performed with a substantial margin of normal tissue all around and beneath the lesion. To facilitate surgical closure and minimize scarring, the incision is usually diamond- or spindle-shaped (often somewhat inaccurately termed elliptical). Mohs surgery is a technique for excising malignant skin lesions in stages, with examination of specimens from each level by frozen section. At autopsy, the pathologist studies the entire skin surface grossly and may take specimens from abnormal areas for microscopic study.

Classification of Skin Lesions

Grossly evident, local cutaneous abnormalities can be reduced to a relatively small number of types. Any of these can occur as a solitary lesion, in one or more clusters, or distributed widely or generally over the skin. Two or more types of lesion may occur together, and one type can evolve into another. A **macule** is a flat spot, of any shape, that differs in color from surrounding skin. This difference may result from an increase or decrease in normal pigment or from the presence of abnormal substances or of normal substances in abnormal amounts. A **petechia** is a macule due to extravasation of blood just beneath the epidermis. A **telangiectasis** is a permanent dilatation of one or more small blood vessels visible through the skin. A **tattoo** is a deposit of foreign material in the dermis that is visible through the epidermis. Besides deliberate injection of inks for decorative purposes, tattooing can result from accidental injury in which foreign material is introduced into the dermis and retained there. A **plaque** is a flat zone varying in texture from surrounding skin (usually it is harder) as well as in appearance.

A **papule** is a small raised area of skin. A **nodule** is a larger and more deeply seated elevation. A still larger mass in the skin may be designated a **tumor**. Papules and nodules vary in shape and may or may not differ in color from surrounding skin. They are solid, not fluid-filled. A papule with a broad, flat base is called sessile, and one with a narrower attachment or stalk is called pedunculated. A cutaneous **horn** is a hard, pointed projection consisting of densely packed keratinous material. A **wheal** is a transitory papule due to local edema and occurring in hives and other conditions.

A **vesicle** is a small, thin-walled, raised zone of epidermis filled with serum, plasma, or blood. A **bulla** (**bleb**) is a similar lesion, but larger. A **pustule** is a vesicle that contains pus. A **cyst** is a thicker-walled abnormal structure containing fluid or semisolid material. A **comedo** is a dilated sebaceous duct or gland containing a keratin plug.

An **erosion** or **excoriation** is a surface defect in the epidermis produced by rubbing or scratching. An **ulcer** is a cutaneous defect of any size or shape extending into the dermis. A **fissure** is a linear defect or crack in the continuity of the epidermis. **Lichenification** refers to a localized thickening and coarsening of the skin as a result of chronic irritation (usually scratching). A **scale** is a visible flake of epidermis, of any size, shape, or color, that is shed from the skin surface. Extensive shedding of scales is called desquamation or exfoliation. A **crust** (scab) is a hard, friable, irregular layer formed of dried blood, serum, pus, tissue debris, or any combination of these on the surface of injured or inflamed skin. An **eschar** is a crust formed on a burn.

Lesions resulting from acute trauma are classified as **incised wounds**, inflicted by sharp objects with relatively little force; **lacerations**, bursting injuries caused by blunt trauma, with more or less crushing of wound edges; **contusions**, due to blunt trauma that does not break the skin; **puncture wounds**, penetrating wounds of very small breadth; and **abrasions**, with mechanical removal of epidermis and even dermis by a scraping movement parallel or tangential to the surface. A cutaneous wound measuring more than 2–3 mm in any direction and penetrating the basal layer of the epidermis usually heals by formation of a **scar** (**cicatrix**). A **keloid** is a hypertrophic scar. A **pit** is a small depression in the skin resulting from focal atrophy or scarring after trauma or inflammation.

The dermatologist uses the term **nevus** for any birthmark—that is, for any congenital cutaneous lesion, whether its color is due to a deposit of melanin or not. In pathology, however, a nevus is a pigmented (melanotic) lesion, whether raised or flat.

Inflammation of the Skin

Dermatitis is a nonspecific term for any inflammatory process involving the skin. Dermatitis can result from acute or chronic trauma by chemical (contact dermatitis) or physical agents; local or systemic infection due to bacteria, viruses, or fungi; allergy or autoimmunity; and unknown causes. Grossly evident changes in acute dermatitis include erythema, edema, vesicle formation, and oozing. The term **eczema**, sometimes used synonymously with dermatitis and sometimes limited to allergic (atopic) dermatitis, means literally "boiling out" and refers to the phenomenon of oozing or weeping. Because itching is also a feature of dermatitis, excoriation and lichenification often follow. Secondary bacterial infection may augment the inflammatory reaction and cause suppuration. By definition, all of the changes in dermatitis are reversible. Some types of dermatitis, however, are exceedingly chronic.

Some cutaneous diseases affect primarily the dermal appendages—nails, hair, sebaceous glands, and sweat glands. Pigmentation or deformity of nails can result from congenital disorders, trauma, systemic diseases or intoxications, fungal infection, and other causes.

Onychomycosis (fungal infection of a nail) causes discoloration, thickening, splitting into layers, and separation from the nail bed. Alopecia (calvities, baldness) may be partial or total, congenital or acquired. It may result from local conditions of the scalp or from systemic disease. Graying of the hair (canities), besides occurring with aging, may also be a feature of vitiligo. Hirsutism (hypertrichosis), or excessive facial and body hair, is nearly always hereditary or constitutional but may accompany adrenal or ovarian disease. In acne vulgaris, overactive sebaceous glands become plugged with thickened secretion, forming comedones. These often progress to a cystic or pustular stage. In seborrheic dermatitis, there is diffuse erythema, with excessive oiliness of the skin and scale formation. Dyshidrotic eczema is a dermatitis accompanied by distention of sweat glands, particularly on the hands. Hidradenitis suppurativa is a deep, spreading, chronic pyogenic infection of sweat glands, usually in the axillae and groins.

Diseases of the Epidermis

Some dermatologic disorders arise in and remain largely confined to the epidermis, while others affect principally dermal structures, but the two levels are so intimately associated that any severe or chronic disease of the skin will eventually produce changes in both. Because the epidermis contains no blood vessels or connective tissue elements, its range of abnormal responses is different from that of many other tissues.

Histologic changes in the epidermis can be divided into abnormalities of keratinocyte growth and development, inflammatory reactions, pigmentary changes, and neoplasms arising from keratinocytes or melanocytes. Various patterns of altered growth can disturb the normal, regular outward migration and keratinization of cells from the basal layer. **Hyperkeratosis** refers to an increased thickness of the stratum corneum, which may be described as compact, lamellated (layered), or in a basketweave pattern. Usually hyperkeratosis is associated with an increased number of cell layers in the stratum granulosum (**hypergranulosis**). When, on the contrary, the stratum granulosum is reduced, and keratinocytes with persistent nuclei are found in the stratum corneum, the condition is known as **parakeratosis**. Any other disorder of keratinization, including those associated with anaplasia and malignant change, may be designated generically **dyskeratosis**. **Acanthosis** is a hyperplasia of the stratum spinosum, which usually causes a change in the shape of the rete pegs, sometimes making them appear more rounded, and at other times creating a sawtooth configuration.

The usual response of the epidermis to irritation or injury is the development of focal or diffuse intercellular edema. In more severe conditions there is also microvesiculation (formation of microscopic fluid-filled clefts among cells), which may progress to production of grossly evident vesicles. **Acantholysis** refers to a loss of intercellular bridges in the prickle-cell layer, with separation and isolation of cells. **Spongiosis** is a patchy intercellular edema of the epidermis, which yields a spongy or porous appearance on microscopic examination and may advance to microvesiculation. In **ballooning degeneration**, basal cells become swollen and vacuolated, and their nuclei undergo a mitotic division to form multinucleate giant cells. **Reticular colliquation** refers to a patchy degeneration of keratinocytes in which adjacent masses of disintegrating cells coalesce to form strands of eosinophilic material in a reticular pattern, the spaces being filled by edema fluid. With **liquefaction degeneration** there is obliteration of the basement membrane, edema of the basal cells and the immediately subjacent dermis, and an infiltrate of inflammatory cells at the junction of dermis and epidermis. Small collections of neutrophils scattered throughout the epidermis are called **microabscesses**. Vesicles, bullae, and pustules appear as open clefts or spaces between layers of the epidermis, or between dermis and epidermis, and may contain eosinophilic traces of plasma, red blood cells, neutrophils, or tissue debris. In some conditions, inflammatory cells migrate into the epidermis from the dermis (transepithelial migration of chronic inflammatory cells).

Neoplasms of the Epidermis

Benign neoplasms arising from keratinocytes are common. Most are of only cosmetic significance, but some undergo malignant degeneration. A **wart** (verruca, condyloma acuminatum) is a benign neoplasm of keratinocytes induced by infection with human papovavirus. Grossly it appears as a rough, friable plaque or papule. Histologically warts display acanthosis and hyperkeratosis with acidophilic and vacuolar change in the cells of the stratum granulosum. A **seborrheic keratosis** is a yellow or brown warty papule or nodule covered with a greasy scale. On microscopic examination it shows hyperkeratosis and melanosis (increased pigment); it is benign. The term **actinic keratosis** (also senile or solar keratosis) is applied to a rough, irregular, usually darkened zone of thickened epidermis typically seen in elderly skin and resulting from prolonged exposure to the sun. On microscopic examination these lesions are found to contain keratinocytes showing varying degrees and combinations of hyperkeratosis, parakeratosis, and dyskeratosis (hyperchromasia, pleomorphism), with increased melanin, infiltrates of mononuclear cells from the dermis, and superficial accumulation of keratinous material. **Leukoplakia** is an analogous lesion on mucous membranes, consisting of whitening and thickening of surface epithelium. Actinic keratosis and leukoplakia can evolve into squamous-cell carcinoma.

Skin cancer is the most common human malignancy, and two types of cancer that develop from keratinocytes account for all but a small fraction of skin cancers. **Basal cell carcinoma**, the most prevalent type, appears on the head or neck in 90% of cases and is more likely to occur in fair-skinned persons. Its gross appearance is somewhat variable but in nearly all cases ulceration eventually occurs, and may result in widespread destruction of tissue (rodent ulcer). A typical gross appearance is of a nodule or cyst with pearly margins and telangiectases. Hyperpigmentation may occur. Histologically a basal cell carcinoma consists of nests or concentric swirls of closely packed, monomorphous oval cells without intercellular spines. Focal edema, hyaline degeneration, and necrosis may modify the microscopic appearance. Though locally destructive, basal cell carcinomas seldom metastasize.

Squamous cell carcinoma is also more common on the head and neck than elsewhere. Grossly this tumor appears as a chronic, non-healing, scaly, crusting, indurated and eventually ulcerated zone surrounded by normal skin. It may develop from actinic keratosis. On microscopic examination, irregular nests of epithelial cells showing malignant changes are found to have invaded the dermis to a variable depth. These cells may be highly anaplastic or they may give evidence of their origin from any of the strata of the epidermis. Epithelial "pearls" of keratinous debris may appear within cell nests. Metastasis is uncommon.

Bowen's disease is a premalignant neoplasm consisting of one or more papules with a rough, keratotic surface and, on microscopic examination, zones of dyskeratosis with large round keratinocytes having pale cytoplasm and large nuclei.

Local and general changes or variations in the degree of pigmentation in the epidermis are due to variations in the activity of melanocytes, rather than to changes in their number. In albinism (congenital absence of melanin), vitiligo (acquired patchy depigmentation, of unknown cause), postinflammatory hypopigmentation, and other leukodermas, melanocytes are present in normal numbers, but do not produce melanin. When increased pigmentation is grossly evident, melanocytes are usually normal in number, but they produce and release more melanin and may be enlarged as a reflection of increased activity.

Increased pigmentation (melanosis or hypermelanosis) is a common feature of many local and systemic conditions and disorders. Heightened melanocyte activity occurs in tanning and in freckles (ephelides) as a result of ultraviolet irradiation, in pregnancy and Addison's disease as a result of hormonal stimulation. Blotchy facial hyperpigmentation seen in pregnancy and other conditions is called chloasma or melasma. Melanosis may accompany or follow any chronic irritation or inflammation in the skin.

Benign pigmented **nevi** (pigmented moles) occur in the skin of virtually all persons except albinos. They are of concern principally because they must be distinguished from malignant neoplasms. The characteristic histologic feature of all pigmented nevi is the nevocyte or nevus cell, a polymorphic pigment-producing cell that may be a modified melanocyte or a cell of different origin. Nevus cells typically occur in clusters or nests, and their location with respect to the dermoepidermal junction forms the basis of the histologic classification of nevi as **junctional** (in the stratum germinativum), **intradermal** (predominantly or exclusively within the dermis), and **compound** (about equally distributed in both areas). In a **blue nevus**, loose aggregations of elongated melanocytes appear in the superficial dermis. A **lentigo** is a macular, freckle-like lesion consisting of an increased number of normal-appearing melanocytes at the dermoepidermal junction. **Lentigo maligna** (Hutchinson's melanotic freckle) contains an irregular proliferation of atypical melanocytes at the junctional zone, and often undergoes malignant change.

Malignant melanoma is a rapidly growing, aggressively malignant neoplasm that may be flat or raised and may appear in previously normal skin or as a development in a lentigo maligna. Grossly, malignant melanoma is characterized by irregularity of shape, border, and pigment distribution, rapid growth, and a tendency to bleed. Histologic examination shows cells of melanocytic origin with typical features of malignant change. Five stages of development are distinguished:

Stage I: Malignant melanoma in situ; malignant cells in epidermis only.

Stage II: Malignant cells in papillary layer of dermis.

Stage III: Malignant cells filling papillary dermis.

Stage IV: Malignant cells in reticular dermis.

Stage V: Malignant cells in subcutaneous fat.

Besides histologic staging of malignant melanoma and verification that all margins of surgically excised tissue are free of neoplastic cells, measurement of the thickness of the primary lesion with an ocular micrometer has proved to be of great importance in predicting the outcome of surgical removal. Invasion beyond a depth of 2.25 mm carries a much less favorable prognosis. Metastasis of malignant lymphoma is by blood and lymph.

Diseases of the Dermis

The proportion of elastic fibers in the dermis varies from person to person. **Hyperelastosis cutis** (Ehlers-Danlos syndrome) is a familial excess of elastic fibers with resultant rubbery texture and exaggerated stretchability of the skin. Abnormal growths of dermal blood vessels (hemangiomas) are among the commoner kinds of birthmark. **Capillary hemangiomas** are pink or red and may be flat (nevus flammeus, port-wine stain) or elevated (strawberry hemangioma). Often they enlarge during the first few months of life but then spontaneously shrink or disappear. They consist of dilated capillaries that on histologic examination appear immature or poorly differentiated. A **cavernous hemangioma** is a more elaborate, mature vascular malformation, often containing arteriovenous shunts. It is of a deeper color and shows no tendency to regress spontaneously.

Any severe acute dermatitis is accompanied by histologic evidence of inflammation in the dermis. Certain infections (leprosy, tuberculosis, syphilis) and certain autoimmune disorders (lupus erythematosus, scleroderma) produce chronic inflammatory changes. Infiltrates of neutrophils or lymphocytes, depending on chronicity, may be junctional, perivascular, patchy, or diffuse in distribution. Mast cells, plasma cells, or eosinophils may be present in significant numbers. Often there is associated hyaline or fibrinoid degeneration of collagen, granuloma formation, or both. **Solar elastosis** (solar degeneration) is a condition induced by chronic exposure to sunlight, with production of spaghetti-like tangles of basophilic connective tissue fibers. **Xanthosis** refers to deposition of cholesterol or similar material in the dermis, with resultant yellow coloration of the skin. This may form flat plaques on the eyelids or elsewhere (xanthelasma) or nodules over the extensor surfaces of the extremities (xanthoma tuberosum). Histologic examination reveals ill-defined nests of lipid-containing histiocytes (foam cells, lattice cells), with sparse inflammatory cell infiltrate and sometimes Touton giant cells with lipid-laden cytoplasm rimmed by nuclei.

Cicatrization is formation of a mass of collagenous fibers to repair a skin wound that has traversed and disrupted the basal cell layer. A **keloid** is a hypertrophic scar, with thick, eosinophilic bands of collagenous fibers, active fibroblasts, and often associated epidermal atrophy.

Neoplasms of the dermis may arise from any of its component cells or tissues, or may extend or metastasize from deeper structures.

Only the commoner dermal neoplasms will be mentioned. **Neuro-fibroma** is a benign nodular lesion derived from nerve sheath (Schwann) cells. The lesion may be solitary, or numerous nodules may form over the whole body surface (neurofibromatosis, von Reckling-hausen's disease of skin). In the generalized form, neurofibromas are accompanied by cáfe-au-lait spots on the skin and by lesions of peripheral nerves.

Mycosis fungoides is a malignant condition in which itchy erythematous patches (premycotic stage) gradually evolve into plaques infiltrated by abnormal lymphocytes with convoluted nuclei called Sézary cells (infiltrative stage) and so on to a tumor stage. Sézary cells also appear in the peripheral blood. **Kaposi sarcoma** consists of solitary or multiple purple nodules usually appearing on the extremities and containing irregular, intercommunicating vascular channels. Histologic examination shows pseudogranulomatous aggregations of cells and infiltrates of lymphocytes and plasma cells. This malignant tumor is much commoner in persons with impaired immunity, such as those with AIDS, in whom visceral spread and fatal outcome are also more likely.

Panniculitis is inflammation of the panniculus adiposus or subcutaneous fat layer. It may result from extension of an inflammatory or infectious process from the skin or may be a reflection of a systemic disorder. Inflammatory nodules and fat necrosis are often found. Infiltrates of inflammatory cells may be primarily in connective tissue septa (septal panniculitis), primarily in fat lobules (lobular panniculitis), or diffusely distributed.

Cutaneous Infections

Numerous infectious diseases cause pathologic changes in the skin. Some of these are purely local processes and others are systemic diseases with cutaneous manifestations. A rash or eruption accompanying a systemic infection is called an **exanthem**. Similar involvement of mucous membranes, as in the mouth and vagina, is an **enanthem**. **Pyoderma** is a general term for any skin condition caused by pyogenic (pus-forming) bacteria, usually *Staphyloccus aureus*. Local infection may follow any event or process that impairs the integrity of the skin surface. The usual portals of entry for bacteria into intact skin are the openings of the sebaceous glands. **Folliculitis** designates an infection largely confined to the pilosebaceous follicles. A **furuncle** is a solitary cutaneous abscess consisting of a focus of purulent material surrounded by a zone of active inflammation with fibrinous exudate and fibroplasia. A **carbuncle** is a deeper and more extensive suppurative process, which may communicate with the surface at several points.

Impetigo is a superficial, rapidly spreading bacterial dermatitis with oozing and crust formation. When the process invades the dermis it is called **ecthyma**. **Erysipelas** is a spreading cellulitis due to streptococci and characterized by marked edema and hyperemia. **Pyogenic granuloma** is a nodule or tumor containing proliferating endothelial vessels, fibrotic reaction, and pus. Systemic bacterial infections with conspicuous cutaneous lesions include anthrax, tularemia, brucellosis, leprosy, tuberculosis, and syphilis.

The characteristic cutaneous lesion of viral infections, whether local or systemic, is the vesicle. However, some viral infections are papular. Common warts (verrucae vulgares) and genital warts (condylomata acuminata) have been mentioned under neoplasms of the epidermis. **Molluscum contagiosum** is a small, pearly nodule, often umbilicated and generally occurring in clusters about the lower trunk and genitalia. Histologic examination shows dense superficial aggregations of large dyskeratotic cells, called molluscum bodies, with shrunken nuclei and light eosinophilic cytoplasm containing inclusions called elementary bodies of Lipschütz.

Herpes simplex is a viral cutaneous infection characterized clinically by a cluster of painful vesicles that soon rupture and slough, leaving still more painful ulcers. Common sites are the lips (herpes labialis, orofacial herpes) and the genitals (herpes progenitalis, genital herpes). Microscopic examination shows hyperplasia of keratinocytes with ballooning degeneration and giant cell formation, neutrophilic infiltrates, and edema of the underlying dermis. Some infected cells show large eosinophilic nuclear inclusions. A Tzanck smear (a stained preparation of vesicle fluid) shows giant cells. Systemic viral infections that cause typical papular or vesicular exanthems include varicella (chickenpox), measles (rubeola), rubella, roseola, erythema infectiosum, Kawasaki disease, cat-scratch disease, and various types of ECHO and coxsackievirus infection.

Superficial fungus infections are commonplace and often of little clinical significance. *Candida albicans* causes a diffuse dermatitis with erythema, edema, thinning of the epidermis due to superficial destruction of epithelial cells, and weeping. Candidal infection of mucous membranes (thrush) is accompanied by formation of dense, firmly adherent, curdlike excrescences consisting of colonies of *Candida*. Candidal infection is more common in diabetes, pregnancy, and immune deficiency. **Tinea** is a general term for any superficial fungal infection causing a round or oval reddened scaly patch with a sharp margin that tends to grow outward with clearing of the center. Various species of *Microsporum, Epidermophyton,* and *Trichophyton* cause tinea capitis (ringworm of the scalp), tinea corporis (ringworm of the body), tinea cruris (ringworm of the groin), and tinea pedis (athlete's foot). Microscopic examination of scales or scrapings from skin or mucous membranes infected with a superficial fungus shows hyphae on or among epithelial cells. The usual practice in preparing a slide of scrapings is to destroy the human tissue by applying potassium hydroxide (KOH) and, in the case of keratinized skin, heating the slide. Deep fungal infections with cutaneous features include actinomycosis, blastomycosis, sporotrichosis, and geotrichosis.

Review Questions

1. What two basic cell types are found in the epidermis?
2. What is a pilosebaceous unit?
3. What are the two principal skin cancers?
4. Define or explain: *alopecia, macule, papule, ulcer, vesicle.*

17

The Breast

Gross and Microscopic Anatomy

The breast, or mammary gland, is by embryonic origin a specialized development of the skin. The glandular tissue of the breast consists of numerous alveoli formed of simple cuboidal epithelium. These are arranged in 15–20 grossly distinguishable lobes, each with its own duct leading to the nipple. The ducts are also made up of cuboidal epithelial cells. The glandular tissue of the mammary gland is under the control of ovarian and pituitary hormones. Its microscopic appearance and activity vary greatly between the lactating and nonlactating state and even between different phases of the menstrual cycle.

The stroma of the breast consists of a framework of fairly dense connective tissue and a substantial amount of fat. Cooper's ligaments are bands of fibrous tissue that extend through the breast to give it support. Fibrous septa also separate the lobes. The glandular parenchyma is further divided into lobules by a more delicate meshwork of connective tissue. Periductal and interlobular connective tissue responds to hormonal stimulation along with glandular epithelium. Breast tissue in the male is rudimentary, being limited normally to a few scattered ductal elements without alveoli or secretory potential.

Surrounding the nipple is a zone of pigmented skin, the areola, containing smooth muscle fibers and modified sebaceous glands called the glands of Montgomery.

Pathologic Study of the Breast

Pathologic study of breast tissue is most often undertaken to explore the possibility of malignancy or to assess its type and extent. Exfoliative cytology of nipple lesions and cytologic smears of nipple discharge may be performed to search for malignant cells. Solid breast masses may be investigated by fine-needle aspiration, needle biopsy, or open biopsy. In the latter case, frozen section is normally done so that more extensive surgery can be performed at once if necessary. After mastectomy the entire breast is submitted for pathologic study, often along with subjacent muscle and dissected axillary lymph nodes. At autopsy the breasts are examined from within after reflection of the skin and subcutaneous fat of the anterior chest.

Developmental and Inflammatory Disorders

Supernumerary nipples occasionally develop in both sexes along the so-called milk line running from axilla to groin on each side and corresponding to the position of nipples in many lower mammals. This condition is called polythelia. Much rarer is the actual development of one or more accessory breasts (polymastia), with or without nipples. Adolescent breast development (thelarche) results from estrogenic stimulation, and may occasionally proceed to extreme overdevelopment (virginal hypertrophy) of one or both breasts. Hypertrophy may occur at any age as a result of functioning neoplasms of the ovary or adrenal.

During the reproductive years, secretory and periductal tissues undergo periodic engorgement and edema as a result of rising progesterone levels during the latter half of each menstrual cycle. In pregnancy, the glandular tissue is further stimulated by chorionic gonadotropin. Actual milk formation (lactation) does not occur until late in pregnancy. A galactocele is a milk-filled cyst developing in an obstructed duct during lactation. Acute inflammation of the breast (acute mastitis) is uncommon except during lactation, when it usually results from bacterial invasion via the ducts or through fissures of the nipple. It may progress to abscess formation.

After menopause, the glandular elements of the female breast normally atrophy. Cystic dilatation of ducts (duct ectasia) often accompanies this process. Gynecomastia (hypertrophy of the male breast) can result from hormonal disorders and from certain drugs. The adipose tissue of the breast may undergo fat necrosis with formation of one or more hard, waxy or soapy nodules, which must be distinguished from neoplasms. Sometimes there is a history of prior trauma. Mondor's disease is acute phlebitis of subcutaneous veins of the breast or adjacent chest wall.

Fibrocystic disease of the breast, also called cystic mastitis and mammary dysplasia, is an exceedingly common disorder, occurring in various forms and degrees, and leading to the development of painful nodules and cysts within the breast substance. It is almost exclusively a disease of the reproductive years and apparently results from inappropriate response of the breast tissue to cyclical variations in hormone levels. Apart from the discomfort it causes, its chief importance arises from the need to distinguish it from malignant disease. Microscopic examination shows hyperplasia of secretory epithelium with duct obstruction, cyst formation, and varying degrees of acute and chronic inflammation. Apocrine metaplasia (formation of secretory cells) may occur in ductal epithelium. Epithelial tissue may spill over into the stroma (adenosis) and may form benign neoplastic nodules (adenomas).

Neoplasms

Fibroadenoma is a solitary, circumscribed, benign proliferation of both secretory epithelium and interlobular connective tissue. The tumor grows slowly and has a distinctive rubbery texture and a pale, granular, homogeneous cut surface. Histologic examination shows variable proportions of dysplastic glandular and connective tissue without malignant changes. **Cystosarcoma phyllodes** is a myxomatous variant that may become quite large and has some metastatic and malignant potential. **Intraductal papilloma** is a benign pedunculated epithelial mass forming within a milk duct beneath or immediately adjacent to the nipple. The lesion is pink and friable. It may lead to ductal obstruction with cyst formation and is a common cause of bleeding from the nipple. Histologic study shows hyperplasia of secretory epithelium in a branching or frondlike pattern, without invasion of the basement membrane.

Breast cancer is the commonest cancer in women, accounting for one-fourth of all malignant disease and one-fifth of all cancer deaths in women. Mammary carcinomas are described as either ductal or lobular depending on their histologic origin. Over 90% arise from ductal epithelium. Both types vary greatly in malignant potential and behavior. They may proliferate extensively in situ or infiltrate surrounding tissues early. Clinically, breast cancer occurs as a solitary, hard, painless nodule, which may grow slowly or rapidly and may invade the overlying skin, the underlying chest wall, and the axillary lymph nodes. Edema of the overlying skin due to invasion of lymph vessels results in a coarse orange-peel (peau d'orange) texture. Fixation to deeper tissues creates a breastplate appearance (carcinoma en cuirasse).

Scirrhous carcinoma, accounting for about three-fourths of all breast cancers, is a very dense, hard tumor showing extensive desmoplasia (hyperplasia of fibrous tissue), while **medullary carcinoma** is composed almost exclusively of epithelial elements with little stroma. In **mucinous carcinoma**, the stroma is converted to a gelatinous, myxoid material. Plugging of ducts with pasty debris results in a form of intraductal tumor called **comedo carcinoma**. A rapidly growing malignancy may be associated with erythema and edema (**inflammatory carcinoma**); this is a bad prognostic sign. Clustered microcalcifications (which are not necessarily microscopic in size) occur in many breast cancers.

Paget's disease of the breast arises from an underlying malignancy of ductal epithelium that invades the nipple, causing a dermatitis that progresses to ulceration and local tissue destruction. Paget's cells are large, bizarre, anaplastic cells with hyperchromatic, vesicular nuclei and vacuolated cytoplasm, which are seen in Paget's disease of the breast. They also occur in extramammary Paget's disease, an exactly analogous primary neoplasm arising from sweat glands of the axillae, genitalia, or face in elderly persons of both sexes.

Mammary carcinomas metastasize to regional and mediastinal lymph nodes, the lungs, liver, bone, and brain. They are staged as follows:

Stage 0: No symptoms.
Stage I: Mass in the breast.
Stage II: Spread to axillary nodes only.
Stage III: Local spread (fixation, supraclavicular nodes, peau d'orange).
Stage IV: Distant metastasis.

Review Questions

1. What is the principal pathologic importance of fibrocystic disease of the breast?
2. What benign breast neoplasm is a common cause of bleeding from the nipple?
3. What is the most striking physical feature of scirrhous carcinoma?
4. Define or explain: *areola, gynecomastia, thelarche.*

18

The Blood-Forming Organs

The cells of the blood were described in Chapter 7. The starting point of a diagnostic investigation of any disorder of the blood or blood-forming organs is an examination of a specimen of peripheral blood, obtained by venipuncture and ordinarily treated with anticoagulant. The procedures included in the complete blood count (CBC) are enumerations of both red and white blood cells in a standard volume of blood; determination of the hemoglobin concentration and hematocrit; and examination of a stained smear to observe the shapes of red and white blood cells and to determine the relative proportions of the various types of white blood cell in the first hundred cells counted. These and other tests of peripheral blood pertain to clinical pathology and are discussed in Chapter 29, where disorders of red blood cells are also described.

As discussed in Chapter 7, red blood cells, granulocytes, and monocytes are formed in bone marrow, while lymphocytes are formed in lymphoid tissue.

Bone Marrow: Gross and Microscopic Anatomy

The shafts of long bones are tubular in structure, and most bones also have cavities that are crisscrossed by reinforcing struts of calcified bone tissue called **trabeculae**. Bone having this trabecular configuration is called spongy or **cancellous**. The cavities of long bones and the hollows of cancellous bone are filled with a soft tissue called marrow, of which two types are distinguished. **Red marrow**, the chief blood-forming tissue in the adult, consists of a framework of reticular cells and fibers in which may be found, in varying numbers and proportions, megakaryocytes (which form platelets) and immature cells of the red blood cell and white blood cell lines. Some fat cells are also normally present. In **yellow marrow**, fat cells completely replace the hematopoietic (blood-forming) cells. Yellow marrow may retain the potential to resume its blood-forming function when needed.

Pathologic Study of Bone Marrow

Marrow aspiration is a diagnostic procedure for obtaining a specimen of red marrow for histologic study. Under local anesthesia a large bore needle is inserted into the marrow space of the sternum or posterior iliac crest, and a quantity of material drawn into a syringe by suction. A larger bore biopsy needle may also be used to obtain marrow without the distortion caused by suction (suction artifact). Marrow specimens are ordinarily smeared and stained, but may be embedded in paraffin, like solid tissue. At autopsy, marrow cavities can be subjected to direct examination by sawing or chiseling into bone.

Diseases of Marrow

Any significant disturbance of the structure or function of the marrow will be reflected in a reduction of circulating red blood cells (anemia), granulocytic white blood cells (granulopenia), platelets (thrombocytopenia), or all of these. It does not follow, however, that all abnormalities in circulating cells are accompanied by visible changes in the marrow.

Various kinds of marrow failure can follow poisoning with heavy metals, organic chemicals, or drugs, or exposure to ionizing radiation. In **aplastic anemia** the production of erythrocytes is principally suppressed, and in such cases examination of the marrow shows reduction in cellularity, with hypoplasia or gelatinous degeneration of erythropoietic elements, or replacement by fat. Formation of white blood cells and platelets may also be impaired. In various types of anemia that are not due to marrow failure, examination of the marrow often shows an increase in red blood cell production (reactive hyperplasia).

Agranulocytosis, a reduction in the number of circulating neutrophils, eosinophils, and basophils, results chiefly from reactions to drugs, including antimetabolites used in the treatment of malignant tumors. Marrow aspiration shows deficiency of cells of the granulocytic series. In myelofibrosis, marrow is replaced by fibrous connective tissue or displaced by hypertrophic bony trabeculae. This condition may result from poisoning but is most often associated with myelogenous leukemia.

Leukemia is a malignancy of tissues that form white blood cells, ordinarily resulting in a great increase in the number of such cells in the circulation. Myelogenous leukemia affects the marrow production of granulocytes and monocytes, lymphatic leukemia the formation of lymphocytes in lymphoid tissue. In **chronic myelogenous leukemia**

the marrow shows a great increase in cells of the granulocytic series (myeloblasts, myelocytes), usually at the expense of erythropoiesis. In **acute myelogenous leukemia**, a higher proportion of immature white blood cells is found, and red blood cell production is even further compromised. Auer's bodies, rod-shaped cytoplasmic granules, are seen in myeloblasts and myelocytes in both marrow and circulating blood in myelogenous leukemias. **Monocytic leukemia** is rare. Two types are distinguished: the Naegeli type, in which the abnormally proliferating cells resemble myeloblasts, and the Schilling type, in which they are more like monocytes (histiocytes). Malignant proliferation of large mononuclear cells with villous cytoplasmic projections is called **hairy-cell leukemia**.

Multiple myeloma is a malignant tumor of marrow arising from plasma cells and forming soft, vascular nodules that may cause local bone destruction and pathologic fracture. Microscopic examination shows diffuse and focal infiltrates of large, round, immature, pleomorphic plasma cells with basophilic cytoplasm and eccentric, hyperchromatic, sometimes double nuclei having several nucleoli. Multiple myeloma is associated with the appearance of an abnormal globulin (M protein) in the blood and of Bence Jones protein, a different abnormal globulin, in the urine. Primary amyloidosis, affecting skeletal and cardiac muscle, may accompany multiple myeloma.

Carcinomas of the breast and prostate frequently metastasize to marrow, particularly that of the vertebrae, ribs, and pelvis. In lymphatic leukemia and Hodgkin's disease, patchy infiltrates of malignant mononuclear cells commonly appear in the red marrow, displacing normal tissue.

Lymphoid Tissue: Gross and Microscopic Anatomy

Like red marrow, **lymphoid tissue** features a stroma of reticular cells and fibers. In addition there are dense aggregations of lymphocytes and their precursors. Lymphoid tissue is widely distributed throughout the body, particularly in the skin and the walls of the digestive tract, but the principal collections of lymphoid tissue are in the lymph nodes, the tonsils, the spleen, and the thymus.

A **lymph node** is a kidney-shaped mass of lymphoid tissue 0.3 to 3 cm in length with a connective-tissue capsule and a hilum where blood vessels enter and leave. One or more lymphatic channels also leave at the hilum, but afferent channels enter around the convex surface of the node. The interior of a lymph node is divided into two zones, a cortex and a medulla. In the **cortex**, connective-tissue elements extend inward from the capsule to form fairly regular trabeculae, and lymphocytes are found arranged in spherical nodules with lighter-staining inner zones called germinal centers. In the **medulla** the connective-tissue trabeculae form an irregular network, and lymphocytes are disposed in cords that branch and rejoin as they course through the stroma. Clefts and spaces among the cells, called **sinuses**, contain lymph. Lymph nodes occur at many sites throughout the body. They are particularly numerous in the subcutaneous tissue of the neck, axillae, and groins, and along the major blood vessels in the thorax and abdomen.

Other lymphoid organs—the tonsils, the spleen, and the thymus— share the general features of lymph nodes but have no lymph sinuses and limited or no connections with lymph channels. The **tonsils** are anatomically discrete aggregations of lymphoid tissue surrounding the pharynx. They are covered by pharyngeal mucous membrane, which dips down to line a variable number of grossly evident clefts or crypts. In the crypts the epithelium may show some degree of keratinization. Together the lingual and pharyngeal tonsils surround the pharynx in a configuration called Waldeyer's ring.

The **spleen** is a large, soft, deep purple, flattened and somewhat pyramidal organ situated in the left upper quadrant of the abdomen and weighing normally 150–175 g in the adult. It has a tough fibrous capsule and a dense stroma of reticular connective tissue containing elastic fibers and smooth muscle in substantial amounts. The tissue of the spleen is distinguishable grossly into **red pulp**, which is found on microscopic study to contain venous sinuses packed with erythrocytes, and **white pulp**, the lymphoid tissue proper, in which lymphocytes form spherical aggregates or follicles called **malpighian corpuscles**. Some of these have lighter-staining germinal centers. The red pulp acts as a filter for the blood, which is subjected to the action of histiocytes and free phagocytes as it trickles through the sinuses. Because the spleen is particularly important in clearing encapsulated bacteria such as *Diplococcus pneumoniae* and *Neisseria meningitidis* from the blood, persons who have undergone splenectomy show heightened susceptibility to infections caused by these organisms. The spleen also acts as a reservoir for blood: by contracting during exercise or after severe hemorrhage, it delivers supplemental numbers of erythrocytes to the circulation. Besides producing lymphocytes, the spleen is a major site of red blood cell production in the fetus.

The **thymus**, located in the upper anterior thorax, is a flat, two-lobed organ consisting entirely of lymphoid tissue. Each lobe is invested by a connective-tissue capsule from which trabeculae extend inward and separate the lymphoid tissue into lobules. In the cortex, lymphocytes are packed densely together without the germinal centers seen in the spleen and lymph nodes. In the medulla, lymphocytes occur in concentric swirls called **Hassall's corpuscles**. The thymus attains its maximum weight of about 35 g around puberty and then regresses. In older adults, no trace of it may remain.

Pathologic Study of Lymphoid Tissue

Material from enlarged or abnormal subcutaneous lymph nodes can be obtained by fine-needle aspiration, or open biopsy may be performed with excision of the entire node. Surgery for the removal of malignant neoplasms often includes extensive lymph node dissection, with removal of many regional lymph nodes that are known or suspected to contain metastatic malignant tissue. Such nodes must be carefully distinguished as to site, so that the pattern and extent of spread of the neoplasm can be accurately mapped.

Percutaneous biopsy of the spleen is not feasible because of the danger of hemorrhage from this highly vascular organ. For the same reason, it is unsafe to attempt to remove part of the spleen by open biopsy. The spleen may be surgically removed in its entirety for various reasons, including hemorrhage resulting from trauma to the organ occurring during surgical operation on an adjacent structure. At autopsy the spleen is routinely examined for evidence of abnormalities in size, shape, and consistency. After being weighed, it is cut into thin sections with a knife for evaluation of its internal structure, and specimens are taken for microscopic study.

Diseases of the Spleen

Congenital absence or malformation of the spleen is rare, but the presence of one or more small accessory spleens is not uncommon. In diseases of bone marrow associated with marked reduction of red blood cell production, the spleen may resume its fetal function of forming red blood cells (extramedullary hematopoiesis). This must be distinguished from **myeloid metaplasia**, in which zones of erythroblastic and myeloblastic activity develop in the spleen (and other organs) from cells that have spread from malignant foci in the bone marrow. When no primary source for such cells can be found, the condition is termed agnogenic myeloid metaplasia.

Splenomegaly (enlargement of the spleen) is a common feature of many infectious, hematologic, and circulatory diseases. Some enlargement of the spleen may occur in any severe acute infection with septicemia, particularly in infective endocarditis. Acute septic splenitis (acute splenic hyperplasia) is a condition of pronounced gross and microscopic change generally associated with disseminated bacterial infection. The organ is moderately enlarged and soft or even mushy in texture. The cut surface is red or reddish gray and bulges. Microscopic examination shows many neutrophils in both pulp and sinuses, and atrophy of follicles with central zones of necrosis. Splenic inflammation and enlargement also occur in typhoid fever, brucellosis, tuberculosis, malaria, leishmaniasis, schistosomiasis, and infectious mononucleosis. The more chronic the process, the larger the spleen becomes, and the greater the extent to which fibrous elements preponderate over lymphoid tissue, making the organ firmer.

Because the spleen is the principal site of red blood cell destruction (hemolysis), many disorders associated with excessive hemolysis lead to enlargement and overactivity of the spleen. This is particularly conspicuous in sickle cell disease, hereditary spherocytosis, and polycythemia vera. In these conditions, there is hyperemia of the splenic pulp and often deposition of hemosiderin as a product of exaggerated hemolysis.

Passive congestion of the spleen in cardiac failure results in mild enlargement. Grossly the organ appears deep purple and has a rubbery feel, and its cut surface looks congested and meaty. Microscopic examination shows engorgement of the sinuses and thickening of the trabeculae. Chronic passive congestion is associated with progressive increase in connective tissue elements and reduction in lymphoid tissue. Similar changes occur in portal hypertension, a local circulatory disturbance (usually due to liver disease) in which there is diminished flow and increased pressure in the portal vein, into which the splenic vein drains. In addition, splenic engorgement due to this cause may lead to focal hemorrhages, which organize and become the site of grossly visible deposits of hemosiderin and calcium called Gandy-Gamna nodules or tobacco nodules. Banti's syndrome consists of splenomegaly, anemia, and ascites as a consequence of portal hypertension.

Rupture of the spleen is the most common cause of fatal hemorrhage after abdominal trauma. It is more likely to occur when the organ is enlarged. Thrombosis or embolization of the splenic artery or one of its branches can result in infarction of the entire spleen or of a cone-shaped wedge of splenic tissue. The infarcted area appears gray or white, with one or more inner zones of hemorrhage and necrosis.

The spleen is the organ most frequently affected in amyloidosis secondary to systemic disease. Amyloid may be diffusely deposited or may be confined to the follicles. In the latter case the deposits are grossly evident on the cut surface as pearly or waxy nodules (sago spleen). Microscopic examination in amyloidosis shows the abnormal protein material to be deposited just beneath the endothelium of blood vessels and sinuses. Large amounts of blood pigment (hemosiderin, hematoidin) may be found in macrophages of the splenic pulp in hemolytic diseases and hemochromatosis. In various disturbances of lipid metabolism (Hand-Schüller-Christian disease, Gaucher's disease, Niemann-Pick disease), accumulations of lipid material may appear in macrophages in the splenic sinuses. Metastasis of malignancies to the spleen is uncommon.

Diseases of Other Lymphoid Organs

The lymph nodes act as filters, removing particulate foreign material, bacteria, and metastatic tumor cells from the lymphatic circulation. Lymphadenitis, inflammation of a lymph node, occurs when filtered material elicits a local reaction. Associated inflammation of lymphatic vessels is called lymphangitis. Any local infection may lead to acute inflammation of regional lymph nodes. The nodes become enlarged and firm, and on microscopic examination infiltrates of neutrophils and monocytes are seen in the sinuses. Suppuration and abscess formation may occur. With longstanding lymphadenitis, the infiltrates contain chiefly mononuclear cells, and fibrous reaction, even calcification, may permanently alter the consistency of the gland. Lymphadenitis is a prominent feature of some acute infections (infectious mononucleosis, rubella, cat-scratch disease, Kawasaki disease, bubonic plague) and of some chronic infections (tuberculosis, brucellosis, lymphogranuloma venereum, toxoplasmosis). The spread of malignant cells to regional lymph nodes is the most common form of metastasis for many tumors, especially carcinomas, and the histologic study of these nodes is of great importance in the diagnosis, staging, and prognosis of many malignancies.

In general, the **tonsils** are subject to the same kinds of pathologic process as the lymph nodes. Acute tonsillitis accompanies any severe pharyngitis. In chronic follicular tonsillitis the tonsils themselves become the primary focus of infection. Proliferation of pyogenic organisms leads to enlargement of lymph follicles due to hyperplasia of their germinal centers, and so to chronic enlargement of the tonsils, with accumulation of exudate and debris in crypts. In addition, infiltrates of inflammatory cells and fibrous reaction are seen throughout the tonsillar stroma. The tonsil may be the site of a squamous cell carcinoma arising from its mucosal surface. The thymus typically atrophies after puberty and is of little clinical significance. Thymoma is a benign neoplasm including lymphoid, epithelial, vascular, and connective tissue elements; it accompanies some cases of myasthenia gravis.

Neoplasms of Lymphoid Tissue

All primary neoplasms of lymphoid tissue are more or less malignant. They are divided into lymphatic leukemias, which result in increased numbers of lymphocytes in peripheral blood (lymphocytosis) without marked enlargement of lymphoid organs, and lymphomas, which are solid tumors of lymphoid tissue not necessarily associated with lymphocytosis. The distinction between these is not absolute. Both are presumably unifocal in origin but often involve many sites (lymph nodes, spleen, nonlymphoid tissue) when first diagnosed, having spread via lymphatic vessels or the blood. Both are associated with anemia, weakness, weight loss, hemorrhagic tendencies, and increased susceptibility to infection.

Acute lymphatic leukemia is a rapidly progressive malignant disease in which significant numbers of lymphoblasts (blast forms) appear in the circulation. This is a disease of children and young adults. In **chronic lymphatic leukemia** the course is more protracted and circulating lymphocytes are mature. The onset of symptoms is usually during middle age, and survival may be 10–15 years. In both forms of lymphatic leukemia the spleen and lymph nodes are enlarged and heavily infiltrated with proliferating mononuclear cells, whose numbers obscure or distort the normal structural features.

The most distinctive lymphoma is **Hodgkin's disease**, in which bizarre lymphocytes called Reed-Sternberg cells appear in spleen and lymph nodes. The Reed-Sternberg cell is large, with a pale acidophilic cytoplasm, a large nucleus showing marginal clumping of chromatin, and a prominent acidophilic nucleolus. Duplication of the nucleus may create the appearance of a normal cell seen together with its mirror image. These cells are also seen in infectious mononucleosis, mycosis fungoides, and other conditions. In addition to Reed-Sternberg cells, variable numbers of eosinophils, inflammatory cells, and fibers may be found in affected tissue. Hodgkin's disease is classified on the basis of histologic features as lymphocyte-predominant, nodular sclerosing, mixed cellularity, and lymphocyte-depleted. As a rule the two latter types are more widely disseminated and have a poorer prognosis. Hodgkin's disease is staged as follows:

Stage I: Confined to one or more lymph nodes in a single anatomic region.

Stage II: Confined to two or more lymph node regions on the same side of the diaphragm.

Stage III: Confined to lymphoid tissue on both sides of the diaphragm.

Stage IV: Involving nonlymphoid tissue on both sides of the diaphragm.

To the stage number is added the letter A if the patient has no systemic symptoms (fever, weight loss, itching, bone pain), the letter B if such symptoms are present.

Non-Hodgkin's lymphomas vary greatly in microscopic appearance and course. They are divided into nodular and diffuse lymphomas according to histologic pattern, and each of these patterns is further divided on the basis of malignant cell type into undifferentiated, lymphocytic, histiocytic (reticulum cell sarcoma), and mixed. Burkitt's lymphoma is a highly anaplastic tumor of lymphoid tissue apparently induced by infection with the Epstein-Barr virus and occurring almost exclusively in Africa.

Review Questions

1. What is the chief source of red blood cells in the adult?
2. What disease is associated with plasma cells, M protein in the blood, and Bence Jones protein in the urine?
3. List the principal lymphoid organs.
4. What is the importance of noting the exact anatomic site of each lymph node removed during an operation for cancer?
5. Name some conditions associated with enlargement of the spleen.
6. Define or explain: *agranulocytosis, leukemia, thrombocytopenia.*

19

The Cardiovascular System

Gross and Microscopic Anatomy

The cardiovascular or circulatory system is virtually coextensive with the body. The term circulation is to be taken literally: a red blood cell leaving the left ventricle of the heart on its way to the tissues will, barring accidents, eventually return to the same point not once but many times during the course of its existence. The blood flows in a closed circuit, taking up oxygen from the lungs and absorbed nutrients from the liver and intestines, delivering these to the tissues while taking up carbon dioxide and nongaseous wastes there, carrying the latter to the kidney to be excreted in the urine, and, on its next pass through the lungs, releasing the carbon dioxide while picking up more oxygen. The circulation also serves as a delivery system for hormones and other chemical agents and for white blood cells.

The circulatory system comprises three specialized types of structure: the heart, the arteries and veins, and the capillaries. The **heart** is a pump, or more precisely two pumps operating in parallel. One of these, the **right ventricle**, after being primed with systemic blood collected by the veins and funneled through the right atrium, sends this blood through the lungs for gas exchange. The other pump, the **left ventricle**, which receives oxygenated blood from the lungs via the left atrium, sends that blood into the systemic circulation by way of the aorta and its branches. Under normal conditions the pumps contract simultaneously, but there is no mixing of the two circulations. The **pericardium**, a serous sac consisting of visceral and parietal layers, completely encloses the heart.

The adult heart weighs 275–350 g. The heart consists almost entirely of cardiac muscle. Its lining, the **endocardium**, is a simple squamous endothelium overlying a layer of loose connective tissue, the subendocardium. The muscle layer or **myocardium** is arranged in

163

spiraling sheets whose fibers run in different directions. The external surface of the heart, called the **epicardium**, consists of a connective-tissue layer covered by visceral pericardium. The blood supply of the myocardium is derived from the coronary arteries, the first branches of the aorta.

The flow of blood through the cardiac chambers is regulated partly by four valves, whose leaflets are specialized folds of endocardium reinforced by connective tissue. Each of the valves is mounted in a dense ring of connective tissue, the annulus fibrosus, which surrounds the orifice controlled by the valve and is intimately joined to the adjacent myocardium. The rhythmic, coordinated contraction of the myocardium is triggered by impulses that arise in the sinoatrial node, located in the wall of the right atrium, and are conducted to the ventricles by the atrioventricular node and the bundle of His. These structures consist of specialized cardiac muscle fibers called Purkinje fibers.

Arteries and veins are the principal conduits for circulating blood. Arteries carry blood away from the heart and veins carry blood toward the heart. Both types of vessel undergo repeated branchings with continuing reduction in both the thickness of their walls and their internal caliber. An artery is typically smaller in caliber than the corresponding vein, but has a thicker wall.

The wall of a representative large **artery** consists of three readily distinguishable coats: a lining or tunica intima of endothelium resting on a layer of connective tissue; a tunica media, a meshwork of spirally arranged smooth muscle and elastic fibers that render the vessel distensible and resilient; and a tunica adventitia, a thin outer sheath of connective tissue that blends with surrounding structures. The innermost layer of elastic fibers in the tunica media is distinguished as the internal elastic membrane. Analogous structures form the walls of a **vein**. However, in a vein the intima and media are thinner than in an artery of corresponding size, and the adventitia is thicker. The media contains circularly disposed smooth muscle fibers, the adventitia both circular and longitudinal muscles and connective tissue. Some of the larger veins are provided with valves to prevent back-flow of blood. Like the cardiac valves, a venous valve is a flap of endothelium reinforced by connective tissue.

Capillaries are microscopic blood vessels. The repeated branching of an artery eventually results in a network of very small vessels whose caliber is barely larger than the diameter of a blood cell and whose walls are formed of a single layer of endothelial cells. In turn, the coalescence of capillaries into increasingly large trunks results in the formation of veins. All exchanges of gases, nutrients, electrolytes, hormones, and cells between the blood and the tissues occur through capillary walls. Capillaries intersect repeatedly with other capillaries to form an anastomosis, a vascular network. Tissues vary in the richness of their capillary supply. Epithelium and dental enamel have none. Moreover, the flow of blood through a capillary bed is regulated by the valvelike action of arterioles, very small arteries in which the tunica media is represented by a single layer of smooth muscle fibers.

In addition to the cardiovascular system, a second set of channels, the **lymphatic vessels**, carries a fluid called lymph through the tissues. Lymph is a colorless fluid much like plasma but containing many lymphocytes. There is no true circulation of lymph; it flows in one direction only, from the tissues to the heart. Lymphatic vessels are similar in structure to veins, but more delicate. They arise from lymph capillaries, which resemble blood capillaries and form networks parallel to them but not communicating with them. Lymph drains into the blood via the thoracic duct, formed by the junction of smaller lymph vessels and entering the left brachiocephalic vein in the neck. The function of the lymphatic system is to maintain fluid balance in the intercellular spaces and to remove invading microorganisms and foreign material from tissues. Some lymph channels pass through lymph nodes on their way to the thoracic duct.

Pathologic Study of the Cardiovascular System

Vascular structures appear in virtually all pathologic specimens. Vascular lesions are the focus of interest in surgical specimens resulting from vascular graft procedures, amputations for peripheral vascular disease, and excision or stripping of thrombotic or varicose veins. Needle biopsy of the endocardium and myocardium can be carried out through a cardiac catheter. At autopsy the pericardium is incised and any fluid or adhesions are noted before the heart is severed from its vascular attachments. The size, shape, and surface of the heart are noted, and it is weighed. The pathologist then opens the chambers in sequence, following the direction of blood flow. The valves and the walls of the chambers are measured, and any deformities or abnormalities of size, color, or texture are noted. The myocardium is cut into thin sections, and serial cross cuts are made through the main coronary arteries.

Developmental Disorders

The **heart** is subject to various **congenital anomalies**, most of them consisting in abnormal communication between two chambers or vessels or in malformation of valves. These anomalies impair, to varying degrees, the function of the circulatory system; some are lethal.

Dextrocardia refers to positioning of the heart on the right side of the thorax rather than on the left. This is of little physiologic consequence when associated with complete mirror-image reversal of thoracic and abdominal viscera (situs inversus), but as an isolated anomaly it may be incompatible with life. Equally catastrophic is anomalous **transposition of the great vessels** (aorta and pulmonary artery) and **persistent truncus arteriosus**, in which these vessels fail to separate during fetal development.

An abnormal opening in the septum between the atria or between the ventricles allows shunting of blood from left (where the pressure is higher) to right, with more or less reduction in the overall efficiency of the circulation. **Patent foramen ovale** is a special case of atrial septal defect, due to failure of the fetal opening to close. **Lutembacher's syndrome** is atrial septal defect with mitral stenosis. **Eisenmenger's complex** refers to the combination of interventricular septal defect with severe pulmonary hypertension. Various forms of stenosis or atresia of one or more of the vessels communicating with the heart, often combined with septal defects, are among the more serious congenital cardiac malformations. **Patent ductus arteriosus** (failure of the fetal ductus arteriosus to close) allows shunting of blood from the aorta into the pulmonary artery. This is the commonest congenital cardiac anomaly resulting from maternal rubella infection. **Tetralogy of Fallot** is interventricular septal defect in combination with stenosis of the pulmonic valve, right ventricular hypertrophy, and overriding of the interventricular septum by the aorta so that it receives some nonoxygenated blood from the right ventricle. **Coarctation of the aorta** is a congenital narrowing of the aorta at some point along its arch.

An **aneurysm** is a localized abnormal dilatation of an artery. Congenital aneurysms can occur in any part of the circulation but are particularly common in the cerebral arteries. Here they appear as small round dilatations (berry aneurysms), which are subject to spontaneous rupture. Cirsoid aneurysm, particularly common in the scalp, is a mass of dilated arteries and veins with numerous direct intercommunications. Cavernous hemangioma is discussed in Chapter 16.

Diseases of Blood Vessels

Acquired aneurysm is usually due to disease of the arterial wall, most often arteriosclerosis. Syphilis was formerly an important cause of aneurysm of the thoracic aorta. Aneurysms are described as saccular (roughly spherical) or fusiform (spindle-shaped). Aneurysms tend to enlarge, to compress or erode adjacent structures, and eventually to rupture. **Dissecting aneurysm** results when circulating blood penetrates the intima of a diseased artery (most often the aorta) and dissects for a variable distance along the media, often reentering the arterial lumen through a second intimal tear. In virtually all cases of dissecting aneurysm the patient is hypertensive and the aorta has undergone cystic medial necrosis. **Arteriovenous fistula** is an abnormal communication between an artery and an adjacent vein, usually developing in an extremity as a result of a penetrating wound. A large fistula may disturb local circulation and even impair cardiac efficiency. Thrombosis and embolism are discussed in Chapter 12.

Veins, including superficial (subcutaneous) veins, are subject to wide variation in location and branching, usually of no great importance. **Varices** (varicosities) are dilated, tortuous veins, whose walls show localized thinning and loss of elastic tissue. Varices occur most often in the saphenous veins in the subcutaneous tissue of the lower extremities, and are usually due to hereditary weakness of vein walls. However, venous obstruction can be a contributing factor. Esophageal varices are mentioned in Chapter 21, varicocele in Chapter 24.

Hypertension is any sustained abnormal elevation of pressure within the systemic arterial circulation. The commonest type, essential hypertension, runs in families and is commoner in blacks, but its cause is unknown. Secondary hypertension embraces all those forms in which elevation of blood pressure is due to some other abnormal condition. By far the most prevalent of these is renal hypertension. A kidney damaged by ischemia or chronic inflammation may produce an excess of renin, an enzyme that catalyzes the formation of angiotensin. This potent vasopressor is responsible for sustained elevation of pressure in renal hypertension. Other causes of secondary hypertension include Cushing's syndrome, aldosteronism, pheochromocytoma, and toxemia of pregnancy. Hypertension is associated with no distinctive pathologic lesion, but is a very frequent cause of arterial degenerative disease and of cardiac dilatation, hypertrophy, and failure.

Acute arteritis generally results from septic embolization or local spread of an infectious process. In **syphilitic aortitis**, the arterial wall is thickened, with necrotic, fibrotic, and inflammatory changes in all coats. **Necrotizing arteritis** (necrotizing angiitis) is a widespread process, generally due to hypersensitivity or autoimmunity, affecting particularly the small arteries (and veins) of the heart, lung, and kidney. Marked edema, inflammation, and necrosis occur in affected vessels, and the outcome is generally fatal. **Periarteritis nodosa** (polyarteritis nodosa), an autoimmune disorder, is characterized by zones of inflammation and fibrinoid necrosis in the tunica media of small arteries, which lead to formation of nodular aneurysms. Many organs and tissues may be involved, but the lungs usually are not.

Hemorrhage and infarction commonly occur. **Temporal arteritis** (giant cell arteritis), a disease of elderly persons also probably caused by autoimmunity, affects the temporal artery and other cranial vessels. The diseased artery and surrounding soft tissues are grossly inflamed and indurated. Microscopic examination shows necrosis of the media, infiltrates of inflammatory cells and multinucleate giant cells in the region of the internal elastic membrane, and eventually fibrosis.

In **thromboangiitis obliterans** (Buerger's disease), which occurs chiefly in young and middle-aged men, small and medium-sized arteries and veins in the extremities undergo gradual narrowing, with resulting gangrene. Intimal proliferation is followed by thrombosis, organization, and eventual obliteration of the lumen by fibrosis. The wavy contour of the internal elastic membrane as seen in cross section is characteristic of the later stages of this disease. **Takayasu's disease** (pulseless disease) is an obliterative arteritis of the main branches of the aortic arch. In **gargoylism** (generalized mucopolysaccharidosis), deposition of myxoid material in the tunica intima of arteries may greatly reduce their lumens. In **cystic medial necrosis**, the tunica media of large arteries degenerates and the muscular and elastic fibers are replaced by a loosely arranged and sparsely cellular connective tissue, with cystic spaces filled by mucinous material. Similar changes are seen in the arteries in Marfan's syndrome.

Arteriosclerosis (hardening of the arteries) is an important cause of disease, disability, and death, particularly in the elderly. Reduction in the caliber of the arteries of the brain, heart, kidneys, and extremities can cause serious functional impairment, infarction, or gangrene. Arteriosclerosis includes various degenerative disorders, of which the most important is **atherosclerosis**. The characteristic lesion of atherosclerosis is a deposition of cholesterol and other lipoid material in the intima. This may appear as grossly visible fatty streaks in the lining of the vessel, and microscopic examination shows subendothelial degeneration with lipoid material in macrophages and cholesterol crystals in tissue clefts. An atheroma is a plaque of lipoid material, with various amounts of fibrous hyperplasia, that forms in the intima, narrowing the lumen. Thrombosis, hemorrhage, and calcification commonly occur.

In **senile arteriosclerosis** (Mönckeberg's sclerosis) the media is principally involved. Fatty and hyaline degeneration of the muscular coat is followed by necrosis and calcification, which may be diffuse (pipestem arteries) or patchy (corduroy arteries). Narrowing of the lumen does not result. **Arteriolosclerosis** occurs chiefly in hypertension and is typified by hypertrophy of the tunica media, with variable amounts of endothelial proliferation. Visceral vessels are principally involved. More than one kind of arteriosclerosis can occur in the same patient and even in the same vessel. Obesity, diabetes, elevated levels of circulating lipids, and the use of tobacco are contributing factors in the development of arteriosclerosis.

Some degree of phlebitis (inflammation of a vein) accompanies any acute local inflammation or infection. **Thrombophlebitis** is an acute inflammatory process in a vein, usually due to local trauma or irritation, which leads to the formation of an obstructive thrombus within the lumen. The wall of the vein shows edema and an infiltrate of inflammatory cells. Although the thrombus is at first firmly attached, part or all of it may break loose and become an embolus. Otherwise, organization and perhaps recanalization eventually occur. Formation of a thrombus in a vein as a result of circulatory stasis or increased coagulability of the blood, without demonstrable inflammation, is called phlebothrombosis. Embolism and thrombosis are discussed in Chapter 12.

Diseases of the Heart

Any disorder affecting the myocardium principally or exclusively may be called **cardiomyopathy**. Cloudy swelling of the heart occurs in acute febrile illness, toxemia, and heavy metal poisoning. The heart is soft and flabby and its cut surface appears gray, granular, and opaque. Hydropic degeneration occurs in beriberi (due to deficiency of thiamine). Fatty degeneration may develop as a further stage of cellular deterioration, with grossly evident streaks of yellow lipid material (tigering) and, on microscopic examination, lipid droplets in myocardial fibers. After prolonged cachexia, the myocardial fibers may atrophy and acquire deposits of yellowish-brown lipofuscin about their nuclei (brown atrophy). Primary amyloidosis causes diffuse or nodular deposition of amyloid in the myocardium, with atrophy of fibers adjacent to deposits. Myxomatous degeneration of the myocardium occurs in myxedema.

Myocarditis (inflammation of the cardiac muscle) occurs in a variety of acute infectious and toxic conditions, including acute rheumatic fever, mumps, diphtheria, typhus, Rocky Mountain spotted fever, coxsackie A virus infection, toxoplasmosis, and carbon monoxide poisoning. The characteristic lesion of **rheumatic myocarditis** is the Aschoff body, a mass of necrotic collagen surrounded by an infiltrate of large, pleomorphic mononuclear cells with occasional giant cells. **Fiedler's myocarditis** (giant cell myocarditis), which occurs in young adults after viral respiratory infection, is marked by granuloma formation, infiltrates of eosinophils, lymphocytes, and plasma cells, and giant cell formation, all confined to the myocardium. Chagas' disease, due to *Trypanosoma cruzi,* is a common cause of myocarditis in areas where it is endemic, as in parts of South America.

Cardiac **dilatation** is stretching or overdistention of the ventricles as a result of cardiac overload or failure. In cardiac **hypertrophy**, the ventricular myocardium actually thickens in response to an increased load, as in hypertension or vascular disease. A massively hypertrophied heart may be called **cor bovinum** ("ox heart"). **Cor pulmonale** is dilatation or hypertrophy of the right ventricle as a result of disease in the lungs or pulmonary circulation. Any enlargement of the heart, whether accompanied by hypertrophy of cardiac muscle fibers or not, is known as cardiomegaly.

Coronary arteriosclerosis is an extremely common cause of disease and death. Reduction in myocardial perfusion due to narrowing of coronary arteries can cause various clinical syndromes, including angina pectoris (episodes of crushing chest pain), arrhythmias (disturbances of heart rhythm), and congestive heart failure, with inefficient pumping action and a rise of venous pressure. Complete occlusion of a coronary artery, usually caused by thrombosis in an arteriosclerotic vessel, leads to myocardial infarction. This condition often culminates in death due to shock, arrhythmia, or severe congestive heart failure. During the healing period, rupture of the heart (cardiorrhexis) may occur, and after healing, a weakened, dilated zone of myocardium may form a ventricular aneurysm.

Grossly an acute myocardial infarct appears as a zone of tan or pale yellow muscle surrounded by hemorrhage. The usual sites of involvement are the left ventricular wall and the interventricular septum. An infarct involving the full thickness of the ventricular wall is called transmural. Microscopic examination shows loss of nuclei from myocardial fibers, hyaline change of cytoplasm, and an inflammatory infiltrate. The type and degree of pathologic change depend on the age of the infarct. When death occurs immediately as a result of arrhythmia or cardiac arrest, changes may be minimal or absent. During healing, infarcted muscle is gradually replaced by a dense patch of fibrous tissue.

Inflammation of one or more heart valves is known as **endocarditis**. Acute endocarditis occurs in rheumatic fever and, rarely, in acute sepsis. **Rheumatic endocarditis** results in formation of verrucous (wartlike) nodules along the closing margins of the affected valves. These are composed of fibrin clot. In healing, they produce a fibrotic distortion of the valve, which often proceeds to calcification. Healed valves may be stenotic (with obstruction to forward flow of blood), incompetent (allowing backflow or regurgitation), or both. The mitral valve is the one most often affected in rheumatic endocarditis. In **Libman-Sacks endocarditis** (atypical verrucous endocarditis), a feature of systemic lupus erythematosus, vegetations consist of necrotic debris and inflammatory cells.

Infective endocarditis (subacute bacterial endocarditis) usually attacks valves that are already deformed, either congenitally or by rheumatic disease. Friable vegetations form on the margins of the valves. On microscopic examination these vegetations are seen to consist of masses of fibrin containing bacteria and surrounding central foci of necrotic tissue. Vegetations frequently break loose to become septic emboli. Infective endocarditis may also occur about the margins of a ventricular septal defect.

Atrial myxoma is a benign tumor of the endocardium consisting of mesenchymal connective tissue and arising usually from the interatrial septum. When pedunculated, it may interfere with cardiac function.

Pericarditis (inflammation of the pericardium) occurs in rheumatic fever, uremia, pneumonia, and other acute infectious and toxic conditions. Acute benign pericarditis (fibrinous pericarditis), the commonest type, may accompany or follow various infections, particularly viral respiratory infection. Visceral and parietal surfaces of the pericardium show shaggy patches of fibrinous exudate (bread-and-butter heart). Although ordinarily this is a benign disease, it may lead to copious pericardial effusion, which can interfere with the function of the heart (cardiac tamponade). Hemorrhage into the pericardium (hemopericardium) due to trauma or vascular or cardiac disease can also cause tamponade.

Bacterial or tuberculous pericarditis generally arises by extension of infection from the lungs or pleura. Organization of fibrinous or purulent pericardial exudate can result in adhesions between the two pericardial surfaces (adhesive pericarditis). Occasionally adhesions are so extensive as to impair cardiac action, particularly when calcification occurs (constrictive pericarditis). This most often follows staphylococcal or tuberculous pericarditis.

Review Questions

1. Name the four chambers of the heart.
2. What are some adverse consequences of arteriosclerosis?
3. Distinguish *cardiac dilatation* from *cardiac hypertrophy.*
4. What is meant by cardiac (or pericardial) tamponade?
5. Define or explain: *aneurysm, capillary, hypertension, pericardium, varices.*

20

The Respiratory System

Gross and Microscopic Anatomy

The respiratory system embraces all the structures concerned with the exchange of oxygen and carbon dioxide between the blood and the atmosphere. For our purposes, this system can be divided into two major components: the lung tissue proper, in which this gaseous exchange takes place, and the respiratory tract, a system of tubes that carry air to and from the lungs.

The **respiratory tract** begins at the lips and nostrils and ends, after much branching, within the substance of the lungs. Throughout most of its length, the respiratory tract is lined by pseudostratified columnar epithelium having a ciliated border. Among the epithelial cells are mucus-secreting goblet cells. Beneath a distinct basement membrane lies a layer of connective tissue, the lamina propria, with abundant elastic fibers and alveolar glands producing serous or mucous secretions. These glands keep the lining of the respiratory tract covered with a film of mucus to protect the surface and trap inspired particulate matter. The cilia of the epithelial surface, by their constant whiplike motion, cause this mucus film to move toward the pharynx, where it is periodically swallowed along with saliva.

Along its course, the respiratory tract shows a number of structural modifications. The nasal cavity and its accessory sinuses make up a system of cavities formed of bone and cartilage and lined by typical pseudostratified columnar epithelium. In the pharynx, wherever two surfaces regularly touch or rub, the pseudostratified columnar cells are replaced by stratified squamous epithelium. The pharyngeal connective tissue contains many aggregations of lymphoid tissue in addition to the tonsils, which are discussed in Chapter 18. The epiglottis and vocal apparatus of the larynx are formed of stratified squamous epithelium over a framework of elastic cartilage. The vocal cords are folds of epithelium covering the vocalis muscles. The pharynx and larynx are supplied with skeletal muscle for swallowing and speech.

The trachea and bronchi, which extend from the larynx to the hila of the lungs, are lined by pseudostratified columnar epithelium among which goblet cells are abundantly interspersed. The walls of these structures are reinforced by incomplete rings of hyaline cartilage, and the lamina propria contains many elastic fibers. With repeated branchings inside the lungs, the respiratory tract forms increasingly numerous ducts of increasingly small caliber and structural modification, the bronchioles. The epithelium becomes thinner, and cartilage elements gradually disappear. But the proportion of elastic fibers in the lamina propria increases as the lumen diminishes, and smooth muscle fibers appear with greater frequency. Terminal bronchioles, their name notwithstanding, branch further into respiratory bronchioles, and these again branch into alveolar ducts, which form part of the lung tissue proper.

The **lungs** are pink in infants and children, but with advancing age they become increasingly darkened by carbon particles absorbed from the atmosphere and trapped in macrophages, so that in older adults they appear slate-gray or black. The normal lung has an elastic, spongy texture, and crackles slightly on being compressed. The right lung normally weighs about 625 g and the left about 575 g. The right lung has three lobes and the left lung has two lobes. Each lung is further divided into bronchopulmonary segments (ten in the right and eight in the left) on the basis of common bronchial, arterial, and venous connections. Segments are divided into lobules.

Lung tissue proper is composed of very thin-walled air cells or pulmonary alveoli. A pulmonary alveolus is a microscopic sac whose wall consists of a single layer of extremely thin squamous epithelium lining a delicate connective tissue framework which contains a rich network of capillaries. The exchange of oxygen and carbon dioxide between inspired air and the blood occurs through the walls of the pulmonary alveoli and adjacent capillaries. Macrophages in the alveolar walls, called dust cells, engulf and remove inspired particulate matter. A cluster of alveoli is known as an alveolar sac, and many such alveolar sacs are grouped about an alveolar duct, which is formed by their inner walls and has no epithelium of its own.

The stroma of the lung is a scaffolding of fibrous and elastic connective tissue which separates the alveoli into segments and lobules. A large part of the substance of each lung is occupied by the branchings of the respiratory tract. The visceral pleura is a layer of mesothelium that covers the lung and is continuous with the parietal pleura lining the chest cavity.

Pathologic Study of the Respiratory System

Specimens of sputum can be examined for pathogenic microorganisms and malignant cells. Pathologic specimens from the upper respiratory tract can be obtained by smear or biopsy techniques under direct vision. Biopsy material can be secured from the larynx through a laryngoscope and from the trachea and bronchi through a rigid or fiberoptic bronchoscope. Tracheobronchial and bronchoalveolar lavage can also be carried out through a bronchoscope to obtain cell washings for cytologic study. Lung biopsy is performed as an open procedure, but pleural biopsy can be done either open or percutaneously. Thoracentesis, the removal of an abnormal collection of fluid from the pleural space, may yield material for microbiologic or cytologic study.

At autopsy the lungs are inspected in situ and any pleural fluid or adhesions noted before the lungs are removed. The size, shape, and surface features of each lung and its degree of inflation are observed. The main stem bronchus and segmental bronchi, as well as the pulmonary artery and its branches, are opened in each lung. The lung tissue is then sectioned with a long knife for examination of internal architecture and a search is made for cavities, abscesses, nodules, and zones of necrosis, hemorrhage, or fibrosis. The character of any fluid or exudate expressed from the cut lung surface is noted.

Diseases of the Larynx, Trachea, and Bronchi

Epiglottitis (epiglottiditis) is a severe acute inflammation of the epiglottis occurring usually in children and caused by *Haemophilus influenzae* in most cases. The epiglottis is markedly edematous and hyperemic. The importance of this condition lies in the risk of airway obstruction.

Papillomas of the vocal cords are irregular nodules, frequently multiple, which are more common in children. They tend to recur after surgical removal but eventually regress spontaneously. Histologic study shows irregular thickening of the cord with mononuclear cell infiltrates. **Laryngeal nodule** (singer's nodule) affects the contacting surfaces of the vocal cords in adults. This lesion too, although benign, tends to recur after surgical excision. Beginning as a polyp with a connective-tissue core covered by normal epithelium, the nodule eventually undergoes hyaline change, with atrophy of overlying epithelium. Sometimes the epithelium shows zones of hyperplasia and dyskeratosis.

Squamous cell carcinoma of the vocal cords begins as a plaque or papillary growth on a cord, expands slowly, and metastasizes late to regional lymph nodes. **Leukoplakia** of the cords, also called pachyderma, is a slowly evolving hyperplastic and acanthotic lesion of cord epithelium with some malignant potential.

Tracheitis is typically an acute, self-limited inflammatory response to infection, inhaled gases, fumes, or dust, or aspirated foreign material. It is a common feature of acute viral respiratory infection. Examination shows edema, inflammatory exudate, and excessive mucus. Bronchitis often accompanies or follows tracheitis. **Acute bronchitis** is a self-limited inflammatory process due to viral or bacterial infection or inhaled irritants. There is hyperemia of the mucosa, and copious mucopurulent exudate appears in bronchial lumens. Microscopic examination shows desquamation of columnar epithelium and neutrophilic infiltration. **Chronic bronchitis** may develop as a consequence of acute bacterial bronchitis, but allergy, tobacco smoke, and atmospheric pollution are also thought to play a part in its genesis. Pathologic study shows thick mucopurulent secretion in respiratory passages, with hyperplasia and hypertrophy of mucous glands and zones of acute and chronic inflammatory cell infiltrates. **Bronchiolitis** is a severe infection of the bronchioles in children, usually due to a virus (influenza, measles, pertussis, respiratory syncytial virus). The bronchioles are distended and filled with fibrinous exudate.

In **cystic fibrosis** (mucoviscidosis), a congenital disorder of exocrine glands affecting the sweat glands and pancreatic acini as well as the lung, abnormally thick mucus plugs the bronchioles, eliciting a chronic inflammatory reaction and leading to collapse and consolidation of alveoli, with heightened susceptibility to infection, particularly due to *Staphylococcus aureus* and *Pseudomonas aeruginosa.*

Bronchiectasis is a chronic necrotizing infection of bronchi and bronchioles, leading to permanent dilatation of their lumens. The walls of the dilated bronchi are thick and rigid because of replacement of the muscular coat by an irregular proliferation of collagenous fibers. Inability of the patient to clear his respiratory tract of secretions results in puddling of purulent, necrotic material and chronic bacterial growth. The epithelium of dilated bronchi may show squamous metaplasia. Bronchiectasis occurs with increased frequency in persons with cystic fibrosis, asthma, and chronic sinusitis.

Bronchial asthma, also called reactive airways disease (RAD), is a syndrome of coughing, wheezing, and dyspnea due to bronchospasm, bronchiolar edema, and production of abnormally tenacious respiratory tract mucus. Attacks of asthma can be induced in susceptible persons by inhaled allergens (pollens, dusts) or irritants (tobacco smoke, ozone), environmental factors (cold or damp air), respiratory infection, emotional stress, or exercise. Asthma may occur in infrequent attacks, or symptoms may be chronic with acute exacerbations. A particularly severe attack of asthma not responding to conventional treatment is called status asthmaticus.

An attack of asthma begins when mast cells in bronchial walls release histamine and leukotrienes, which cause bronchospasm, and other active substances including prostaglandins. The ensuing inflammatory response includes infiltration of neutrophils, eosinophils, and basophils, which release substances that cause necrosis and sloughing of ciliated epithelium, thus impairing the normal centripetal flow of respiratory tract mucus and eliciting further inflammation. The lungs in asthma are grossly dilated, the mucosa of the smaller bronchi is hyperemic and edematous, and their lumens are full of thick mucous exudate. Microscopic examination shows distention of alveoli, hypertrophy of the bronchial musculature, and submucosal infiltrates of neutrophils, eosinophils, and mononuclear cells. In longstanding asthma the basement membrane of the bronchial epithelium undergoes hyaline change, and subepithelial collagen deposition and fibrosis lead to irreversible reduction in bronchiolar caliber. Laënnec's pearls and Curschmann's spirals are small plugs of inspissated mucus formed in the bronchioles in asthma and expelled in the sputum. The sputum may also contain Charcot-Leyden crystals, elongated doubly pyramidal structures apparently derived from deteriorated eosinophils.

Diseases of the Lungs

Atelectasis is loss of air space by collapse of lung tissue, generally as a result of absorption of air distal to an obstruction (as by a mucus plug or tumor). It can also result from pneumothorax (presence of air inside the pleural cavity). Atelectasis may affect a small zone of lung tissue, a segment, a lobe, or an entire lung. Grossly the atelectatic lung appears shrunken and dull purple, with a wrinkled pleura. The lung parenchyma is compressible but it does not crackle. On microscopic examination, alveoli and alveolar ducts are seen to be collapsed or filled with mucus or exudate.

Pulmonary emphysema is overinflation of the lungs with enlargement of air spaces due to a breakdown of alveolar septa. Emphysematous lungs are pale and have a pillowlike consistency. They remain expanded when the thorax is opened. On microscopic examination, air spaces are enlarged and irregular. In centrilobular emphysema, distended, intercommunicating, saclike spaces are seen at the center of lobules, while in panlobular emphysema there is diffuse involvement throughout the lobule. About 10% of persons with emphysema have hereditary deficiency of the plasma protein alpha$_1$ antitrypsin, and about 20% develop peptic ulcer. Bullous emphysema refers to the formation of very large open spaces, usually in the apex of the lung, which are not lined by epithelium. An emphysematous bleb is a pocket of air that forms between the lung parenchyma and the visceral pleura.

Pulmonary congestion arises from an increase in pressure in the pulmonary arteries, usually due to valvular disease or congestive heart failure affecting the left ventricle. Engorgement of pulmonary vessels leads to perivascular edema and transudation of fluid into the alveoli. Severe acute left heart failure results in **acute pulmonary edema**, in which pulmonary gas exchange may be dangerously compromised. In **chronic passive congestion** of the lung, fibrin-rich exudate favors development of infection in lower lobes (hypostatic pneumonia). The combination of fibrosis in passively congested lung tissue with phago-cytosis of extravasated red blood cells by lung histiocytes leads to a condition called brown induration of the lung. Mononuclear cells with phagocytized hemosiderin (heart failure cells) may appear in the sputum. **Pulmonary hypertension** is a rise in the pressure in the pulmonary artery due to disease in the lung, generally emphysema, pulmonary fibrosis, or pneumoconiosis. It may lead to arteriosclerotic change or thrombosis in the pulmonary vessels.

Pulmonary embolism is blockage of a pulmonary artery or one or more of its branches, generally by a thrombus migrating from veins of the lower extremities (95%) or pelvis, less often by amniotic fluid, fat, or air. Emboli may be multiple. Acute pulmonary embolism is often rapidly fatal because of acute right ventricular failure (acute cor pulmonale). Infarction of lung tissue follows pulmonary embolism only when the bronchial circulation is compromised as well. The infarct appears as a pyramidal hemorrhagic zone. A fibrinous exudate may coat the overlying pleura. Microscopic examination shows ischemic necrosis, manifested by loss of cellular detail, and extravasa-tion of red blood cells. Healing of a pulmonary infarct is by fibrosis.

Pneumonitis

The causes of pneumonitis (pneumonia), inflammation of the lung, are many and various, and the symptoms and pathologic changes vary accordingly. **Acute pneumonitis** can be caused by inhalation or aspiration of irritant substances or by infection with bacteria, rick-ettsias, viruses, fungi, or parasites. Bacterial pneumonias are divided into those that cause consolidation and those that do not. Consolidation is defined as a pathologic process in which normally aerated lung tissue is converted into a dense, airless mass by a com-bination of interstitial edema and exudation of fibrin-rich fluid into alveolar spaces. Consolidative pneumonia due to pneumococcus (*Streptococcus pneumoniae*) and *Klebsiella pneumoniae* tends to be lobar in distribution—that is, it eventually spreads to involve the entirety of one lung lobe but may spare all other lung tissue. The pathologic changes in **pneumococcal pneumonia** are divided into four stages. In the stage of **congestion**, the lung tissue is soggy with edema, and a central zone of consolidation gradually expands toward the periphery of the affected lobe. The tissue appears reddish gray and exudes a frothy, bloody fluid. In the stage of **red hepatization**, edema fluid is replaced by a richly cellular exudate containing fibrin and extravasated red blood cells. The lung is heavy and firm, and its cut surface appears dull red, granular, dry, and friable. Microscopic examination shows alveoli to be uniformly filled with exudate. There is no necrosis or disruption of alveolar septa. In the stage of **gray hepatization** the lung assumes a gray color as extravasated red blood cells are broken down. Both grossly and microscopically the lung tissue looks like liver, hence the term hepatization. In the stage of **resolution**, alveolar exudate is liquefied by tissue enzymes, and healing follows, occasionally accompanied by severe fibrosis.

Friedländer's pneumonia, caused by *Klebsiella pneumoniae,* also progresses to lobar consolidation. This infection is commoner in chronic alcoholics and debilitated persons. The affected lung tissue is mottled gray and red, with patchy zones of purulent and hemorrhagic exudate. Microscopic examination shows inflammatory cell infiltrates and alveolar necrosis.

In contrast with the lobar distribution of pneumococcal and Friedländer's pneumonia, most other infections of lung tissue are patchy and diffuse, involving parts of all lobes. This distribution of pulmonary infection is called **bronchopneumonia**. Some degree of consolidation occurs in bronchopneumonia due to staphylococci, *Mycoplasma, Legionella,* and influenza. **Staphylococcal pneumonitis** is characterized by hemorrhage, abscess formation, and a tendency toward cavitation—that is, formation of large open spaces in lung tissue through coalescence of smaller spaces created by necrosis of alveolar septa. **Mycoplasmal pneumonia** also causes patchy zones of hemorrhagic consolidation. Bronchi and alveoli contain mucopurulent exudate but abscess formation does not occur. In **influenza** there are patches of hyperemia, edema, and consolidation alternating with zones of normal lung. Alveolar septa are thickened by edema and contain cellular infiltrates. Alveoli may become lined by a hyaline membrane, and septal necrosis may occur. **Legionella pneumonia** (legionnaires' disease) produces a patchy, multifocal involvement but may progress to lobar consolidation and cavitation.

The term **interstitial pneumonitis** refers to pulmonary infection in which inflammatory changes in alveolar septa are prominent. **Q fever**, caused by *Coxiella burnetii,* a rickettsia, is an interstitial pneumonitis with mononuclear cell infiltrates in alveolar septa and copious fibrin-rich exudate. **Interstitial plasma cell pneumonia**, due to *Pneumocystis carinii,* a protozoan parasite, occurs chiefly in infants and persons with impaired immunity. There is mononuclear cell infiltrate of alveolar septa and foamy exudate in the air spaces. Oval or helmet-shaped parasites may be identified by special stains containing silver.

Chronic pneumonic processes have varying etiologies, including bacterial and fungal infection, hypersensitivity, and inhalation of irritant dusts. Most of these processes are associated with granuloma formation and gradual replacement of alveolar tissue by fibrosis. **Pulmonary tuberculosis** is the most typical and most serious expression of infection with *Mycobacterium tuberculosis*. In the primary or exudative phase, organisms reaching the lung through the air passages cause a local infection with hyperemia, edema, neutrophilic infiltration, and fibrinous exudate. Mononuclear cells that have ingested invading organisms, called epithelioid cells because of their resemblance to cuboidal epithelium, form dense aggregations. These gradually evolve into microscopic granulomatous tubercles of highly characteristic appearance. In the center is a zone of caseous necrosis, a mass of eosinophilic, lipid-rich material without cellular detail. Surrounding or adjacent to this central zone are Langhans giant cells, each a circular or horseshoe-shaped syncytium derived from monocytes, with its nuclei ranged around the periphery. A dense, irregular infiltrate of lymphocytes encloses the tubercle. Coalescence of microscopic tubercles leads to formation of grossly visible nodules. Simultaneous appearance of many small nodules throughout both lungs, an uncommon development due presumably to hematogenous spread with diminished tissue resistance, is called miliary tuberculosis.

Pulmonary tuberculous infection typically spreads to regional lymph nodes. Both the primary focus and the infected nodes eventually undergo fibrosis and calcification. Infection is not arrested, however, and reactivation of the primary lesion may lead to a secondary stage with more extensive and more severe tissue damage. Large areas of lung tissue may be replaced by fibrosis. Cavities may be formed by necrosis of tissue, and fatal hemorrhage may result from erosion of blood vessels. Infection may spread to other tissues, the bone, gastrointestinal tract, genitourinary system, and central nervous system being most vulnerable. Organisms of the *Mycobacterium avium* complex (MAC) can cause fulminant tuberculosis in persons with AIDS.

Fungal infections of the lungs produce pathologic changes similar to those of pulmonary tuberculosis. Actinomycosis, blastomycosis, coccidioidomycosis, and histoplasmosis are all chronic granulomatous infections due to fungi in which focal lesions showing giant cells and central caseation or microabscess formation coalesce to form nodules that eventually become fibrotic and calcify. Miliary spread and cavitation may also occur.

Sarcoidosis (Boeck's sarcoid) is a systemic disease of unknown cause, whose most severe manifestation is granulomatous pneumonitis. Noncaseating tubercles of epithelioid cells form and coalesce, eventually being replaced by fibrous tissue. Lesions also occur in the skin, spleen, and lymph nodes. Marked enlargement of hilar lymph nodes is characteristic. These nodes do not calcify and eventually return to normal size. In **Goodpasture's syndrome**, an autoimmune disorder, inflammation and fibrinoid degeneration occur in both the lungs and the kidneys. Pulmonary changes include hemorrhages within alveoli and collagenous deposits in alveolar septa. **Pulmonary alveolar proteinosis**, a disorder of unknown cause, consists of filling of distal alveoli by a proteinaceous material that interferes with gas exchange. Signs of inflammation are absent. Extensive fibrosis may follow. In **hyaline membrane disease**, which affects newborns, alveoli are lined by a layer of eosinophilic hyaline material. Extensive atelectasis usually occurs also and the condition is frequently fatal. **Aspiration pneumonitis** results from entry of liquid material, usually vomitus, into the lower respiratory tract. There is acute inflammation with edema and exudation and often also hemorrhage and abscess formation. **Lipoid pneumonitis**, due generally to excessive use of oily nose drops, is marked by the appearance of foamy lipoid material and lipoid-laden macrophages in bronchioles. Alveolar septa are replaced by inflammatory cells and fibrosis.

Hypersensitivity pneumonia (extrinsic allergic alveolitis) is a pulmonary inflammation caused by allergy to various inhaled microorganisms, principally molds. Bagassosis results from sensitivity to *Thermoactinomyces sacchari,* a mold found in bagasse, a sugar-cane product. Farmer's lung is due to sensitivity to *Microsporum faeni,* found in moldy hay. Pigeon-breeder's lung is due to molds in avian excreta. In each of these conditions, an acute stage with alveolar wall edema, cellular infiltration, and exudation may be succeeded by a stage of progressive and widespread pulmonary fibrosis.

Pneumoconiosis is a chronic inflammatory process due to prolonged inhalation of mineral dusts, chiefly in an occupational setting. Typically there is a very gradual fibrotic reaction, which may in time lead to severe impairment of pulmonary function. **Silicosis**, due to chronic inhalation of silicon (sand) particles, produces widespread fibrotic nodules, which may coalesce. Microscopic examination shows a characteristic concentric onionskin configuration of collagenous fibers, which may have undergone hyaline change. Persons with silicosis show heightened susceptibility to pulmonary tuberculosis. **Anthracosis** (black lung) is due to coal dust. Massive deposits of carbon are grossly evident. Besides nodular fibrosis there may be zones of alveolar necrosis with emphysema or cavitation. **Asbestosis**, due to inhalation of asbestos fibers, causes extensive pulmonary fibrosis, particularly in the lower lobes. Microscopic examination shows asbestos bodies—fibers of asbestos covered with a protein material—surrounded by macrophages. Fibrotic plaques may also form in the pleura and eventually calcify. **Berylliosis**, due to inhalation of beryllium dust, is a granulomatous pneumonitis resembling sarcoidosis in pathologic features. Noncaseating nodules contain multinucleate giant cells and are surrounded by lymphocytic infiltrate.

Neoplasms of the Respiratory System

Bronchogenic carcinoma, arising from columnar epithelium lining bronchial passages, is the principal malignancy of the lung. It is a common neoplasm, accounting for one-third of all cancer deaths in men and one-fifth of all cancer deaths in women. The risk of bronchogenic carcinoma is increased by cigarette smoking. Carcinomas arising from bronchial epithelium assume various histologic forms. Adenocarcinoma shows features of secretory epithelium, including some attempt at gland formation and mucus secretion. Squamous cell carcinoma of the bronchus consists of malignant stratified squamous cells arising apparently by metamorphosis of columnar epithelium. Oat cell carcinoma is a highly malignant variant composed of small oval cells with scanty cytoplasm. Small round cell carcinoma contains cells reminiscent of lymphoid cells. Still more anaplastic, undifferentiated carcinomas also occur. Besides extensive local invasion, bronchogenic carcinoma can cause bronchial stenosis, with resultant atelectasis or pneumonitis or both, and hemorrhage by erosion of blood vessels. Metastasis is principally to regional lymph nodes, the opposite lung, the liver, and the brain. Bronchogenic carcinoma, particularly of the oat cell variety, may produce hormonelike substances capable of inducing Cushing's syndrome, hypercalcemia, or inappropriate secretion of antidiuretic hormone.

Metastasis of malignant tumors from other organs to the lung occurs frequently. Spread is generally lymphatic. Tumors of the kidney, breast, colon, and cervix uteri are particularly likely to spread to the lung, but as many as one-half of all fatal malignant tumors are found at autopsy to have spread to the lung. Metastatic tumors of the lung tend to occur in the lower lobes and to have a smooth or lobulated contour. Frequently they are multiple.

Diseases of the Pleura

Inflammation of the pleura (**pleuritis**, pleurisy) accompanies any acute or chronic inflammatory process affecting the periphery of the lung, and may also result from trauma to the chest wall. Healing of fibrinous pleuritis may give rise to fibrous pleural adhesions. **Empyema**, a pocket of pus between visceral and parietal pleura, is generally a complication of bacterial pneumonitis. **Hemothorax** (effusion of blood in the pleural cavity) and **pneumothorax** (air in the pleural cavity) often result from blunt or penetrating trauma to the chest and may occur together. Spontaneous pneumothorax results generally from rupture of an emphysematous bleb. Mesothelioma is a highly malignant tumor arising from pleural mesothelium and invading the chest wall.

Review Questions

1. What is the function of cilia on the lining of the respiratory tract?
2. What structural feature keeps the trachea and bronchi from collapsing when the air pressure inside them is reduced?
3. What is the usual source of a pulmonary embolus?
4. Distinguish *lobar pneumonia* from *bronchopneumonia*.
5. Of what type of pulmonary infection are epithelioid cells, caseous necrosis, and Langhans giant cells characteristic?
6. Define or explain: *atelectasis, bronchial asthma, bronchiectasis, pleurisy, pneumoconiosis, pneumothorax, pulmonary emphysema.*

21

The Digestive System, Liver, and Pancreas

The digestive system includes a number of specialized organs and tissues whose collective function is the ingestion, digestion, and absorption of nutrients and the disposal of associated wastes. Reduced to its simplest terms, the digestive system consists of a single unbranched tube, the alimentary canal, which runs from the lips to the anus, and several specialized glandular structures—the salivary glands, the liver, and the pancreas—which produce digestive fluids and deliver them to the alimentary canal via ducts. The teeth and the tongue are also regarded as digestive structures.

The Alimentary Canal: Gross and Microscopic Anatomy

The structure of the alimentary canal follows the same general plan throughout its length. The lining **mucosa** consists of simple or stratified epithelium with a well-defined lamina propria and, beneath that, a layer of smooth muscle, which is called the muscularis mucosae (for lamina muscularis tunicae mucosae). A **submucosa** of areolar connective tissue lies between these mucosal structures and the principal muscle layer of the digestive tract, called the **muscularis externa** to distinguish it from the muscularis mucosae. Typically the muscularis externa includes an inner layer of circularly disposed smooth muscle fibers and an outer longitudinal layer. Outside the muscular coat is another layer of connective tissue. When this blends into surrounding tissue it is called a (tunica) **fibrosa**, and when it is covered by mesothelium (i.e., peritoneum) it is called a (tunica) **serosa**. Autonomic nerve tissue is represented throughout the alimentary canal, beginning in the esophagus, by Auerbach's myenteric plexus between the layers of the muscularis externa and Meissner's plexus in the submucosa.

The mucous membrane of the **mouth** is covered by stratified squamous epithelium. Over the gums and hard palate this epithelium shows some degree of keratinization (loss of nuclei in outer cell layers), as in the skin, and beneath it is a layer of tough connective tissue with coarse collagenous fibers. The upper surface of the tongue is covered by numerous small projections called papillae, which are classified by shape as filiform (threadlike), fungiform (mushroomlike), and vallate or circumvallate (surrounded by a groove). Most of the substance of the tongue is skeletal muscle.

The **esophagus** is lined by stratified squamous epithelium and its submucosa contains alveolar mucous glands. At the junction of the esophagus with the stomach, the surface of the mucosa changes abruptly to simple columnar epithelium. The lining of the **stomach** is thrown into grossly evident folds or rugae. In the lamina propria are simple tubular glands that discharge their secretion to the surface through minute pores called foveolae or gastric pits. These glands contain three types of secretory cells: chief cells, which produce the digestive enzyme pepsin; parietal cells, which produce hydrochloric acid; and mucous cells.

Most absorption of nutrients takes place through the mucosa of the **small intestine**. The absorptive surface of the small intestinal mucosa is greatly increased by being thrown into minute fingerlike projections called villi, which give the surface a velvety look and feel. Each villus consists of a core of connective tissue over which the simple columnar epithelium is stretched. Each villus contains a lymphatic vessel or lacteal, which absorbs fatty material, and a network of capillaries which absorb other nutrients. The crypts of Lieberkühn are simple tubular glands that lie in the lamina propria and open between the villi. They consist of goblet cells secreting mucus and Paneth cells, which produce digestive enzymes.

Each division of the small intestine has its histologic peculiarities. In the duodenum the villi are leaf-shaped, and the submucosa contains tubuloalveolar glands, called Brunner's glands, which empty into the crypts of Lieberkühn. The villi of the jejunum are rounded. In the ileum the villi are club-shaped and the lamina propria and submucosa contain aggregations of lymphoid tissue called Peyer's patches.

The principal functions of the **colon** are the absorption of water from digestive wastes and the production of mucus. Its lining has no villi and its crypts of Lieberkühn contain exclusively goblet cells. The epithelium is simple columnar. The appendix is a projection of the cecum or first portion of the colon, and its structure closely resembles that of the colon. It differs in having prominent lymphoid nodules in its lamina propria.

The mucous and serous glands found in the walls of the alimentary canal are supplemented by larger aggregations of glandular tissue lying outside the canal and communicating with it by ducts—the salivary glands, the pancreas, and the liver. The **salivary glands** are small discrete structures situated in the mouth and producing saliva. They contain alveoli lined with cuboidal glandular cells, and branching duct systems lined with columnar epithelium, in a connective-tissue stroma. The parotid gland contains only serous elements; the submaxillary and sublingual glands contain serous, mucous, and mixed alveoli. Serous cells in the salivary glands contain prominent secretory granules and produce enzymes for the digestion of starches.

Pathologic Study of the Alimentary Canal

Material can be obtained from the digestive tract for cytologic or histologic study in a variety of ways. Exfoliative cytology can be performed in the mouth by simple scraping of the mucosa, and from other parts of the alimentary canal by washing or brushing or both through suitable instruments. Mucosal lesions can be biopsied if they can be reached with a snare or biopsy forceps passed through an endoscope. For some regions and some types of lesion, open biopsy is preferable. Any tissue removed during surgery on the digestive system is submitted for pathologic study, whether malignant disease is suspected or not. At autopsy, the entire digestive tube from pharynx to rectum is inspected externally for perforations, adhesions, nodules, and other gross abnormalities. It is then opened longitudinally from end to end, its contents noted, and the mucosa examined for ulceration, inflammation, hemorrhage, scarring, and other lesions. Specimens are taken for microscopic study as appropriate.

Developmental Disorders of the Alimentary Canal

The digestive tube is subject to a variety of congenital developmental anomalies, some of them having little clinical significance and others life threatening. Only the more common will be mentioned. **Cleft lip** (harelip, cheiloschisis) is a failure of midline fusion in the upper lip. When the cleft extends back through the palate the condition is termed **cleft palate** (uranoschisis). **Macrognathia** refers to abnormal size and prominence of the mandible, **micrognathia** to hypoplasia of the mandible. Micrognathia is a feature of several congenital syndromes, including Pierre Robin syndrome (which includes cleft palate) and Treacher Collins syndrome (mandibulofacial dysostosis). **Macroglossia** is overdevelopment of the tongue, a feature of cretinism.

A **thyroglossal duct cyst** lined by ciliated columnar epithelium may develop along the course of the thyroglossal duct, an embryonic passage tracing the migration of the thyroid gland from the root of the tongue to the neck. Depending on its location, the cyst may rupture to the skin surface near the anterior midline of the neck, or to the root of the tongue, producing a fistula in either case. A **branchial cleft cyst** occurs laterally in the neck, near the angle of the jaw, as a result of failure of the second branchial cleft to close. It is lined by squamous or columnar epithelium and contains a watery or mucoid secretion. It may be associated with a fistula passing from the pharynx to the skin surface.

Atresia refers to the congenital absence of a lumen or passage in some part of a normally hollow or tubular structure. Atresia of a segment of the esophagus occurs fairly frequently. Often the patent segment above the area of atresia communicates by a fistula with the trachea. Atresia of the bowel is less common. When it occurs in the distal rectum the condition is termed imperforate anus. Abnormal narrowing of a tube or passage is called stenosis. **Pyloric stenosis** is a congenital narrowing of the gastric pylorus due to hypertrophy of the muscularis. It is commoner in male infants and usually does not cause obstruction and vomiting until the third or fourth week of life.

An abnormal bulge, pocket, or pouch formed from a tubular or hollow structure is known as a **diverticulum**. Congenital diverticula of the bowel, particularly the duodenum, are relatively common and of little significance. Because they usually cause no symptoms, congenital diverticula are often discovered incidentally, and may be difficult to distinguish from acquired diverticula. **Meckel's diverticulum** occurs in the ileum about 30 cm proximal to the ileocecal valve (in adults) and represents a partial persistence of the embryonic omphalomesenteric duct. It rarely exceeds 6 cm in length and is similar in structure to the ileum. Often, however, it contains islands of gastric mucosa and sometimes also zones of pancreatic tissue; inflammation (Meckel's diverticulitis) and ulceration may occur.

Malrotation refers to a failure of the bowel to undergo the expected rotation during fetal development. This is of little importance except that it places the appendix in an unexpected part of the abdomen and may complicate the diagnosis of acute appendicitis. **Congenital megacolon** (Hirschsprung's disease) is a dilatation and hypertrophy of the colon resulting from sustained contraction of the muscular coat of the rectosigmoid, due to degenerative changes in sympathetic ganglion cells of Meissner's and Auerbach's plexuses. Because symptoms commonly appear soon after birth, the condition is thought to arise from a congenital abnormality in these cells.

Diseases of the Alimentary Canal

Stenosis, diverticula, and fistulas may be acquired as a result of traumatic, inflammatory, degenerative, or neoplastic disease of the digestive tract or adjacent structures. Stenosis or stricture of the esophagus usually results from the ingestion of lye or other corrosive material. Stenosis can occur in any part of the digestive tract as a consequence of fibrotic reaction after inflammation.

Acquired diverticula are largely limited to the esophagus and the colon. **Esophageal diverticula** are classically divided into two types. The more common **pulsion diverticulum**, due to increased pressure from within the esophagus, consists of a gradually enlarging pouch of esophageal mucosa and submucosa that bulges through the muscular coat. Usually this occurs just below the pharynx, where it is called **Zenker's diverticulum**. Trapping of food and obstruction to swallowing may eventually occur. The **traction diverticulum** was so named because it was thought that the shrinkage of healing tuberculous lymph nodes in the mediastinum pulled out a segment of the esophageal wall. There is now some doubt about this etiology. This type of diverticulum involves all the layers of the esophagus and can occur at any level. Symptoms and complications are less frequent than with pulsion diverticula.

Colonic diverticula commonly occur with aging and may be asymptomatic, even when quite numerous. Typically their walls consist of mucosa and serosa without any intervening muscle tissue. They rarely exceed 1 cm in diameter, but because their communications with the bowel lumen are often smaller than their diameters, feces tends to accumulate within them and predisposes to inflammation (diverticulitis). This may lead to hemorrhage, perforation with abscess or fistula formation, or stricture due to fibrosis.

A **fistula** is an abnormal passage through tissue, which places one hollow or tubular organ or cavity in communication with another or with the body surface. An acquired fistula can result from trauma, foreign body, infection, inflammation, degeneration, necrosis, or neoplastic disease.

Intestinal obstruction is a serious, often fatal condition, leading to impairment of circulation in the affected portion of the bowel, sequestration of intestinal contents, distention of the bowel with gas and fluid, and absorption of toxic products. Hemorrhage, shock, and intestinal perforation may occur. True **mechanical obstruction** can result from an abnormal substance or material within the lumen (obturator obstruction, due to foreign body, gallstones, or worms), disease of the bowel wall (edema, fibrosis, neoplasm), or external constriction (peritoneal adhesions, adjacent neoplasm, volvulus, intussusception, or hernia). Some of these causes require explanation. In volvulus, two segments of bowel become twisted around each other, the segment between them being converted into a closed loop. Intussusception occurs when a segment of bowel advances into the segment distal to it. Often this results from peristaltic traction on a pedunculated tumor within the lumen.

A condition similar to intestinal obstruction occurs when normal intestinal motility is impaired. **Ileus** refers to a cessation of normal peristalsis, with obstructive consequences. Adynamic (or paralytic) ileus is atony or paralysis of the muscularis, due to drugs, toxemia, trauma, surgery, or other local or general cause. Dynamic (or spastic) ileus results from spastic contraction of a segment of bowel.

Inflammatory Disorders

Both the epithelial lining of the digestive tube and its muscular and connective-tissue elements are subject to numerous inflammatory disorders, some of them (such as herpetic stomatitis, cholera, and pseudomembranous enterocolitis) due to infection or other clear-cut causes and others (such as peptic ulcer, Crohn's disease, and ulcerative colitis) of dubious or unknown etiology. Any interruption in the continuity of a body surface not due to acute trauma may be called an **ulcer**. Ulceration of the gastrointestinal mucosa can occur as part of an inflammatory process affecting any portion of the digestive tract. Ulcers of the digestive tract can assume a wide variety of forms: they may be solitary or numerous; shallow or deep; round, oval, or linear; sharp-edged ("punched out") or ragged; surrounded by healthy or by diseased mucosa; symptomatic or asymptomatic.

Cheilitis is inflammation of the **lips**. The lips are a common site of herpes simplex infection (herpes labialis). Hyperkeratotic thickening and fissuring of the skin at the corners of the mouth, usually associated with repeated licking, is called cheilosis or perlèche. The **buccal mucosa** is subject to various forms of inflammation (stomatitis), most of them due to trauma or infection. An aphtha (aphthous ulcer) is a shallow, painful, punched-out mucosal ulcer surrounded by a narrow zone of erythema and having a shaggy yellow base. Microscopic examination shows destruction of the mucosa and a chronic inflammatory cell infiltrate in the submucosa. Trauma is probably the usual cause, but some persons are subject to recurrent attacks of several aphthae at a time. Vincent's infection (necrotizing gingivitis, trench mouth), due to fusiform and spirochetal bacteria acting synergistically, causes edema and necrotizing ulceration of the gums and buccal mucosa. Herpes simplex can also cause ulcerative stomatitis and pharyngitis. Thrush, due to overgrowth of *Candida albicans* in the oral mucosa, causes patches of white or gray material consisting of cellular debris and fungal organisms. Other infectious diseases with oral lesions include coxsackie A virus infection (herpangina), hand, foot, and mouth disease, measles, and varicella.

Periodontitis (pyorrhea alveolaris) is an inflammation of the **gums** accompanied by degeneration of periodontal tissues and resorption of alveolar bone. Epulis is a nodular mass forming on a gum and consisting of highly vascular granulation tissue, infiltrates of neutrophils, lymphocytes, plasma cells, hemosiderin deposits due to hemorrhage, and variable amounts of fibrosis.

Glossitis (inflammation of the tongue) can occur as part of any inflammatory process affecting the mouth or pharynx. Atrophy and destruction of lingual papillae resulting in a beefy red appearance of the tongue and accompanied by an infiltrate of chronic inflammatory cells in the lamina propria occur in pernicious anemia, pellagra, and other nutritional disorders. A deeply erythematous tongue (strawberry tongue) is a characteristic feature of scarlatina.

Infection of the **salivary glands** with the mumps virus (epidemic parotitis) causes gross enlargement of one or both glands due to interstitial edema and distention of glandular acini. Histologic study shows degenerative changes in ductal epithelium, periductal infiltration of lymphocytes and mononuclear cells, and distention of acini with atrophy or necrosis of secretory epithelium. Acute suppurative parotitis, usually due to *Staphylococcus aureus,* occurs occasionally as a complication of systemic infection or major surgery. An acute suppurative process, initially periductal, extends to the parenchyma and may cause abscess formation and widespread destruction of glandular tissue. Sjögren's syndrome (keratoconjunctivitis sicca), an autoimmune disorder of middle-aged and elderly women, includes dysfunction of lacrimal and salivary glands and connective-tissue disease such as rheumatoid arthritis, scleroderma, or systemic lupus erythematosus. The salivary glands are enlarged and their function is impaired. Histologic examination shows perivascular infiltrates of chronic inflammatory cells, atrophy of secretory epithelium, and fibrous proliferation. Mikulicz's syndrome is a similar condition or variant in which lymphoid tissue replaces secretory acini in salivary glands.

Pharyngitis (inflammation of the pharynx, sore throat) is usually due to viral infection but in a significant minority of cases is caused by group A hemolytic streptococci. Tonsillitis is discussed in Chapter 18. Occasionally suppurative infection extends to the deeper structures of the oral and pharyngeal wall and beyond, creating severe swelling and pain and endangering the airway. **Peritonsillar abscess** (quinsy) extends from the tonsil and its capsule to surrounding soft tissues. **Retropharyngeal abscess** involves the lymphoid tissue in the posterior and lateral pharyngeal walls. **Ludwig's angina** is a severe cellulitis of the floor of the mouth often due to oral trauma or dental infection.

Esophagitis usually results either from ingestion of irritant or corrosive chemicals or from reflux of acid gastric juice from the stomach. Candidal infection of the esophagus is not common but occurs with increased frequency among persons whose immune defenses are impaired. **Acute gastritis** may result from ingestion of irritants, including alcohol, aspirin, and other drugs, or may be a feature of an acute viral infection involving the intestine as well (acute gastroenteritis). Chronic gastritis is divided into two classes. In **hypertrophic gastritis**, thickening of the rugae is grossly evident, and microscopic examination shows hypertrophy of the gastric glands and chronic inflammatory cell infiltration in the lamina propria. **Atrophic gastritis**, which occurs in pernicious anemia, pellagra, and other deficiency syndromes, features thinning of the mucosa with loss of rugae and, on microscopic study, atrophy of the chief and parietal cells, fibrosis in the lamina propria, hypertrophy of the muscularis mucosae, and scattered lymphocytes and plasma cells. This condition is commonly associated with achlorhydria—lack of hydrochloric acid in the gastric juice—and with increased risk of gastric carcinoma.

An ulcer occurring in any part of the gastrointestinal tract that is exposed to acid gastric juice (esophagus, stomach, duodenum, Meckel's diverticulum) is called a **peptic ulcer**. Peptic ulcer may occur in the lower esophagus either because of an abnormal reflux of acid gastric juice or because of the presence of ectopic gastric epithelium there (Barrett's esophagus). Presumably peptic ulceration of the stomach and duodenum results from the failure of some natural mechanism to protect the gastrointestinal mucosa from its own digestive secretions. Although emotional stress, diet, alcohol, nicotine, and caffeine have often been implicated in the genesis of peptic ulcer, the exact etiology remains unknown. In many cases of chronic gastritis and peptic ulcer, infection or colonization by *Helicobacter pylori,* a gram-negative bacillus, seems to increase vulnerability of the mucosa. Eradication of this organism greatly reduces the likelihood of recurrent peptic disease. On the other hand, many persons infected with *H. pylori* have no evidence of the disease.

Acute peptic ulcer is a relatively uncommon lesion, usually resulting from some sudden disturbance of physiologic balance, e.g., severe burns (Curling's ulcer), intracranial trauma or disease (Cushing's ulcer), or treatment with adrenocortical steroid. Acute ulcers typically occur in the stomach, are often numerous, and may progress rapidly to hemorrhage, perforation, or both.

Chronic peptic ulcer results from a poorly understood anatomic, physiologic, or constitutional aberration whose lifelong duration and widespread effects are reflected by the term peptic ulcer disease. The majority of chronic peptic ulcers occur in the duodenum, and most of the rest occur in the gastric pylorus. The typical chronic peptic ulcer is solitary, nearly round, and 1–2 cm in diameter. The margin is punched-out or slightly cratered, not heaped up or undermined. The base is granular and beefy, often with a thin film of fibrinous exudate. The ulcer may extend into the muscularis and even the serosa, where extensive fibrosis may occur, producing thickening, deformity, or fixation to adjacent structures. Microscopic examination shows destruction of mucosa and submucosa; a base of granulation tissue with neutrophils and macrophages near the surface and lymphocytes, eosinophils, and plasma cells at deeper levels; and variable amounts of fibrosis. After healing, a patch of fibrous tissue remains at the site of the ulcer. The mucosal surface is covered with simple columnar epithelium having no glands. The principal complications of peptic ulcer are hemorrhage, perforation, and obstruction. Postmortem digestion of the gastric mucosa is distinguished from peptic ulceration by the absence of inflammatory reaction.

Inflammation of the small bowel (enteritis), the colon (colitis), or both (enterocolitis) is usually mild, acute, and self-limited, the commonest cause being a virus. Chemical poisons such as mercury and arsenic can cause acute enteritis with edema, hyperemia, and mucosal ulceration. Enteric involvement in acute bacterial infections may be due to invasion of the bowel wall by bacteria, but is usually the effect of toxins elaborated by bacteria. Infection with *Campylobacter jejuni* causes generalized edema and mucosal ulceration of the jejunum and ileum. Microscopic examination shows epithelial necrosis, neutrophilic infiltration of the lamina propria with variable numbers of mononuclear cells and eosinophils, and crypt abscesses. *Yersinia enterocolitica* also causes toxic necrosis of intestinal mucosa, with hemorrhage and mesenteric lymphadenitis. Toxigenic strains of *Escherichia coli* produce a similar enteritis, characterized by hypersecretion in the small bowel. **Pseudomembranous enterocolitis**, which typically occurs after antibiotic treatment, is due to toxins elaborated by *Clostridium difficile*. Gross examination shows closely adherent plaques (mushroom caps) of a shaggy gray mucuslike substance. Hemorrhage and toxemia commonly occur.

Severe acute enteritis is a feature of cholera, bacillary dysentery, and typhoid fever. In **cholera**, which is due to *Vibrio cholerae,* the entire bowel shows mucosal destruction and submucosal congestion. Hemorrhage may occur but ulcers are not found. Severe diarrhea may lead to dehydration, acidosis, shock, and early death. **Bacillary dysentery**, caused by *Shigella* organisms, shows necrosis and ulceration of the epithelium, principally in the colon. Destruction may extend to the muscularis and is accompanied by infiltrates of polymorphonuclear cells, fibrin deposition, and formation of granulation tissue. Intestinal involvement in **typhoid fever** (due to *Salmonella typhi*) is just one feature of a systemic infection having cardiac, respiratory, cutaneous, and constitutional manifestations as well. The enteric lesion is a hyperplasia of Peyer's patches in the distal ileum which progresses to necrosis and ulceration. The ulcers are deep, with raised edges, and elongated in the direction of the bowel length. Microscopic examination shows lymphoid hyperplasia, infiltrates of macrophages, and much necrotic debris.

Chronic enteric infection is uncommon. Tuberculosis can cause caseating granulomas and ulcerations in Peyer's patches. Lymphogranuloma venereum produces fibrosis of perirectal tissues, particularly in women. In many forms of parasitic infestation the intestine is the principal focus of disease. **Amebic dysentery** results from invasion of the colonic mucosa by *Entamoeba histolytica,* a protozoan. Grossly there are small ulcers with shaggy, overhanging margins (flask-shaped ulcers) surrounded by normal mucosa. Microscopic examination shows coagulation necrosis in the crypts of Lieberkühn, neutrophilic infiltrates about the margins of the ulcers, and amebas within tissues. Complications include secondary bacterial infection, perforation, and amebic abscess of the liver. Intestinal amebiasis may exist in a mild, even asymptomatic form. Infestation with *Giardia lamblia,* another protozoan, may also be asymptomatic. Giardia invades the mucosa of the small bowel, interfering with absorption of certain nutrients, and may cause flatulence and diarrhea. Both amebiasis and giardiasis are commoner in male homosexuals. Infestation with round worms and tapeworms may interfere with nutrition and can even lead to intestinal obstruction, but often there are no symptoms.

Acute appendicitis is a common and life-threatening disease. Obstruction of the appendiceal lumen by hyperplasia of submucosal lymphoid follicles or by a mass of inspissated feces (fecalith) results in distention of the lumen with mucus, lymphedema, bacterial proliferation and invasion, circulatory impairment due to passive congestion, and eventually gangrene and rupture. Progress is rapid and without prompt surgical intervention the outcome is often fatal. The gross appearance of an acutely inflamed appendix depends on the speed with which the diagnosis has been made. Early in the course of the disease, the appendix appears normal. Later, distention, edema, congestion, subserosal hemorrhage, and fibrinous exudation are evident on external inspection, and the lumen may show a purulent exudate and mucosal ulceration. Still later, a deeply discolored or black zone of gangrene, or frank perforation, may be seen. Microscopic examination shows inflammation and ulceration of the mucosa and submucosa, with a neutrophilic infiltrate and purulent exudate. Lymphoid hyperplasia with microabscess formation in lymphoid follicles is often seen.

The term **inflammatory bowel disease** refers to two similar but apparently unrelated chronic and usually progressive disorders of the intestine, which are of unknown cause and which can have widespread systemic effects. **Crohn's disease** (regional enteritis, regional ileitis) can affect any part of the small or large intestine but shows a predilection for the ileocecal area. Segmental distribution (disease in several areas with "skip areas" of normal bowel in between) is common. Inflammation involves all layers of the bowel wall and often extends to adjacent mesentery and lymph nodes. Gross examination shows thickening of the bowel wall due to edema and fibrosis. The mucosa has a cobblestone appearance due to the presence of small submucosal nodules, and may show deep, punched-out, longitudinally disposed ulcers with normal mucosa surrounding them. Microscopic examination discloses infiltrates of neutrophils, lymphocytes, plasma cells, and eosinophils. The most specific pathologic finding is the presence of noncaseating granulomas in the lamina propria. Clinically the disease is manifested by abdominal pain, weight loss, and diarrhea. Stenosis of the bowel and formation of abscesses and fistulas, particularly anal, are common complications.

The inflammatory changes in **ulcerative colitis** are limited to the colon and specifically to the colonic mucosa. The rectum is nearly always involved, and skip areas of normal bowel between zones of inflammation are not found. Fistulas and obstruction do not occur. The affected mucosa is edematous, granular, and friable. Ulcers are shallow and irregular, and surrounded by mucosa that shows pathologic changes. Proliferation of epithelium between ulcers may lead to the formation of pseudopolyps. The most distinctive lesion on histologic examination is the crypt abscess, an intense local inflammatory reaction within a crypt of Lieberkühn, with an infiltrate of polymorphonuclear and mononuclear cells and an accumulation of exudate within the crypt. The usual presenting symptom of ulcerative colitis is bloody diarrhea. The disease is associated with an increased risk of colonic cancer.

Proctitis (inflammation of the rectum) may be the principal or sole manifestation of ulcerative colitis. Proctitis due to *Neisseria gonorrhoeae* occurs in male homosexuals. Anal fissure is an ulcer of the anal canal. Acute fissure, usually due to trauma, is superficial and heals rapidly. Chronic fissure extends deeper and is accompanied by signs of chronic inflammation.

Degenerative Disorders

The musculature of the tongue is a common site of amyloid deposition in primary amyloidosis; this may result in enlargement and stiffening of the tongue. In the form of scleroderma called CREST syndrome (calcinosis cutis, Raynaud's phenomenon, esophageal dysfunction, sclerodactyly, telangiectasia), esophageal dysfunction results from atrophy of the muscularis and fibrosis of the submucosa. Achalasia of the esophagus (inability of the smooth muscle layer to relax) is due to degeneration or absence of nerve cells of Auerbach's plexus, and leads to dilatation of the esophagus and severe difficulty in swallowing. Bleeding from one or more longitudinal lacerations at or above the gastroesophageal junction induced by vomiting is called Mallory-Weiss syndrome. Esophageal varices are lower esophageal veins that have dilated as a consequence of portal cirrhosis or thrombosis of the portal vein. Rupture of esophageal varices generally leads to massive hemorrhage.

Occlusion of a mesenteric artery or vein as a result of thrombosis, embolism, or vascular disease produces infarction of the bowel, often extensive. Hemorrhagic necrosis occurs early, and the situation is complicated by bacterial invasion and adynamic ileus. With or without perforation, peritonitis quickly ensues.

Melanosis coli, an irregular pigmentation of the colonic mucosa that can be detected endoscopically, occurs in persons who regularly use anthracene laxatives such as cascara and senna. It is benign and reversible.

Hemorrhoids are dilated anal veins, whose pathogenesis continues to elude explanation. Hemorrhoidal disease is common and seldom serious, though chronic bleeding from hemorrhoids can lead to severe anemia. Hemorrhoids may be internal (developing above the pectinate line and hence covered by mucosa) or external (developing below the pectinate line and covered by skin). In a thrombosed hemorrhoid, blood within the dilated vessel clots and there is local inflammation. Healing is by organization of the thrombus with fibrotic obliteration of the hemorrhoid.

Neoplasms

Benign and malignant tumors can arise from any of the cell types found in the gastrointestinal tract. Most malignancies of the lips, tongue, gums, buccal mucosa, pharynx, tonsils, esophagus, and anus are **squamous cell carcinomas**. About half of all malignancies of the oral cavity are squamous cell carcinomas arising on the tongue. The behavior of these squamous cell carcinomas depends on their location and their degree of anaplasia and invasive potential. Typically the lesion begins as a hyperkeratotic plaque, which evolves into an ulcer with heaped-up margins due to neoplastic invasion of the submucosa. Metastasis to regional lymph nodes and extension to adjacent structures occur early. The use of tobacco, including smokeless tobacco, heightens the risk of squamous cell carcinoma of the lip, oral and pharyngeal structures, and esophagus.

Leukoplakia is a focal hyperplasia of the oral mucosa, similar microscopically to actinic keratosis of the skin and, like it, regarded as a premalignant lesion. Grossly the lesion is a plaque of whitened, thickened, fissured mucosa. There may be several adjacent or coalescent plaques, and ulceration may occur. Microscopically leukoplakia displays hyperkeratosis, acanthosis, epidermal anaplasia, and mild inflammatory reaction in the dermis.

Most malignant tumors of the stomach and intestine arise from secretory epithelium and are therefore classed as adenocarcinomas. Over half of all carcinomas of the stomach begin in the pylorus. **Gastric carcinoma** usually presents as an ulcerative lesion, which may be mistaken for a peptic ulcer. Distinctive features of malignant gastric ulcer are its appearance in the midst of an elevated plaque (niche en plateau), its irregular, often scalloped shape, and its elevated margins. Invasion as far as the serosa is common. Less often, gastric carcinoma presents as a fungating, cauliflower-like polyp extending into the gastric lumen, and still less often as a diffuse thickening of the gastric wall with loss of rugae and shallow mucosal erosions rather than deep ulceration. When invasion of the wall is extensive, this type of carcinoma is called linitis plastica ("leather bottle stomach"). Metastasis from gastric carcinoma commonly occurs to regional lymph nodes, the peritoneum, and the liver.

The great majority of intestinal malignancies are **adenocarcinomas** arising in the **colon**, particularly the distal colon and rectum. Typically the tumor begins as a raised zone of mucosa, which eventually ulcerates. Meanwhile, malignant cells invade the submucosa, advancing peripherally with a tendency to encircle the bowel and to involve all layers of the bowel wall. Localized constriction of the colon by encircling tumor is called a napkin-ring lesion. Microscopically, colonic adenocarcinoma often displays irregular glandlike formations of mucus-secreting cells. Metastases are to regional lymph nodes and liver. Invasion of adjacent tissue commonly occurs early. Hemorrhage, perforation, obstruction, and formation of gastrocolic, rectovaginal, and rectovesical fistulas are the principal complications.

Although adenocarcinomas occur in the salivary glands, most salivary gland neoplasms are mixed tumors consisting of irregular aggregations of highly pleomorphic secretory epithelium along with myoepithelial cells and stromal proliferation. Vacuolation and myxomatous or hyaline degeneration occur frequently, as well as formation of pseudocartilage. Though this is ordinarily a benign tumor, malignant change sometimes occurs. It is considered to be derived from embryonal cells.

A significant minority of gastric and intestinal malignancies are **lymphosarcomas**, arising from lymphoid tissue in the submucosa, including Peyer's patches in the ileum. Diffuse infiltration and ulceration are typical. **Carcinoid tumor** (argentaffinoma) arises from the argentaffin cells of Kultschitzky. More than half develop in the appendix, and carcinoid tumor is the most common neoplasm developing in the appendix. Grossly a carcinoid tumor appears as a firm, rubbery nodule with a pale yellow color. Microscopic examination shows irregular nests of argentaffin cells. Though histologically benign, carcinoid tumors often invade locally and metastasize to the liver. The chief importance of carcinoid tumors not arising in the appendix lies in their production of serotonin, which causes cardiovascular and respiratory symptoms, the so-called carcinoid syndrome. **Adenomatous polyps** of the colon are common and may be sessile or pedunculated. Most contain functioning mucinous acini. Some undergo malignant change, with ulceration, hemorrhage, and extension into the surrounding epithelium before deeper invasion.

The Teeth

The teeth are not often subjected to pathologic study because of their hardness. A tooth consists of a crown—the part extending above the gum—and a root, which is anchored in the bone of the jaw. Its outer layer or enamel is the hardest substance in the body. Beneath this lies a material called dentin, similar in composition but less brittle. Both dentin and enamel consist of a framework of organic fibers in which calcium salts have been deposited. Within the dentin layer is a hollow pulp chamber containing cells that form dentin and a rich blood and nerve supply that enters through the root canal.

Hypoplasia of the enamel may occur as a congenital defect or may result from a disturbance of calcium metabolism. A dentigerous cyst forms around the crown of an unerupted tooth as a result of aberrant enamel production. Caries is a breakdown of enamel and underlying dentin by enzymes produced in adherent mucinous films containing bacteria and called plaques. Infection of the pulp chamber, usually resulting from caries or injury to a tooth, is called pulpitis. Odontoma is a mixed tumor arising from undifferentiated tissue of a tooth bud, while ameloblastoma (adamantinoma) is derived from enamel-forming cells. Both occur primarily in children and adolescents and though benign may be locally destructive.

The Liver and Biliary Tract:
Gross and Microscopic Anatomy

The liver is the largest gland in the body. Like the pancreas, it has functions unconnected with its role as a source of digestive fluid. The liver is a large, lobed structure of a dark reddish-brown color lying in the right upper quadrant of the abdomen. Its average weight in the adult is about 1400 g. It is partly covered by serosa. Beneath this it is entirely surrounded by a delicate connective tissue envelope, the capsule of Glisson. At the hilum or porta, four tubes—the hepatic artery, the hepatic vein, the portal vein, and the hepatic or bile duct— enter the liver.

The internal architecture of the liver is distinctive and complex. A fine connective tissue framework divides the glandular tissue into cylindrical lobules. Each lobule consists of plates or cords of polygonal liver cells or hepatocytes radiating from a central vein. Between these plates are open spaces lined with endothelium, also radially disposed, called sinusoids, through which blood filters toward the central vein. Scattered about the walls of the sinusoids are star-shaped macrophages called Kupffer cells. In the interstitial connective tissue between lobules, and typically grouped together, are branches of the hepatic artery, the portal vein, and the hepatic duct—the so-called portal triad. The tissue space through which such a triad courses is called a portal canal.

Blood enters the liver through two different systems of vessels. The hepatic artery delivers freshly oxygenated blood, while the portal vein carries absorbed nutrients and other materials from the digestive tract. Blood from both sources trickles through the sinusoids and leaves by the central veins, which join to form the hepatic vein. During the passage of the blood through the sinusoids, the liver cells pick up nutrients for processing or storage, release other nutrients and hormones into the circulation, and discharge wastes for disposal by the lungs or the kidneys. At the same time, bile formed in the liver cells is collected by an extremely delicate system of channels or canaliculi, which conduct it to branches of the hepatic duct. These branches coalesce to form right and left hepatic ducts, which carry the bile out of the liver.

The hepatic duct is lined with cuboidal epithelium and has connective tissue and smooth muscle layers. A special modification of the hepatic duct, the gallbladder, acts as a reservoir for bile and also serves to concentrate bile by reabsorbing water and electrolytes from it. The normal gallbladder measures about 2.5 × 10 cm and has a capacity of about 35 mL. The gallbladder has a lining of columnar epithelium, a well-defined muscularis, and a serosa. Its epithelium is thrown into villi, which lend it a velvety appearance and feel.

Pathologic Study of the Liver and Biliary Tract

Liver tissue may be obtained for study by needle biopsy or open biopsy. At autopsy the liver is dissected free from its attachments, note being taken of any adhesions to adjacent structures. The organ is weighed and observed for abnormalities of shape, color, texture, or other surface features. It is cut into thin slices and the color, consistency, and tissue pattern of the cut surfaces are examined. Specimens are taken for histologic study.

The gallbladder most often comes to the attention of the pathologist as a surgical specimen after cholecystectomy, with or without stones. At autopsy the gallbladder and biliary tract are inspected, palpated, and opened.

Diseases of the Liver

The highly versatile secretory epithelial cells of the liver are also highly sensitive to damage by metabolic, toxic, infectious, or circulatory insult. On the other hand, they have remarkable regenerative powers. Cloudy swelling, resulting from febrile illness, toxemia, or other systemic causes, is manifested by enlargement of the liver, with stretching of its capsule. The texture is softer than normal and the cut surface appears pale and more opaque. On microscopic examination the cells appear swollen, with pale cytoplasm. In secondary amyloidosis the liver is a principal site of amyloid deposition. The amyloid liver is enlarged, firm, and pale in color. Compression of liver cells by amyloid deposits results in atrophy and necrosis.

Fatty change in the liver accompanies both obesity and malnutrition and is also found in chronic alcoholism, diabetes, chemical poisoning, Reye's syndrome, and other metabolic disorders. Deposition of fat may be confined to hepatic cells or may also appear in the stroma. The fatty liver is enlarged and tense, its cut surface pale, greasy, and bulging. Deposits of hemosiderin in hepatic cells and Kupffer cells appear in hemolytic disease and in hemochromatosis. Extensive deposits may impart a grayish-brown color to the liver. When the glycogen content of the liver cells is increased, as in diabetes and glycogen storage diseases, the glycogen may appear in hepatic cell nuclei, causing enlargement, vacuolation, and margination of chromatin.

Causes of hepatitis (inflammation of the liver) include viral and bacterial infection and parasitic infestation. Viral hepatitis is classified on the basis of the causative virus. **Hepatitis A** (infectious hepatitis), an acute, self-limited infection, generally causes mild symptoms. The virus is transmitted chiefly by the fecal-oral route. **Hepatitis B** (serum hepatitis), a more severe infection which, in some cases, becomes chronic, is transmitted chiefly via the blood stream and also by sexual contact. After recovery some patients become carriers. **Hepatitis C**, the major cause of post-transfusion hepatitis, typically causes mild clinical illness but becomes chronic in at least half of all cases. **Hepatitis D** occurs only in persons previously infected with hepatitis B, although it is due to a distinct virus. **Hepatitis E**, which occurs chiefly in the tropics, resembles hepatitis A in that it is transmitted by the fecal-oral route and does not become chronic or lead to a carrier state, but has a much higher mortality.

The liver in acute hepatitis is soft, dark, and congested. On histologic examination, cellular edema, ballooning degeneration, and necrosis of liver cells are evident, with infiltrates of inflammatory cells at the periphery of the lobules. Hepatitis lasting more than one year is designated chronic. In **chronic active hepatitis**, an autoimmune complication of viral infection, inflammation remains intense and spreads to periportal areas, with plasma cell infiltrates. The prognosis is poor. Cirrhosis eventually ensues, with progressive liver failure and an increased risk of hepatocellular carcinoma. **Chronic persistent hepatitis** is a milder process, without extension to periportal areas or serious sequelae.

Hepatic abscess can follow inoculation of liver tissue with pyogenic organisms from the systemic circulation, the portal circulation, the biliary tract, or adjacent structures. Amebic abscess occurs as a complication of colonic amebiasis. Liver flukes are trematode worms of the genera *Clonorchis, Fasciola,* and others that pass part of their life cycle in the liver. They may cause extensive inflammation, fibrosis, and biliary obstruction. Hydatid disease of the liver is caused by the formation of one or more larval cysts by tapeworms of the genus *Echinococcus*. These may expand enormously and cause symptoms by compressing or displacing tissue.

Alcoholic hepatitis is an acute inflammatory process due to ethanol intoxication. Besides fatty change, polymorphonuclear infiltrates, and degeneration and necrosis of liver cells, this condition causes the formation of a characteristic irregular eosinophilic hyaline inclusion body (alcoholic hyalin) in hepatocytes.

The term **cirrhosis** refers to a group of chronic, progressive inflammatory disorders in which destruction of liver cells is followed by nodular regeneration and fibrotic proliferation of the stroma, with loss of normal microscopic architecture. Portal cirrhosis (Laënnec's cirrhosis, nutritional cirrhosis, micronodular cirrhosis), the most common type, is usually due to chronic alcoholism. Early in its course the liver cells show fatty change and degeneration, with hyaline cytoplasmic material (Mallory bodies), and inflammatory infiltrates are present. Nodular regeneration of hepatic cells produces a hobnailed appearance of the liver surface. Along with fibrous proliferation in periportal areas, this nodular regeneration is responsible for distortion of normal cellular organization and for obliteration of portal venous channels. This leads to portal hypertension, splenomegaly, ascites, and formation of collateral venous channels, including esophageal varices. Late in the course of cirrhosis, the liver becomes shrunken and hard, and hepatic cellular function is severely impaired. Cirrhosis also occurs in hemochromatosis and Wilson's disease, after prolonged obstruction of the bile ducts (biliary cirrhosis, which has an autoimmune component), in chronic congestive heart failure (cardiac cirrhosis), after acute viral hepatitis or exposure to hepatotoxic chemicals (postnecrotic cirrhosis), and in chronic active hepatitis.

Necrosis of liver cells is classified according to its distribution as focal, zonal, and diffuse. **Focal necrosis,** caused by various toxemias, consists of randomly distributed patches of degenerating and necrotic cells with inflammatory cell infiltrates. Zonal necrosis is subdivided into central, midzonal, and peripheral, depending on the portions of the lobules in which degeneration and atrophy of cells are most pronounced. **Central** (centrilobular) **necrosis,** the commonest type, results from ischemia, drugs, and chemical poisons, particularly halogenated hydrocarbons (chloroform, carbon tetrachloride). **Midzonal necrosis** is typical of yellow fever and **peripheral necrosis** is seen in phosphorus poisoning and toxemia of pregnancy. **Diffuse necrosis,** sometimes called acute yellow atrophy, is a widespread, catastrophic destruction of liver cells precipitated by severe poisoning, toxemia, or infection with hepatitis B virus (less often, hepatitis A).

Chronic passive congestion of the liver regularly accompanies chronic right ventricular failure. The liver is enlarged, soft, and deep purple. Its cut surface bulges and exudes dark blood, and in well-established chronic passive congestion it displays a characteristic nutmeg pattern due to centrilobular congestion and fatty infiltration of the peripheral lobular parenchyma. Microscopic examination shows engorgement of sinusoids, atrophy and centrilobular necrosis of hepatic cells, deposits of hemosiderin in Kupffer cells, and periportal fibrosis. Primary adenocarcinoma of the liver is an uncommon neoplasm in the United States. Hepatic cirrhosis is a predisposing factor. Most hepatic carcinomas arise from hepatic cells (hepatocarcinoma) and contain abortive hepatic lobules. Less commonly, carcinoma develops from bile duct cells (cholangiocarcinoma). With its dual blood supply the liver is particularly subject to metastatic invasion by tumor cells. Hepatic metastases occur in about one-third of all cancers and are especially likely in cancer of the stomach, intestine, genitourinary organs, and breast. Metastatic nodules in the liver are distinguished from primary tumors by their irregular shape, their tendency to be multiple, and often by umbilication due to central necrosis.

Diseases of the Gallbladder

Cholecystitis (inflammation of the gallbladder) may be acute or chronic. Acute inflammation without prior gallbladder disease begins at the mucosa and travels outward, causing mucosal destruction, interstitial edema, submucosal hemorrhage, and formation of a purulent exudate in the lumen. In chronic cholecystitis the wall of the gallbladder is thickened by fibrosis. On microscopic examination, outpouchings of the mucosa, the sinuses of Rokitansky-Aschoff, are seen extending along blood vessels into the muscularis. Chronic cholecystitis is usually associated with cholelithiasis (formation of gallstones), either as cause or effect. Gallstones contain varying proportions of bilirubin, cholesterol, and calcium carbonate depending on whether they form as a result of changes in the composition of bile, bile stasis, or chronic inflammation of the gallbladder or bile ducts. Gallstones frequently obstruct the biliary tract. When the level of cholesterol in bile is elevated, deposits of this material in the gallbladder mucosa (cholesterolosis) cause grossly visible yellow streaking, the so-called strawberry gallbladder. Most malignancies of the gallbladder arise from columnar duct epithelium. More than 90% occur in gallbladders containing stones.

The Pancreas: Gross and Microscopic Anatomy

The pancreas is a flat, tongue-shaped, fleshy organ lying against the posterior abdominal wall in the left upper quadrant, between the duodenum and the spleen. It is 12–15 cm in length, 5–6 cm in greatest width, and weighs 45–90 g. It is a ruddy buff in color and its lobular structure is grossly apparent. Its secretion passes into the duodenum by the duct of Wirsung. The pancreas lies outside the peritoneal cavity and has neither a distinctive capsule nor a serosa. Its alveoli (acini) are all serous and their secretion contains enzymes for the digestion of carbohydrates, fats, and proteins. In addition, the pancreas contains spherical masses of specialized endocrine cells, the islets of Langerhans, some of which are large enough to be grossly visible. The islets of Langerhans produce the hormones glucagon and insulin, essential for carbohydrate metabolism. These are taken up by the blood and do not enter the duct system of the pancreas. Glucagon is produced by A or alpha cells, which have acidophilic granules, and insulin is produced by B or beta cells, which have basophilic granules. The delta or D cells, which also have basophilic granules, produce somatostatin.

Pathologic Study of the Pancreas

Material from the pancreas can be obtained for pathologic study by fine-needle percutaneous aspiration or open biopsy. Part or all of the pancreas may be excised for malignant or other diseases. At autopsy the pancreas is exposed, dissected free from the posterior body wall, and opened for examination of its internal structure and duct system.

Diseases of the Pancreas

Acute interstitial pancreatitis is an occasional feature of mumps. **Acute hemorrhagic pancreatitis**, a severe and often fatal disease, results from widespread release of pancreatic digestive enzymes into the substance of the gland as a consequence of chronic alcoholism, biliary tract disease, or abdominal trauma. The pancreas is enlarged, generally firm but sometimes with mushy areas of necrosis, and hemorrhagic or frankly gangrenous in gross appearance. Microscopic examination shows extensive necrosis of secretory epithelium with loss of acinar organization, interstitial hemorrhage, and variable amounts of fat necrosis. A pseudocyst filled with fluid and necrotic debris may form between the pancreas and adjacent structures. **Chronic pancreatitis**, a smoldering process apparently due to chronic or recurrent obstruction of the pancreatic duct, leads to extensive replacement of acini with fibrous overgrowth of stroma and consequent failure of glandular function. Calcification often occurs.

Pancreatic carcinoma forms a hard, sometimes multinodular mass which on microscopic examination is seen to be composed of ductal (less often acinar) cells in irregular ductal (or glandlike) formations. Two-thirds of carcinomas arise in the head of the gland (the right half), where they often obstruct the biliary tract because the pancreatic and hepatic ducts enter the duodenum together. The prognosis is poor in pancreatic carcinoma. **Insulinoma**, a benign tumor of beta cells, produces excessive insulin, which may cause severe, even fatal depression of blood sugar. **Gastrinoma**, arising from non-beta cells of the islets of Langerhans, produces gastrin (normally secreted only by the stomach) and is associated with multiple peptic ulceration (Zollinger-Ellison syndrome).

In **cystic fibrosis** (mucoviscidosis), congenital inability of pancreatic acini to secrete chloride leads to production of abnormally thick mucus, which plugs acinar ducts and eventually leads to atrophy of secretory epithelium and extensive fibrosis of the gland.

Diabetes mellitus is a congenital or acquired disorder in which insulin production by the beta cells of the islets of Langerhans is inadequate for normal needs. Insulin is necessary for the transport of glucose, fatty acids, and amino acids into cells and the incorporation of these materials into metabolic processes. In type I diabetes mellitus (insulin-dependent diabetes mellitus, IDDM), the deficiency of insulin is life-threatening and must be made up by administration of insulin by injection. This form of diabetes mellitus typically begins early in life and is associated with more severe symptoms and complications. Histologic study of the pancreas shows hyalinization and fibrosis of the islets of Langerhans. Persons with type II diabetes mellitus (non-insulin-dependent diabetes mellitus, NIDDM) have less severe disease and can be successfully treated without administration of insulin. Gestational diabetes occurs during pregnancy and usually disappears afterwards. Hemochromatosis may lead to impairment of insulin secretion (bronze diabetes), and so may chronic pancreatitis. Total pancreatectomy induces an insulin-dependent diabetes mellitus.

In all forms of diabetes mellitus, abnormality of glucose metabolism gradually leads to degenerative and obstructive disease of small blood vessels (microangiopathy), with widespread organ and tissue damage. Aberrant metabolism of fats in untreated or undertreated insulin-dependent diabetes mellitus causes the appearance of ketone bodies in the circulation and associated biochemical imbalances (ketoacidosis), which may culminate in coma (diabetic coma), shock, and death.

The Abdominal Wall and Peritoneum

An abnormal bulging of the contents of a structure through a weakness or defect in its wall is called a **hernia**. Most hernias of medical importance are due to weakness in some part of the myofascial envelope containing the abdominal and pelvic organs. Most hernias are traceable to congenital defects, but symptoms may not appear until middle life or later.

Hiatal hernia is an upward shifting of the stomach through the esophageal hiatus of the diaphragm. Often it causes no difficulty but it may result in peptic esophagitis or peptic ulceration of the esophagus due to reflux of acid gastric juice. An **umbilical hernia** protrudes through the umbilicus. Hernias in the groin area may protrude at various anatomic sites. **Direct inguinal hernia** is a local weakening of the lower abdominal wall associated with aging. An **indirect inguinal hernia** passes down the inguinal canal toward or into the scrotum. **Femoral hernia** occurs through the femoral canal. Virtually all groin hernias contain loops of intestine. The chief complications are incarceration (inability to reduce the hernia, with ensuing obstruction) and strangulation (impairment of blood supply to the sequestered loop of bowel).

The relations of the abdominal and pelvic organs to the peritoneum are described in Chapter 8. **Acute peritonitis** usually follows inflammation or rupture of an abdominal or pelvic organ or a penetrating wound of the abdominal wall. Chemical irritation by leaking digestive fluids and blood is quickly complicated by bacterial infection. Intense inflammatory reaction with edema and exudation of fibrin-rich fluid may successfully limit the spread of infection (localized peritonitis). Localized accumulation of infected and necrotic material may constitute an abscess, particularly under the diaphragm (subphrenic abscess) or in the rectouterine pouch (pelvic abscess). Otherwise generalized peritonitis may follow, with paralytic ileus, toxemia, and shock. Healing of acute peritonitis may generate fibrotic adhesions. Primary neoplasms of the peritoneum are uncommon, but implantation of metastatic foci from abdominal malignancies may be extensive. The condition of pseudomyxoma peritonei results from widespread implantation of jelly-like material from a myxomatous tumor.

Review Questions

1. What three types of cells are found in the gastric mucosa?
2. Why is intestinal obstruction a life-threatening condition?
3. Distinguish *atrophic* from *hypertrophic gastritis*.
4. Where do most peptic ulcers occur?
5. State several points of difference between Crohn's disease and ulcerative colitis.
6. What is the commonest type of intestinal malignancy, and in what part of the intestine does it most often arise?
7. Mention some conditions associated with fatty change in the liver.
8. Distinguish *type I* from *type II diabetes mellitus*.
9. What are the principal types of groin hernia?
10. Define or explain: *crypts of Lieberkühn, diverticulum, fistula, portal triad, rugae, villi*.

22

The Excretory System

Gross and Microscopic Anatomy

The excretory system includes the kidneys, the ureters, the bladder, and the urethra. The function of this system is to regulate the composition of the blood by disposing of wastes and excessive amounts of water, electrolytes, and other substances. The **kidneys** lie in the upper abdomen behind the peritoneal cavity, protected by cushions of fatty tissue. They are a reddish tan to warm brown in color. Each is 10–12 cm in length and weighs about 150 g. Each has a pronounced hilum at which an artery, a vein, and a ureter are attached. The kidney is covered by a tough capsule of connective tissue. Beneath this capsule the surface of the kidney is smooth and deep red.

On section the kidney is seen to consist of two zones, a dark brown, granular cortex and a lighter, striated medulla, arranged concentrically around an inner cavity, the renal sinus. The cortex is not of uniform thickness. Wedges of cortical tissue, the columns of Bertin, extend down through the medulla to the margin of the renal sinus. The medulla is disposed in conical masses, the renal pyramids, whose apices, or papillae, protrude into the sinus. The sinus is thus scalloped in contour, and several recesses called minor and major calyces extend from it into the medulla. The funnel-shaped cavity between the calyces and the origin of the ureter is termed the renal pelvis.

The renal cortex contains many thousands of microscopic filtration units called malpighian corpuscles. The medulla is largely composed of a system of radially oriented ducts carrying urine toward the sinus. Each malpighian corpuscle consists of a tangle of capillaries called a glomerulus and a two-layered sheath of squamous epithelium called Bowman's capsule, which surrounds the glomerulus. Urine filtered from the capillaries composing the glomerulus enters Bowman's capsule and passes into a tortuous tubule whose chief divisions are called the proximal convoluted tubule, the loop of Henle, and the distal convoluted tubule. The proximal convoluted tubule is lined by low columnar cells having a brush border. In parts of Henle's loop the epithelium is of the squamous type. The cells of some parts of the duct system actively excrete materials into the urine or reabsorb materials from it. The term nephron refers to a functional unit of renal tissue: a glomerulus with its associated Bowman's capsule and tubule.

The vessels leading to and from the glomerulus are called, respectively, the afferent arteriole and the efferent arteriole. The side of the glomerulus on which these vessels enter is called its vascular pole, and the opposite side, where the renal tubule arises from Bowman's capsule, is the urinary pole. Between the afferent and efferent arterioles lies the polar cushion (Polkissen), an aggregation of specialized secretory cells which, along with similar cells in the vicinity, forms the juxtaglomerular apparatus. These structures produce renin, which is involved in the regulation of blood pressure.

The renal pelvis, ureters, and bladder are lined by a type of epithelium called transitional: it appears squamous when the organ is distended with urine, cuboidal at other times. The mucosa of the ureter and bladder is thrown into deep folds. The lamina propria contains many elastic fibers. In the muscularis, smooth muscle fibers are arranged in both longitudinal and circular layers. In microscopic features, the urethras of the two sexes do not differ greatly. The urethra is lined by stratified squamous epithelium except where it emerges from the bladder, where a transitional type is more usual. The branched tubular glands of Littré in the connective tissue below the lining epithelium produce mucus.

Pathologic Study of the Excretory System

Percutaneous needle biopsy of the kidney is a standard procedure. Biopsy specimens of the ureter, bladder, and urethra can be obtained through an endoscope. Centrifuged urine or washings of the bladder or renal sinus can be subjected to cytologic study. The entire kidney is submitted as a surgical specimen after nephrectomy. Other parts of the urinary tract excised in the course of surgery for trauma or malignant disease may become pathologic specimens. Stones removed from the kidney, ureter, or bladder are submitted for examination and chemical analysis. At autopsy the kidneys are removed and weighed, and their color, size, texture, and surface features are noted. The capsule of each kidney is incised along its greater curvature and peeled away from the cortex. Normally it strips with ease, although the stripping tears a delicate fibrovascular network between capsule and kidney. The kidney is next bisected in the frontal plane and the cortex, medulla, and sinus are inspected for abnormalities. The ureters and bladder are opened and examined for stones, obstruction, or signs of inflammation.

Developmental Disorders

Various developmental anomalies may affect the gross or microscopic structure of the kidney. Some of these are of little clinical importance, even when both kidneys are affected. Since one healthy kidney suffices for normal excretory needs, hypoplasia or even agenesis of the other is ordinarily of no medical consequence. Fusion of the kidneys across the midline by either renal tissue or a fibrous band is called **horseshoe kidney**. In 90% of cases of horseshoe kidney, the kidneys are fused at their lower poles. Reduplication of a ureter or even of a kidney is not uncommon. These anomalies may cause disturbances in urine drainage. **Polycystic kidney** refers to a hereditary malformation in which much of the renal tissue is replaced by grapelike clusters of cysts containing clear or hemorrhagic fluid. Renal function is severely impaired. Infantile and adult forms are recognized, the former often being accompanied by congenital anomalies of other organs, the latter arising in middle life. In **medullary sponge kidney**, also hereditary, there is grossly evident cystic dilatation of collecting tubules in the renal medulla. Histologic examination shows the cysts to be lined by flattened cuboidal epithelium. Calculi may form in some cysts. Often there is little or no impairment of renal function. **Exstrophy of the bladder** is a congenital deformity resulting from failure of fusion of pelvic structures in the anterior midline, so that the bladder opens on the surface of the lower abdomen.

Glomerular vs. Tubular Disease

The type and degree of impairment of excretory function caused by kidney disease depend on the part or parts of the kidney that are involved. The glomerulus and Bowman's capsule act as a filter, allowing passage of water, electrolytes, urea, glucose, and other substances of low molecular weight, but normally holding back plasma proteins. In glomerular disease, these proteins, chiefly albumin, may be irrecoverably lost from the plasma into the urine. The resulting decline in serum albumin leads to osmotic edema, which may be severe and may be accompanied by a rise in plasma lipids (nephrotic syndrome).

The renal tubules actively reabsorb certain substances (water, glucose, chloride) from the glomerular filtrate and actively secrete others (urea, creatinine, potassium). When tubular function is impaired, the kidney loses its ability to conserve water and to excrete potassium, phosphorus, and nitrogenous wastes such as urea and creatinine. Retention of potassium may interfere with the function of skeletal and cardiac muscle fibers. Retention of phosphorus leads to calcium depletion and with it a state of heightened neuromuscular excitability called tetany. Retention of hydrogen ions leads to metabolic acidosis. **Uremia** (azotemia) refers to increased levels of urea, creatinine, and other nitrogen-containing waste products of protein metabolism. Persons with severe uremia may have cerebral edema, seizures, pericardial effusion, pulmonary edema, anemia, and increased susceptibility to infection. Since both glomeruli and tubules are likely to be injured in many forms of severe renal disease, uremic and nephrotic types of excretory failure often occur together.

Several hereditary and acquired biochemical disorders affect the function of the renal tubules without causing gross or microscopic lesions, although they may occur in association with polycystic kidneys and other anomalies. **Renal tubular acidosis** occurs in both infantile and adult forms. Progressive uremia and inability to conserve water may lead to death, or spontaneous recovery may occur. In **renal osteodystrophy** (renal rickets, renal dwarfism), which usually occurs in childhood, the inability of the kidney to conserve calcium leads to osteomalacia, dwarfism, and skeletal deformities. The essence of the **Fanconi syndrome** is a failure of renal tubules to absorb amino acids, glucose, and phosphorus from glomerular filtrate. As in renal rickets, osteomalacia and skeletal malformations may result.

Inflammatory and Degenerative Diseases of the Kidney

Acute glomerulonephritis is a generalized inflammation of glomeruli induced by antibody formed in response to infection (usually pharyngeal) with nephritogenic strains of betahemolytic streptococci or, less often, occurring as an autoimmune disorder. Clinically it is characterized by edema, hypertension, bloody urine, and acute renal failure. The kidneys are enlarged, with tense capsules. The outer surfaces may show punctate hemorrhages. The cut surface bulges, and the cortex appears pale and cloudy while the medulla is dull red and engorged. Microscopic examination shows enlargement of many or most glomerular tufts with endothelial proliferation, infiltrates of inflammatory cells, thrombi in some capillaries, and fatty or hyaline degeneration of renal tubules.

Chronic glomerulonephritis may develop as a consequence of acute glomerulonephritis or may occur as a distinct disease, perhaps related to systemic disease. Chronic glomerulonephritis usually leads to progressive deterioration of renal function. The kidneys are shrunken and coarsely granular in texture, their capsules firmly adherent. The cortices are thinned and the demarcation between cortex and medulla is obscured. There is a reduction of renal parenchyma and often cystic dilatation of renal tubules. Microscopic examination shows eosinophilic deposits in glomerular capillary basement membranes (membranous glomerulonephritis), mesangial cell proliferation (proliferative glomerulonephritis), or both (membranoproliferative glomerulonephritis). Many glomeruli are wholly replaced by hyaline material. Atrophy of tubular cells, increased interstitial connective tissue, and intimal and medial proliferation of arterioles are also seen.

Patchy or diffuse chronic glomerulonephritis occurs in 75% of cases of systemic lupus erythematosus (**lupus nephritis**). Endothelial proliferation of glomerular capillaries occurs, along with hyaline thickening of basement membranes, yielding a wire-loop appearance. In **Goodpasture's syndrome**, an autoimmune disorder, circulating antibodies bind with the glomerular basement membrane, producing hyaline change and leading to progressive renal failure. Pulmonary lesions also occur.

Interstitial nephritis is a general term for any inflammatory or degenerative process of the kidney manifested by interstitial infiltrates of inflammatory cells. It may be due to septicemia, heavy metal intoxication, gout, or any parenchymal disease capable of eliciting an inflammatory response. In the acute stage, the kidney is enlarged and pale, with a thickened cortex. Infiltrates of neutrophils, lymphocytes, plasma cells, and eosinophils are seen focally or diffusely among glomeruli and tubules. Glomerular changes are generally absent but some tubular degeneration usually occurs, with impairment of renal function. The process may become chronic, in which case atrophy of functioning tissue and its replacement by fibrosis are accompanied by progressive decline in renal function.

Pyelonephritis is a suppurative infection of renal parenchyma also involving the renal pelvis and usually the ureter. Staphylococci and gram-negative colon bacilli are the usual causative organisms. Pyelonephritis may arise from infection, with or without obstruction, in the lower urinary tract (ascending pyelonephritis), or it may begin in the cortex of the kidney as a blood-borne infection (hematogenous or descending pyelonephritis). In the acute stage the kidney is enlarged, soft, and congested, with venous stasis and focal hemorrhages. Leukocytic infiltrates are seen in the cortex and the pelvis, and abscesses of renal tissue may be grossly or at least microscopically evident. In the chronic stage the kidney becomes firm and contracted, with an adherent capsule. The cortex is granular, with scattered foci of suppuration and necrosis. The tubules atrophy and glomeruli are replaced by fibrosis. Lymphocytic infiltrates are widespread.

Papillary necrosis (necrotizing papillitis) is a severe complication of pyelonephritis occurring most often in diabetics and others with vascular disease. Its incidence is also increased in persons with sickle cell anemia and after excessive use of phenacetin. The renal papillae become infarcted and necrotic, and their apices may slough into the renal pelvis. The papillae appear red or yellow and are covered by a grayish purulent exudate. A line of demarcation between healthy tissue and the necrotic apex of the papilla is grossly evident, and on microscopic study is found to consist of an intense neutrophilic infiltrate with many bacteria visible in tissue.

Renal amyloidosis affects the glomeruli predominantly and may be of sufficient extent to impair renal function. Amyloid material is deposited between the basement membrane and endothelial lining of glomerular capillaries.

Degenerative disorders of the renal tubules in which the glomeruli are spared are known generically as nephroses. Acute septicemia, toxemia, inflammatory bowel disease, and other acute and chronic disorders may cause cloudy swelling, hyaline or fatty degeneration, or necrosis of tubular epithelium. In Armanni-Ebstein disease (glycogen nephrosis), a complication of diabetes mellitus, there is glycogen vacuolation within the proximal convoluted tubules and loops of Henle.

Tubular damage may be caused by toxic substances contained in glomerular filtrate: bilirubin in jaundice, hemoglobin in transfusion reactions, myoglobin in crushing injury, uric acid in gout, and mercury and other heavy metals in acute poisoning. In **acute tubular necrosis** (lower nephron nephrosis), which occurs as a result of shock (shock kidney), crushing injury (crush kidney), transfusion reaction, or severe ischemia of the kidney, there is generalized tubular damage with almost complete suspension of excretory function (renal shutdown, acute renal failure). The kidneys are edematous, with pale cortices and dusky medullae. Renal tubular epithelium shows albuminoid, hyaline, or lipid degenerative changes and areas of frank necrosis. Tubular lumens contain pigmented casts and interstitial tissues show edema and inflammatory cell infiltrates. Regeneration occurs from the basement membranes of proximal convoluted tubules.

The kidney is subject to a number of circulatory disorders. These are medically important not only because they may diminish the excretory capacities of the kidney but also because an ischemic kidney produces excessive renin. This enzyme catalyzes the formation of angiotensin, a potent vasopressor responsible for renal hypertension, the most common form of secondary hypertension. Renal parenchymal disease, including pyelonephritis, and obstructive uropathy also occasionally lead to renal hypertension.

Arteriolar nephrosclerosis is a degenerative disease of small arteries and arterioles in the kidney, associated with hypertension. The glomeruli show thickening, hyaline change, and atrophy, and the tubules also undergo degeneration and necrosis. Hypertension may initially be responsible for the vascular changes but the ensuing renal ischemia leads to further elevation of blood pressure and further vascular damage. In malignant hypertension, a rapidly progressive condition, there is a necrotizing arteriolitis in the kidneys and other organs. **Kimmelstiel-Wilson disease** (glomerulosclerosis, diabetic nephropathy) occurs in 25% of persons with insulin-dependent diabetes mellitus. The distinctive lesions of this disorder are rounded nodular hyaline masses at the periphery of glomerular tufts, which arise from capillary basement membranes.

Bilateral cortical necrosis is a coagulative infarction of the kidneys due to shock, renal ischemia, septicemia, or toxemia, in which changes are most striking in renal cortices. The kidneys are swollen and soft, and their surfaces are mottled red and yellow. The cut surface bulges and the cortices show irregular yellowish opaque infarcts bordered by hemorrhagic zones. On microscopic examination, glomeruli, tubules, and interstitial tissue are all seen to be affected by hemorrhagic necrosis in affected areas.

Deleterious consequences of blockage to the flow of urine are known collectively as **obstructive uropathy**. Obstruction can occur at any point between the renal pelvis and the distal urethra. External compression of the urinary tract by a tumor or pregnant uterus, inflammation or scarring within the tract, congenital anomalies, and urinary calculi are the most frequent causes of obstruction, which may be partial or complete, intermittent or constant. Damming of urine causes dilatation of the renal pelvis and calyces (hydronephrosis) and, when the obstruction is below the renal pelvis, dilatation of the ureter (hydroureter). Obstruction at or below the level of the bladder affects both ureters and both kidneys. Hydronephrosis rapidly arrests kidney function as the pressure within the urinary tract approaches glomerular filtration pressure. After prolonged hydronephrosis the renal pelvis becomes greatly enlarged while the renal parenchyma undergoes atrophy and fibrosis, being reduced to a thin shell of nonfunctioning tissue. Stagnation of urine above an obstruction is typically followed by infection (pyelonephritis, cystitis).

The formation of calculi within the urinary tract (**urolithiasis**) results from either local disease or alteration in the composition of the urine. A zone of inflammation or necrosis in some part of the renal sinus, most often near the apex of a papilla, can become the site of a superficial deposit of calcium. This in turn can serve as a nidus of stone formation as successive layers of material are added by crystallization of urinary solutes. Probably some such mechanism is involved even when stone formation results from an abnormally high concentration of a solute such as uric acid (in gout), magnesium ammonium phosphate (in chronic urinary tract infection due to organisms that break down urea to ammonia, particularly *Proteus*), or calcium (in hypercalcemia due to renal tubular acidosis, sarcoidosis or parathyroid disease). Two-thirds of renal calculi are composed of calcium oxalate. Cystine stones form in persons with cystinuria, a hereditary disorder of renal tubular absorption of the amino acid cystine.

Upon attaining a certain size a renal calculus ordinarily breaks loose and passes into the ureter, where it may cause pain (ureteral colic) and obstruction. Very small stones (gravel) may be passed painlessly. A stone that remains attached to the kidney tissue until it is too large to enter the ureter may take the shape of the renal calyx in which it has formed (staghorn calculus).

Neoplasms of the Kidney

By far the commonest renal malignancy is **hypernephroma** (renal cell carcinoma), a disease of middle age. This tumor usually occurs near the upper pole of the kidney. It is of an intense yellow color and grows rapidly, with a tendency to necrosis, hemorrhage, and cyst formation. Although sharply defined and even apparently encapsulated, it invades aggressively and metastasizes by the blood to bone, lungs, and liver. Histologic sections show renal tubular cells in various configurations—cords, sheets, and even glandlike structures. A renal cell carcinoma may produce erythropoietin and thus stimulate excessive red blood cell production (polycythemia). **Wilms tumor** (nephroblastoma) occurs in late fetal life or early infancy. It develops from undifferentiated mesodermal cells which form rosettes or abortive renal tubules. Growth is rapid and hematogenous spread occurs to the lungs and brain.

Diseases of the Bladder

Cystitis (inflammation of the bladder) usually occurs as an acute infection due to colon bacilli or, less often, gram-positive cocci. The incidence of cystitis is much higher in women, in whom it usually arises from urethral or genital infections, often as a result of sexual trauma. Cystitis may occur in either sex as a consequence of urethral obstruction or foreign bodies inserted into the bladder. In acute cystitis the bladder is hyperemic and edematous. There may be one or more shallow ulcers representing zones of epithelial necrosis and sloughing. A fibrinous or purulent membrane may cling to the surface, and extensive ulceration may lead to marked bleeding into the urine (hemorrhagic cystitis). Ascending pyelonephritis can complicate untreated cystitis. Interstitial cystitis is a more chronic process affecting chiefly postmenopausal women. The bladder wall is thickened and the submucosa shows lymphocytic infiltration and fibrosis. A chronic mucosal ulcer (Hunner's ulcer) may be found in conjunction with this disorder.

Hypertrophy of the bladder usually results from chronic partial obstruction to the outflow of urine by prostatic enlargement. Bands of hypertrophic smooth muscle form a coarse meshwork of trabeculae visible on the mucosal surface. Bulging of mucosa between trabeculae may result in the formation of numerous diverticula. In contrast, congenital diverticula are usually solitary and always composed of all layers of the bladder wall.

Most **carcinomas of the bladder** arise from transitional epithelium. Smoking and industrial exposure to aromatic amines increase the risk of this malignancy, which occurs chiefly in middle-aged men. The tumor may appear as a solitary nodule, as a flat plaque which tends to ulcerate, or as numerous warty, friable papillomas covering the entire inner surface of the bladder. Besides metastasizing to regional and distant lymph nodes, bladder carcinoma invades contiguous structures aggressively.

Review Questions

1. Distinguish the operations of glomeruli and renal tubules.
2. How is the kidney involved in the origin of some cases of hypertension?
3. Name some conditions that favor formation of kidney stones.
4. Define or explain: *nephron, nephrotic syndrome, pyelonephritis, uremia.*

23

The Female Reproductive System

Gross and Microscopic Anatomy

The female reproductive system consists of the ovaries, the uterus and tubes, and the vagina. Each **ovary** has a broad cortex containing microscopic ovarian follicles in a dense stroma of collagenous fibers, and an ill-defined vascular medulla. Normally but one follicle matures each month. An immature follicle contains a developing **ovum** or oocyte surrounded by a nest of low cuboidal cells having a well-defined basement membrane but no other connective tissue envelope. With maturation the follicle enlarges and develops a double sheath whose layers are the fibrous theca externa and the vascular theca interna. Estrogen, the principal female sex hormone, is produced by the cells of the theca interna. Follicles that begin to develop but then regress and degenerate are said to undergo atresia.

The formation of an ovum involves a variation on mitosis called meiosis or reduction division. Instead of each ovum receiving a full number of 46 chromosomes, as in mitosis, each receives only half that number. The same process occurs in the formation of spermatozoa in the male. Thus the union of spermatozoon and ovum results in just the normal complement of 46 chromosomes rather than double that number.

A mature follicle measures about 1 cm in diameter and is called a **graafian follicle**. Within this follicle the ovum rests in a fluid medium called the liquor folliculi, surrounded by cuboidal epithelial cells forming the membrana granulosa. Small collections of deeply eosinophilic fluid within this cell layer are called Call-Exner bodies (or vacuoles). The graafian follicle lies immediately below the capsule of the ovary and at ovulation the surface gives way to allow the ovum to extrude into the peritoneal cavity. After ovulation the ruptured follicle evolves into a **corpus luteum**, whose lining cells enlarge and develop prominent yellow granules. These cells are the source of a

214

second hormone, progesterone, which prepares the uterus and other tissues for pregnancy. If pregnancy ensues, the corpus luteum continues to develop and produce progesterone until delivery. Otherwise it rapidly deteriorates, and this abrupt withdrawal of progesterone is responsible for the induction of menstruation. A deteriorated corpus luteum is called a corpus albicans.

Upon being released into the peritoneal cavity, a mature ovum enters the open end of the nearer uterine tube, by which it is conducted to the interior of the uterus. The paired **uterine tubes** (fallopian tubes, oviducts) are lined by simple columnar epithelium, some cells of which are ciliated and some not. There are also a lamina propria of loose connective tissue, a heavily developed muscularis, and a serosa. The lining of the tube is continuous with that of the uterine cavity, which is called the endometrium. The endometrium consists of nonciliated simple columnar epithelium and its lamina propria blends into the myometrium or muscular coat, which makes up the bulk of the uterine wall. Outside the muscular layer is a serosa.

The lining of the uterus undergoes cyclical changes coincident with phases of the menstrual cycle. After each menstrual period, there ensues a **proliferative stage** in which the endometrium rapidly regenerates. Straight tubular glands penetrate the stroma and the vascular supply increases. In the **secretory stage** the endometrium develops further and the glands become large and coiled. At this point the endometrium is prepared for the implantation of a fertilized ovum. If this does not take place, a **menstrual stage** follows, in which the built-up endometrium rapidly breaks down and sloughs away, leaving only a thin layer of tissue inside the myometrium. Regeneration begins anew with the next proliferative stage.

Fertilization typically occurs in a uterine tube, and considerable embryonic development has already occurred before implantation takes place. The embryo, surrounded by an epithelial layer called the trophoblast, penetrates the secretory endometrium and becomes firmly attached to its lamina propria. The trophoblast develops into a plate-like membrane, the chorion, which draws nourishment from the underlying endometrium by way of fingerlike projections called villi. The chorion becomes the fetal component of the placenta. A second fetal membrane, the amnion, forms a sac that encloses the developing fetus in a fluid medium, the amniotic fluid. The part of the uterine wall where the chorion is attached undergoes structural adaptation and forms the decidua basalis, the maternal component of the placenta. The remainder of the endometrium also undergoes modification during pregnancy to become the decidua parietalis. The placenta communicates with the fetal circulation by way of the umbilical cord, which normally contains two arteries and one vein surrounded by an immature type of mucous connective tissue called Wharton's jelly.

The **cervix** is a necklike prolongation of the uterus that extends downward into the vagina. Its hollow interior, the endocervical canal, establishes continuity between the vagina and the uterine cavity. The endocervical canal is lined by high columnar cells, some ciliated and some secreting mucus. Tubular mucous glands are also situated in the lamina propria. As the endocervical canal opens out at the external cervical os, the lining epithelium shows an abrupt transition to stratified squamous epithelium, which is characteristic of the vaginal portion of the cervix and of the vagina itself. The mucosa of the **vagina** is thrown into transverse folds. The lamina propria contains a high proportion of elastic fibers and scattered aggregations of lymphoid tissue. The muscularis contains chiefly longitudinal muscle fibers. The fibrosa blends in with surrounding structures.

Pathologic Study of the Female Reproductive System

Material can be obtained from the female genital tract for cytologic study by scraping the vaginal walls and the cervix with a wooden or plastic spatula, by aspirating vaginal secretions with a pipette, and by inserting a cotton swab or bristle brush collector (Cytobrush) into the endocervical canal. These methods are used routinely to obtain material for the Papanicolaou (Pap) smear. Since 1988 the Bethesda system for reporting findings on the cervical and vaginal Pap smear has been generally adopted, and Papanicolaou's original Roman-numeral classification of findings has been abandoned because of widespread inconsistency and confusion in its application and interpretation. According to the Bethesda system, every cytologic report includes an estimate of the adequacy of the specimen, with particular attention to the presence or absence of columnar (endocervical) cells. Descriptive diagnoses are included for benign changes (atrophy, inflammation, evidence of viral infection, presence of organisms such as *Candida* or *Trichomonas*); changes in squamous and glandular epithelium (atypia, dysplasia, neoplasia); and hormonal effect.

Because squamous epithelial cells of the cervix and vaginal mucosa undergo structural changes in response to changing hormone levels, the cytologic smear can provide information about estrogen production, ovulation, and menstrual phase. Three types of vaginal epithelial cells are identified. **Superficial cells** are large, irregular in outline, and platelike, with very small (pyknotic) nuclei. Their numbers are increased in response to high levels of estrogen, and the higher the estrogen, the more eosinophilic their cytoplasm. Superficial cells predominate in a smear taken between the end of one menstrual period and the succeeding ovulation. **Intermediate cells** are similar in form but smaller, and their edges often appear curled or folded in prepared smears. Their nuclei are larger than those of superficial cells and often vesicular. These cells are seen to predominate when progesterone levels are high, between ovulation and menstruation and also during pregnancy. **Basal cells** are small and round, with large nuclei showing prominent chromatin material. Predominance of these cells in a smear implies a reduction in the numbers of superficial and intermediate cells and hence absence of estrogen and progesterone effect, as after the menopause.

When the Pap smear or examination with a colposcope (a low-power microscope used to inspect the cervix) raises a suspicion of dysplasia, malignancy, or human papillomavirus (HPV) infection, solid pieces of tissue can be snipped from the cervix with a biopsy forceps for histologic study. In a more extensive procedure called conization, a cone-shaped piece of cervix is removed, the base of the cone representing most of the mucosal surface of the cervix. Endometrial tissue is obtained by dilatation and curettage (D&C) or by suction (Vabra aspiration). Specimens can be removed from the ovary, tube, body of the uterus, or pelvic peritoneum through a laparoscope (a tubular instrument inserted into the pelvic cavity through a small incision near the umbilicus) or at open surgery.

Developmental Disorders

Developmental defects of the female reproductive system range from minor structural variants to failure of sexual differentiation, in which biological gender can be determined only by cytogenetic study. Many of these defects are associated with sterility (inability to reproduce) or infertility (impaired ability to reproduce). In **Turner's syndrome**, the ovaries are either absent or represented by mere streaks of hypoplastic ovarian tissue in the broad ligaments. Other reproductive structures are present but hypoplastic, and menstruation does not occur. The underlying defect is a lack or irregularity of one X chromosome. Short stature and other somatic abnormalities (webbed neck, cubitus valgus, cardiac anomalies) may be associated.

Structural malformations of the uterus and vagina arising from faulty midline fusion include reduplication of one or both of these structures, partial separation (bicornuate uterus), complete separation of one or both by a septum, gynatresia (occlusion of the vagina and sometimes of the uterus), and imperforate hymen (complete closure of the vaginal introitus).

Women exposed in utero to diethylstilbestrol (DES), formerly prescribed for various complications of pregnancy, may display a number of developmental anomalies of the genital tract, including deformities of the cervix (hood, coxcomb), transverse vaginal bands, and vaginal adenosis (zones of endocervical epithelium on the vaginal mucosa). There is also an increased incidence of clear cell carcinoma of the vagina and cervix among DES daughters.

Intersexuality refers to ambiguous external genitalia or physical features of both sexes united in one person. True hermaphroditism—the presence in one person of functioning ovarian and testicular tissue—is rare. In such cases, the ovary and testis may be separate, or both forms of tissue may be united in a single structure called an ovotestis. More common is pseudohermaphroditism, in which gonads of one sex are present in combination with internal and external genitalia of the opposite sex.

Endometriosis is a condition in which functioning endometrium is located ectopically, most often on the pelvic peritoneum and in the ovaries. Adenomyosis refers to ectopic endometrium within the myometrium. The origin of this aberrant tissue is unknown. Menstrual changes occurring in it may cause severe pelvic pain. Microscopic examination shows a well-developed endometrial stroma and functioning glands. Hemorrhage and cyst formation are common. In the ovary, endometrial cysts contain brown fluid derived from degenerated blood (chocolate cysts).

Cysts and Neoplasms of the Ovary

Non-neoplastic cysts in the ovary may also arise from germinal follicles. **Follicular cysts** form from unruptured, atretic follicles. On microscopic examination they are seen to be lined with a single layer of cuboidal or columnar epithelium. In the Stein-Leventhal syndrome (polycystic ovary syndrome), many such cysts occur in both ovaries, in association with hirsutism and failure to ovulate. The **corpus luteum cyst** develops from a normal germinal follicle after expulsion of the ovum and formation of a corpus luteum. A serous fluid gradually replaces the blood normally found in a corpus luteum, and if the lesion remains for a long time without spontaneous rupture it may become quite large, its walls of luteinizing theca cells being replaced by fibrosis. **Thecalutein cysts** are similar but are multiple lesions in both ovaries induced by excessive levels of chorionic gonadotropin formed in functioning tumors of the chorion (hydatidiform mole, choriocarcinoma). **Germinal inclusion cysts** are small invaginations of germinal epithelium from the ovarian surface, found generally in postmenopausal women and of no clinical significance.

Neoplasms of the ovary are of two types: teratomas, which take origin from germ cells, and tumors of nongerminal origin. A teratoma, developing from highly undifferentiated and pluripotential cells, may incorporate virtually any kind of tissue. Epithelium and other structures of ectodermal origin (hair, teeth, nerve cells) are usually present, and cartilage, bone, and glandular formations may also be found. In **cystic teratoma** (dermoid cyst), ectodermal elements preponderate, and the lesion consists largely or entirely of a multiloculated cyst lined by stratified squamous epithelium and filled with semisolid sebaceous debris. The less common **solid teratoma** contains a greater diversity of tissue. Struma ovarii is a solid ovarian teratoma containing a preponderance of thyroid gland tissue. The cells and tissues composing some teratomas remain highly undifferentiated; these tumors are more likely than other teratomas to undergo malignant change (teratocarcinoma).

The most important ovarian tumor arising from nongerminal tissue is cyst adenocarcinoma, a bulky, nodular malignancy containing many cysts. Two forms are distinguished. In **serous cystadenocarcinoma**, thin-walled cysts are lined with cuboidal epithelium and filled with serous fluid. In **mucinous cystadenocarcinoma** the cysts contain mucoid material and are lined with mucin-secreting columnar cells. These tumors typically occur during or after middle age, and may arise either as malignant tumors or by malignant change in histologically benign serous or mucinous cystadenomas. They may become very large and typically invade contiguous structures and the pelvic wall besides metastasizing to distant sites.

Other primary ovarian neoplasms are the Brenner tumor, a generally benign cystic or solid tumor containing nests of radially disposed cells with pale cytoplasm and longitudinally grooved nuclei; granulosa cell tumor, consisting of clusters of cells with large nuclei, resembling primordial follicles (with Call-Exner bodies) and producing excessive estrogen; and arrhenoblastoma, containing cordlike arrangements of cells resembling testicular structures and producing androgen. Meigs' syndrome consists of ascites and sometimes pleural effusion (usually on the right side) developing in association with a benign ovarian fibroma and disappearing after removal of the tumor.

Malignancies metastatic to the ovary originate most often in the stomach (Krukenberg tumor). Other common sites of origin are the intestine, the uterus, and the breast.

Diseases of the Uterus and Tubes

The term **pelvic inflammatory disease** (PID) denotes a symptom complex of fever, pelvic pain, and evidence of inflammation in the uterine tubes (salpingitis), endometrium (endometritis), or both, along with focal pelvic peritonitis. Salpingitis usually occurs by extension from the lower genital tract. The primary infection is either a sexually transmitted disease due to gonococcus or *Chlamydia* or a complication of childbirth, abortion, or instrumentation of the uterine cavity. Gonococcal salpingitis is manifested by hyperemia, edema, neutrophilic infiltrates and purulent exudate. The tube may become grossly dilated with pus (pyosalpinx), and infection may extend to the ovary (tubo-ovarian abscess), the pelvic peritoneum, and even the upper abdominal quadrants (Fitz-Hugh-Curtis syndrome or gonococcal perihepatitis). Repeated infections lead to fibrotic thickening of the tube, with stenosis or occlusion of its lumen. Peritoneal scarring may lead to formation of fibrotic bands (banjo-string or violin-string adhesions). Salpingitis due to *Chlamydia trachomatis* is similar to gonococcal infection but elicits less inflammation and suppuration and is less likely to result in late complications.

Scarring of the uterine tube after chronic or recurrent salpingitis leads to infertility or sterility and predisposes to **tubal pregnancy**. Tubal pregnancy occurs when a fertilized ovum becomes implanted in the uterine tube because its expected migration to the endometrial cavity has been delayed. The trophoblast and chorionic villi invade the tubal wall, including the muscularis, and eventually cause hemorrhage, perforation, or both. Other possible sites of ectopic pregnancy are the ovary and the abdominopelvic cavity (with implantation on the peritoneum).

The myometrium is frequently the site of **fibromyomas** (fibroids), benign tumors containing both muscular and fibrous elements. These neoplasms are spherical, firm, and well-circumscribed though not encapsulated. Often several fibroids appear in the same uterus. The typical location is intramural (within the muscular wall), but subserosal and submucosal tumors also occur frequently. Enlargement of fibroids often takes place during pregnancy. Microscopic examination shows bundles of smooth muscle in tight but erratic swirls and tangles, and variable amounts of fibrous connective tissue. The muscle fibers may undergo hyaline degeneration, and after menopause fibroids often calcify.

Endometrial adenocarcinoma, a disease primarily of the postmenopausal years, is more common in women with hypertension, diabetes mellitus, thyroid gland disorders, and carcinoma of the breast, and in those who have never been pregnant. The risk is also increased by prolonged administration of estrogen. The tumor occurs in both diffuse and localized forms, sometimes being limited to a single polyp, so that diagnostic curettage often proves curative. Microscopic examination shows numerous, tortuous endometrial glands with an abnormally scanty stroma. The epithelial cells display pleomorphism, large nuclei, hyperchromasia, and numerous mitotic figures. The tumor invades the myometrium, may spread to the tubes, ovaries, and vagina, and metastasizes to pelvic lymph nodes, lung, bone, and brain.

Sarcoma botryoides is a malignant tumor of mixed mesodermal origin arising in the cervix or vagina, less often in the bladder. The tumor occurs usually in children and appears as a grapelike cluster of rapidly growing tumor nodules. Hematogenous metastasis occurs early, particularly to the lung, and the prognosis is poor.

Diseases of the Cervix

Benign lesions of the uterine cervix are common and their chief importance lies in the need to distinguish them from malignant neoplasms. **Cervical polyps** are single or multiple, sessile or pedunculated masses consisting of a fibromyxomatous stroma and covered by benign hyperplastic epithelium. This lesion is more common during pregnancy. A **nabothian cyst** is a small yellowish mass consisting of a dilated endocervical gland and appearing generally at the external cervical os. Condylomata acuminata, ulcers of herpes simplex, and syphilitic chancres may appear on the cervix. **Cervical erosion** denotes a condition in which part of the normal squamous epithelium has been destroyed and replaced by columnar epithelium. This may be difficult to distinguish from **cervical eversion** (or ectropion), in which endocervical mucosa pouts out of the external cervical os. **Squamous metaplasia** is a focal or diffuse replacement of mucus-secreting surface and glandular epithelium by squamous epithelium, which may grow into and completely line glands (epidermidization).

Squamous cell carcinoma of the uterine cervix is still an important cause of morbidity and mortality in women, despite the possibility of detecting dysplastic changes by means of the Papanicolaou smear years before invasive carcinoma develops. Infection with human papillomavirus (HPV), which causes genital warts, a highly contagious sexually transmitted disease and the most prevalent one caused by a virus, has been implicated as a major cause of dysplastic and neoplastic changes in the cervix as well as in other parts of the female genital tract and in the male genitalia, particularly the penis. HPV types 16 and 18, which cause flat genital warts rather than the more common condylomata lata, are associated with highly malignant genital neoplasms in both sexes. Other risk factors for cervical carcinoma are genital herpes simplex, early age of first intercourse, and repeated intercourse with an uncircumcised partner.

Cervical intraepithelial neoplasia (CIN) denotes dysplastic changes confined to the epithelial layer of the cervix. Foci of anaplastic cells with altered, erratic polarity and large, hyperchromatic, irregular nuclei may be found throughout the epithelium, but stromal invasion does not occur even though extension into endocervical glands is common. This lesion is most likely to occur at the squamocolumnar junction. Cervical intraepithelial neoplasia is classified on the basis of depth as follows:

CIN I: Up to ½ of the epithelial thickness (mild dysplasia).

CIN II: From ½ to ¾ of the epithelial thickness (moderate dysplasia).

CIN III: From ¾ to full thickness (severe dysplasia; carcinoma in situ).

Typically a latent interval of years elapses between the development of CIN and evidence of invasion. Invasive squamous cell carcinoma may present as a flat, infiltrating lesion, as an ulcer, or as a nodular excrescence. Microscopic study shows proliferation of moderately well-differentiated, generally nonkeratinizing epithelium. The tumor spreads to the pelvic wall, vagina, bladder, rectum, and regional lymph nodes. The FIGO (International Federation of Gynecologists and Obstetricians) staging of cervical carcinoma is as follows:

Stage 0:   Carcinoma in situ.

Stage I: Carcinoma invading basement membrane but confined to cervix.

Stage II: Carcinoma extending beyond cervix but not to pelvic wall or lower third of vagina.

Stage III: Invasion of pelvic wall and lower third of vagina, bladder, rectum, extrapelvic structures.

Diseases of the Vagina

Vaginitis (inflammation of the vagina) and **vulvitis** (inflammation of the vulva) often occur together and are usually due to infection. The most frequent vaginal pathogens are the fungus *Candida albicans,* the protozoan *Trichomonas vaginalis,* and the bacterium *Gardnerella vaginalis.* Serous, mucous, or purulent exudation is evident, along with hyperemia, edema, and occasionally ulceration of the cervix and vulva. *Neisseria gonorrhoeae* may cause infection of the cervix, vagina, and urethra. Condylomata acuminata (genital warts), syphilitic chancre, and lesions of herpes simplex may appear on the cervix, vaginal mucosa, or external genitalia. Squamous cell carcinoma of the vagina, a relatively uncommon malignancy, occurs in middle or later life. It may develop as an infiltrating plaque, an ulcer, or a fungating mass. Both local extension and lymph node metastasis occur frequently.

Disorders of Pregnancy

Abnormalities of pregnancy develop often, many of them resulting in fetal loss. **Spontaneous abortion** is defined as an accidental termination of pregnancy before the time of fetal viability. Although it may be due to infection, trauma, hormonal disorders, or other causes, spontaneous abortion most often results from some inherent abnormality of the fertilized ovum (blighted ovum). An aborted fetus is usually expelled along with its membranes, but by exception it may remain within the uterine cavity indefinitely (missed abortion). A lithopedion is a retained dead fetus that has calcified.

The placenta is subject to various disorders of formation and implantation, some of which pose severe threats to mother, fetus, or both. **Placenta previa** is a placenta so implanted as to obstruct the internal cervical os partially or completely. Separation of such a placenta before or during labor frequently leads to severe hemorrhage. Another source of dangerous obstetrical hemorrhage is **abruptio placentae**, separation of a normally positioned placenta after the twentieth week of gestation but before birth. Abnormal adherence of the placenta to the uterine wall may be due to attachment of chorionic villi directly to myometrium at a site where the decidua is deficient or absent (placenta accreta); penetration of uterine muscle by villi (placenta increta); or growth of villi all the way to and through the uterine serosa (placenta percreta).

Marginal insertion of the umbilical cord on the placental disk (battledore placenta) is of no clinical significance. The presence of only two blood vessels (one artery and one vein) in the umbilical cord, however, frequently betokens other developmental anomalies in the fetus. Contrary to popular belief, coiling of the umbilical cord around the fetal neck seldom has untoward effects.

Hydatidiform mole is an infrequent development from a fetus that has died before four weeks of gestation. The chorionic villi display an extreme stromal overdevelopment, while the fetus undergoes degeneration and necrosis. The hypertrophic villi form a friable mass consisting of a grapelike bunch of small transparent vesicles attached to the endometrium. Microscopic examination shows irregular trophoblastic proliferation and hydropic degeneration of chorionic tissues. Malignant change in a hydatidiform mole (or, rarely, in the chorion of a normal pregnancy) generates a neoplasm called choriocarcinoma (chorioepithelioma). In this tumor, chorionic villi are absent, and masses of malignant chorionic epithelial cells invade locally and metastasize to lungs, brain, and liver.

Review Questions

1. Distinguish *meiosis* from *mitosis*.
2. Define or explain: *CIN, endometriosis, fibroid, pelvic inflammatory disease.*

24

The Male Reproductive System

Gross and Microscopic Anatomy

In the male, the urethra serves a reproductive function besides carrying urine out of the bladder. The other parts of the male reproductive system are the testicles, the spermatic ducts, the prostate, the glands of Cowper, and the penis. Each **testicle** has a tough capsule, the tunica albuginea, from which incomplete septa descend to divide the organ into lobules. Each lobule contains a number of coiled seminiferous tubules consisting of several strata of cuboidal spermatogenic or germ cells and relatively few tall columnar supporting or sustentacular cells, the cells of Sertoli. In the connective tissue between the lobules lie large oval or polygonal cells, the interstitial cells of Leydig, which produce the hormone testosterone.

As in the formation of ova in the female, spermatozoa (spermatocytes) arise by meiosis rather than mitosis, each having 23 rather than 46 chromosomes. Mature spermatozoa pass from the seminiferous tubules into larger channels lined by cuboidal or columnar epithelium. These freely anastomose in a network called the rete testis. Beyond the rete testis, the coalescence of sperm ducts results in the formation of a single duct from each testis. This duct first passes through an elongated body, the epididymis, which lies adjacent to the testicle, before forming the vas deferens (spermatic cord) and leading through the prostate to the urethra. The duct of the epididymis and the vas deferens are lined by pseudo-stratified columnar epithelium with a ciliated border and conspicuous granules. There is a thick muscularis with both longitudinal and circular fibers.

The testis originates as an abdominal organ and descends into the scrotum around the 28th week of fetal development. The front and sides of each testicle and its epididymis are invested by a double layer of serous membrane, the tunica vaginalis, which develops from the pelvic peritoneum and becomes separated from it after the descent of the testicle.

The function of the **prostate** is to produce the fluid component of semen and to close off communication between the bladder and the urethra at the time of ejaculation. The prostate is a mass of tubulo-alveolar glands packed in a very prominent stroma containing elastic fibers and smooth muscle. The acini are lined by simple cuboidal epithelium. A few are generally found to contain spherical concretions of protein material called corpora amylacea. The seminal vesicles and glands of Cowper are small structures adjacent to the urethra that contribute to the seminal fluid. They contain alveolar glands, ducts lined by cuboidal or columnar cells, and much smooth muscle and elastic connective tissue in their stroma.

The **penis** contains two cylindrical masses of erectile tissue, the corpora cavernosa, which lie side by side and dorsal to the urethra. Each corpus cavernosum consists of a vascular plexus in a stroma rich in elastic fibers and smooth muscle. Lacunae called cavernous veins fill with blood to distend the organ during erection. The corpus cavernosum is covered by a tough fibrous capsule or tunica albuginea. The corpus spongiosum, which surrounds the urethra, is similar in structure to the corpus cavernosum but its capsule is thinner and its erectile function less prominent.

Pathologic Study of the Male Reproductive System

Tissue can be obtained from the urethra through a urethroscope and from the prostate by needle biopsy via the rectum. Fluid expressed from the prostate by massage can be examined for inflammatory or malignant cells. Surgical specimens from the male reproductive tract include the foreskin after circumcision, the testicle after orchiectomy, the prostate after complete resection of the gland, and prostatic shavings after transurethral resection.

Developmental Disorders

Klinefelter's syndrome, a genetic disorder arising from an error of sex chromosome distribution (typically the pattern is XXY but other variants occur), consists of above-normal stature, feminine habitus with gynecomastia, and small testes showing hyalinization of seminiferous tubules and no spermatogenesis. In the **testicular feminization syndrome**, female external genitalia are formed during fetal development despite the presence of (abdominal) testes and the absence of uterus, tubes, and ovaries.

Cryptorchidism (undescended testicle) is a condition in which the descent of one or both testicles from the abdominal cavity during fetal development is arrested. The testicle may lie in the abdominal cavity or in the inguinal canal, but cannot be manipulated into the scrotum. At puberty an undescended testicle generally fails to develop as expected. Spermatogenesis ordinarily does not occur, and the parenchyma eventually atrophies, with a real or apparent increase of Leydig cells. There is an increased risk of malignancy in undescended testicle.

Hypospadias is a malformation of the urethra in which it opens on the lower surface of the penis instead of at the tip of the glans. In **epispadias** the urethra opens on the upper surface of the penis. Congenital diverticulum of the urethra is usually of little significance. **Hydrocele** is a cystic mass of the spermatic cord, testicle, or both consisting of a loculation of serous fluid between the two layers of the tunica vaginalis. Congenital hydrocele may communicate with the abdominal cavity and may be associated with indirect inguinal hernia.

Diseases of the Testicle and Associated Structures

Orchitis, inflammation of the testicle, usually arises by extension of infection from the urethra, bladder, or prostate, and is typically accompanied by **epididymitis**, inflammation of the epididymis. The inflamed testicle is firm, swollen, and cyanotic. Pathologic examination discloses punctate hemorrhages, neutrophilic infiltrates, and perhaps foci of necrosis. Inflammation of the epididymis is manifested by interstitial congestion and edema, neutrophilic infiltrates, and suppuration. When the process is severe it may lead to necrosis of tubules with eventual fibrotic scarring. In mumps, a viral orchitis (often unilateral) may occur with signs of focal inflammation, edema, and marked distention of the tunica albuginea. Atrophy of some testicular parenchyma may ensue but sterility rarely results.

Nearly all neoplasms of the testicle are **teratomas**, tumors of variable malignancy derived from germ cells. These typically occur in adults before age 50, and their incidence is much higher in undescended testicles. By producing high levels of chorionic gonadotropin, they may induce feminization (gynecomastia, loss of body hair). Teratomas may contain zones corresponding to two or more of the following tumor types. Seminoma, the most frequent and least malignant, consists of cords or tubules formed of large round or cuboidal cells, monotonous in their regularity, with large and centrally located nuclei. Embryonal carcinoma is a small, invasive tumor of highly variable gross and microscopic appearance. It contains anaplastic epithelial cells with large, hyperchromatic nuclei. Choriocarcinoma contains more differentiated somatic tissues, including cells resembling those of the trophoblast that forms the fetal chorion. Mature teratoma consists of a chaotic array of fetal and adult structures—keratinizing squamous epithelium, cartilage, smooth muscle, and nerve. Teratocarcinoma, the most malignant germ cell neoplasm of the testicle, is small, soft, often cystic, with zones of hemorrhage and necrosis. It contains both highly anaplastic cells and differentiated elements including tissues of ectodermal, mesodermal, and endodermal origin. Malignant teratomas of the testicle invade locally, often causing obstruction of one or both ureters, and metastasize to regional lymph nodes.

Acquired hydrocele may result from trauma or inflammation of the tunica vaginalis. When of long standing it may lead to fibrous thickening of the tunica with bandlike adhesions and calcification. **Varicocele** denotes dilatation and tortuosity of the pampiniform plexus, the system of anastomosing veins accompanying the vas deferens. It may result from obstruction to venous drainage by edema, scarring, or neoplastic disease within the pelvis. A primary form, common in young men and generally resolving spontaneously, invariably involves the left spermatic cord. **Torsion** (twisting) of the spermatic cord results from abnormal mobility of the testicle, usually due to some anatomic variant. The condition runs in families. Impairment of venous drainage by twisting of the cord leads to edema, which prevents spontaneous untwisting. Without surgical intervention the arterial supply to the testicle becomes compromised, and infarction, degeneration, and necrosis may follow within a few hours.

Diseases of the Prostate

Acute prostatitis (inflammation of the prostate) usually represents extension of pyogenic or gonococcal infection from some other part of the genital tract (bladder, urethra, epididymis), but may arise by the hematogenous route in septicemia. The acutely inflamed prostate is hyperemic and edematous. Desquamated cells and purulent exudate appear in the tubules, inflammatory cells infiltrate the stroma, and frank abscess formation may occur. **Chronic prostatitis**, more common in older men, may evolve from acute prostatitis or may result from stasis of secretions. The gland is enlarged and boggy. Microscopic study shows patchy or diffuse infiltration of lymphocytes and plasma cells. Inflammatory reaction about the acini, which are filled with cellular debris, culminates in proliferation of fibrous connective tissue. Corpora amylacea, calculi, or both are often found in acini and ducts, but whether they contribute to stasis of secretions and chronic inflammation or result from them is not known.

Benign prostatic hyperplasia, often miscalled hypertrophy, occurs very frequently with aging and presumably reflects hormonal influences. The gland is enlarged to two to four times its normal weight of about 20 g. Its surface may be smooth or nodular and its texture is firm but not hard. Early in the course of enlargement, the cut surface may appear homogeneous, reflecting predominantly fibromuscular proliferation. Later the texture becomes nodular and the cut surface exudes a milky fluid. Microscopic examination at this stage shows increased size and number of acini, which contain epithelial debris and may undergo cystic dilatation. Increased mitoses are not seen. Benign enlargement of the prostate often causes urinary obstruction with resultant dilatation and hypertrophy of the bladder, diverticulum formation, and urinary tract infection.

Adenocarcinoma of the prostate usually occurs after age 60. It is the commonest malignancy in adult males. Foci of prostatic carcinoma often accompany benign hyperplasia, and may be found in about half of all autopsy specimens from men over 50. The posterior lobe is the site of origin in three-quarters of cases. The gland is seldom greatly enlarged but the enlargement is usually asymmetrical and the texture woody or stony. Microscopic examination shows adenocarcinoma with variable degrees of differentiation. Acinar cells may have large nuclei with prominent nucleoli but mitotic figures are scarce. There are generally distortion of acinar architecture, reduction of stromal elements, and invasion of the capsule and blood vessels by malignant cells. Metastasis occurs chiefly to the bones of the spine and pelvis and to regional nodes. As a rule, bony metastases are osteoblastic rather than osteoclastic.

Diseases of the Penis and Urethra

Urethritis in the male is nearly always due to sexually transmitted infection with *Neisseria gonorrhoeae, Chlamydia trachomatis,* or *Ureaplasma urealyticum.* Urethritis causes hyperemia, edema, and sometimes ulceration of the urethral mucosa, with a mucous or purulent discharge consisting of neutrophils and cellular debris. In gonorrheal urethritis, gonococci are seen within neutrophils. Repeated episodes of gonococcal urethritis may lead to fibrotic stricture of the urethra, with urinary obstruction. In Reiter's syndrome, urethritis due to *Chlamydia* or other organisms elicits noninfectious conjunctivitis and arthritis, presumably as an autoimmune phenomenon.

Phimosis denotes inability of the foreskin to be retracted from the glans. It may stem from a congenitally small aperture in the foreskin or from fibrosis after infection. Paraphimosis is inability of the retracted foreskin to be replaced over the glans. **Balanitis** (inflammation of the glans penis), posthitis (inflammation of the foreskin), or, more often, balanoposthitis, commonly results from pyogenic infection. Balanitis xerotica obliterans (erythroplasia of Queyrat) is an intraepidermal carcinoma of the glans consisting of an elevated, sharply circumscribed, red or pink plaque with a velvety texture. Microscopic examination shows epithelial atrophy, acanthosis, edema of the dermis, and infiltrates of lymphocytes, plasma cells, and histiocytes, and squamous cell carcinoma in situ.

The skin of the penis or scrotum may be the site of lesions of herpes simplex, condyloma acuminatum (genital warts), syphilitic chancre, and chancroid. Squamous cell carcinoma of the penis seldom develops in circumcised men. The tumor grows slowly, invading deeper tissues and metastasizing late to inguinal lymph nodes. In Peyronie's disease (induratio plastica penis), a chronic inflammation of unknown cause leads to the formation of solitary or multiple nodules or plaques of fibrous hyperplasia in the stroma of the corpora cavernosa, which may distort the penis, particularly during erection, and may ultimately calcify.

Review Questions

1. What is the function of the prostate?
2. What is the commonest malignancy in adult males?
3. Define or explain: *cryptorchidism, hydrocele, phimosis.*

25

The Endocrine Glands

Endocrine glands are those that release their secretions, called hormones, directly into the circulation. Arrived at its target (or end) organ, a hormone exerts some stimulant (occasionally suppressant) action on a specific type of cell or tissue. The chief importance of diseases of the endocrine glands lies in the effect they can have on the level of hormones in the circulation. Degenerative or destructive lesions of a gland may lead to a deficiency of its hormone, while functioning neoplasms of glandular tissue often produce excessive levels of hormone.

The islets of Langerhans, endocrine tissue in the pancreas that produces glucagon and insulin, are discussed in Chapter 21, and the hormone-secreting functions of the ovary and the testicle are discussed in Chapters 23 and 24, respectively. The liver, the walls of the alimentary canal, and some nerve tissue also contain secretory cells that send chemical products directly into the blood. Five anatomically discrete endocrine glands—the pituitary gland, the thyroid gland, the parathyroid glands, the adrenal glands, and the pineal gland—remain to be discussed.

The Pituitary Gland

The pituitary gland, also called the hypophysis, is situated beneath the brain in a bony receptacle on the floor of the skull called the sella turcica. It consists of two entirely distinct masses of tissue, one derived embryonically from the central nervous system and one from the pharynx, which have fused to form a single organ. The smaller **posterior lobe** or neurohypophysis, an extension of the part of the brain known as the hypothalamus, contains modified nerve cells (called pituicytes) with lipid secretory granules. These produce two simple polypeptide hormones: oxytocin, which stimulates the contraction of the uterine muscle during labor; and vasopressin or antidiuretic hormone (ADH), which promotes reabsorption of water in the renal tubules.

The **anterior lobe** of the pituitary gland contains cords of cuboidal or polygonal cells that branch and rejoin to enclose vascular channels called sinusoids, like those of the liver. Three general classes of cells are distinguished on the basis of the staining properties of their granules. Acidophils produce growth hormone and prolactin, a hormone involved in lactation. Basophils produce hormones that regulate the function of the thyroid gland (thyroid stimulating hormone, TSH), the adrenal cortex (adrenocorticotropic hormone, ACTH), and the gonads (follicle-stimulating hormone, FSH; luteinizing hormone, LH). Chromophobe cells, whose granules take up acidic and basic stains poorly, have no known secretory function.

Ectopic pituitary tissue, often found in the submucosa of the roof of the pharynx (pharyngeal pituitary), has no apparent clinical significance. In empty sella syndrome, the pituitary gland is flattened against the hypothalamus instead of appearing in its normal location in the sella turcica. This condition may be associated with increased, normal, or decreased glandular function.

Panhypopituitarism (Simmonds' disease) denotes a deficiency of all hormones produced by the anterior lobe of the pituitary gland. Withdrawal of normal stimulation to the thyroid gland, the adrenal cortices, and the gonads results in a general decline in the function of these glands, with ensuing cachexia, reduction of body hair and skin pigment, and impairment of response to stress and resistance to infection. Total pituitary failure occurring in infancy or childhood also results in dwarfism. Panhypopituitarism may be caused by infarction of the pituitary, destruction by a neoplasm, or surgical removal.

Panhypopituitarism coming on in the postpartum period as a sequel to obstetrical shock is called Sheehan's syndrome. Hyperplasia of the gland during pregnancy makes it vulnerable to infarction if hemorrhagic shock occurs during labor and delivery. The gland becomes pale and opaque, undergoing coagulation necrosis. Microscopic examination shows widespread thrombosis of arteries. Eventually the necrotic parenchyma is replaced by fibrosis. Rarely, depression of pituitary function is due to sarcoidosis, amyloidosis, or xanthomatosis (Hand-Schüller-Christian disease).

Diabetes insipidus is a condition of excessive diuresis caused by deficiency of antidiuretic hormone from the posterior lobe of the pituitary gland. Trauma, tumor, and degenerative disease causing interruption of the neurohypophyseal tract of the hypothalamus are the most likely causes of this condition.

Functioning pituitary tumors derived from acidophil or basophil cells cause symptoms due to excessive levels of hormone. **Acidophil adenoma** is a reddish, globular tumor with a distinct capsule. Histologically it consists of small, well-differentiated acidophilic cells arrayed in dense sheets and occasionally showing papillary formations. There may be zones of infarction and necrosis. An excess of growth hormone, due to acidophil adenoma, leads to pituitary gigantism (excessive length of long bones) when it occurs in childhood, and acromegaly when it occurs after closure of growth centers. Besides bony overgrowth, excess of growth hormone causes enlargement of the tongue (macroglossia), heart (cardiomegaly), and abdominal viscera (splanchnomegaly).

Basophil adenoma is usually a small tumor consisting of well-differentiated polygonal cells with typical basophilic granules. Basophil cells elsewhere in the pituitary gland may be replaced by a homogeneous hyaline material (Crooke's hyaline change) when a basophil adenoma is present. An excess of adrenocorticotropic hormone due to basophilic adenoma induces a condition called Cushing's disease, which is due to overactivity of the adrenal cortices. Cushing's disease is discussed later in this chapter.

Non-hormone-producing neoplasms of the pituitary produce symptoms by displacing the pituitary parenchyma, by disturbing the flow of cerebrospinal fluid through the third ventricle, or by compressing the optic chiasm, the structure formed by the junction and partial crossing of the optic nerves just in front of the pituitary gland. **Chromophobe adenoma**, a benign tumor arising from chromophobe cells, is the commonest pituitary neoplasm. It may cause no symptoms, but often becomes quite large, eroding the sella turcica, compressing the third ventricle, and inducing degeneration and gliosis of the optic chiasm, with impairment of vision. In addition, panhypopituitarism and diabetes insipidus may result from more or less complete destruction of normal secretory tissue of the pituitary gland. The tumor is soft, sometimes highly vascular, and often containing areas of hemorrhagic infarction, degeneration, and cyst formation. Microscopically it consists of polygonal chromophobe cells in sheets or random arrangements, sometimes with papillary projections, and a fibrovascular stroma. As many as 10% of cases of gigantism and acromegaly occur in persons with chromophobe rather than acidophil adenomas.

Craniopharyngioma, typically a disease of childhood and adolescence, is a benign tumor developing from epithelial nests persisting from the embryonic primordium of the nasopharynx. It is a grayish-white, multilocular, cystic mass. The cysts are filled with a cloudy fluid containing crystals of cholesterol and calcium. Grossly evident zones of necrosis and calcification may occur in the solid portions of the tumor. Histologic sections show blocks, strands, or columns of anaplastic epithelial cells varying from columnar to squamous. Compression of the pituitary gland may lead to hypopituitarism and, in early life, pituitary dwarfism.

The Thyroid Gland

The thyroid gland is a flattened, shield-shaped structure incompletely divided into right and left lobes and situated in the front of the neck just above the breast bone. It has a definite connective-tissue capsule, a stroma consisting of septa and trabeculae, and a rich blood and lymph supply. The parenchyma of the gland consists entirely of microscopic follicles or acini. Each follicle is formed of wedge-shaped secretory cells (principal cells) enclosing an interior cavity that contains a gel-like fluid called colloid. A few parafollicular cells (C cells) are also found; these produce the hormone calcitonin, which affects calcium balance by acting as an antagonist to parathyroid hormone (discussed in the next section). The principal hormonal secretion of the gland, thyroxine, regulates tissue metabolism.

Thyroid tissue can be obtained for study by needle biopsy, but most specimens consist of whole glands or lobes removed for the treatment of thyroid hyperfunction or malignancy.

Deficiency of thyroid hormone (hypothyroidism) beginning before or shortly after birth causes cretinism, a syndrome of physical and mental retardation associated with coarseness of the skin, macroglossia, and skeletal malformations. When thyroid deficiency begins later in life, the result is myxedema. In this condition the pulse and blood pressure are low, the skin coarse and dry, the hair thinned, the face and hands puffy, speech hoarse, slow, and slurred, mental functioning retarded, gonadal function impaired, and serum cholesterol elevated. The characteristic pathologic lesion is a deposition of mucoid material in subcutaneous tissue and in or between the fibers of smooth muscle (especially in the bowel wall) and skeletal muscle. The heart becomes dilated, flabby, and pale, and on microscopic examination shows hydropic, vacuolar degeneration of the sarcoplasm (myxedema heart). Histologic sections of skin show hyperkeratosis and increased numbers of mast cells. In adulthood the commonest causes of myxedema are surgical removal of the thyroid gland and drug treatment of an overactive thyroid gland.

Goiter (struma) is a general term for enlargement of the thyroid gland. A goiter may be symmetrical or irregular, smooth or nodular, slight or massive, and associated with normal, increased, or decreased thyroid gland function. **Colloid goiter** (nodular, nontoxic goiter) is an enlargement of the gland that occurs usually in adolescent girls and is not associated with disturbance of hormone production. The thyroid gland is enlarged in a diffuse or nodular fashion. The cut surface shows a pale gray, gelatinous or glassy appearance due to colloid accumulation. Microscopic study shows many large follicles lined by an inactive glandular epithelium and distended by colloid.

Endemic goiter is a reactive hyperplasia of the thyroid gland due to a deficiency of iodine in soil and water. Hypothyroidism does not occur unless iodine deprivation is extreme. The thyroid gland is enlarged, soft, and rubbery, with increased vascularity. Microscopic examination shows hypertrophy and hyperplasia of acinar cells, with papillary projections into acinar lumens and formation of nodules resembling adenomas.

Acute thyroiditis, an uncommon condition, is caused by various bacteria and viruses, including the mumps virus, and typically occurs in a gland that is already diseased. It is a self-limited disorder marked by diffuse enlargement of the gland and inflammatory changes including giant-cell formation. Various forms of subacute or chronic thyroiditis occur, all of them much commoner in women. The commonest of these, **Hashimoto's disease**, is an autoimmune disorder. There is uniform or slightly nodular enlargement of the gland, which has a firmer texture than normal. Fibrous trabeculae are visible on the cut surface. Microscopically there is atrophy of parenchyma with diffuse infiltration of lymphocytes (some forming lymphoid follicles with germinal centers) and considerable interstitial fibrosis.

In **Riedel's struma** (chronic fibrous thyroiditis), part or all of the thyroid gland displays a woody firmness. Enlargement of the gland, often extreme and asymmetrical, may compress the trachea and esophagus. Histologically the tissue presents a similar picture to that of Hashimoto's disease, but the dominant finding is a dense fibrotic reaction replacing atrophic parenchyma. Lymphocytic infiltration is less pronounced and follicle formation does not occur. **De Quervain's disease** (subacute granulomatous thyroiditis), possibly viral in origin, causes a diffuse enlargement of the gland, which becomes pale and firm. Histologic study shows patchy degeneration of thyroid follicles, infiltration of leukocytes, giant cells, and fibroblasts.

Graves' disease (exophthalmic goiter, toxic goiter), a relatively common disorder of young and middle-aged women, runs in families and appears to be due to circulating autoantibodies that simulate the effects of TSH on the thyroid gland. The level of circulating TSH is normal or low. There is diffuse enlargement of the thyroid gland, which becomes firmer than normal and highly vascular. The cut surface is beefy, friable, and glistening. Microscopic sections show hyperplasia of secretory elements. The follicles are lined by tall columnar epithelial cells with vesicular nuclei, which may form papillary projections into the lumens. Colloid is reduced and intrafollicular spaces increased, with scattered lymphocytic infiltrates. The increased production of thyroid hormone causes symptoms of hyperthyroidism (thyrotoxicosis): tachycardia, flushing, sweating, weight loss, and emotional instability. The exophthalmos that accompanies this condition is due to a focal edema of the orbital contents induced by circulating antibodies to extraocular muscle. In iatrogenic hyperthyroidism (due to administration of an excessive dosage of thyroid hormone), the thyroid gland is not enlarged and exophthalmos does not occur.

Carcinoma of the thyroid occurs during early and middle life and is twice as common in women. A history of x-ray treatment of head or neck lesions increases the risk of thyroid carcinoma. The tumor arises from glandular epithelium and grows slowly but metastasizes early to cervical lymph nodes and eventually to lungs and bone. Papillary, follicular, and undifferentiated forms are recognized. **Papillary carcinoma**, accounting for half of all thyroid cancers, tends to occur at an earlier age. The tumor appears as a small, firm, solitary mass with a shaggy, gray cut surface. Hemorrhages and cyst formation are common. Microscopically there are delicate papillary formations consisting of fibrous connective tissue covered by columnar epithelium. The epithelial cells are somewhat larger than normal, with abundant cytoplasm and small nuclei. Their histologic appearance is often benign, though zones of anaplasia may appear. Concentrically laminated concretions called psammoma bodies often occur in these tumors.

Follicular carcinoma of the thyroid gland also appears as a firm gray nodular tumor. Microscopic examination shows small but well-formed follicular structures, some containing colloid, as well as papillary elements as in papillary carcinoma. Follicular cells are large and anaplastic. **Undifferentiated carcinoma** of the thyroid is a bulky tumor, which grows rapidly and metastasizes early. Histologic sections show solid masses of highly anaplastic cells among which follicular and papillary structures may appear. Giant cells are also seen.

Hürthle cells are large cuboidal cells with abundant, deeply eosinophilic, granular cytoplasm sometimes found in the thyroid gland and apparently representing rests of parathyroid tissue. Occasionally they form benign or malignant tumors (Hürthle cell adenoma, Hürthle cell carcinoma).

The Parathyroid Glands

Attached to the thyroid capsule but structurally distinct from the thyroid gland are the four parathyroid glands. Each gland has a capsule and stromal elements of connective tissue. The parenchyma consists of cords of cells, most of them chief (principal) cells but a few of the larger oxyphil (acid-staining) type. The latter are not normally found in children. The secretion of the parathyroid gland, parathormone, regulates calcium and phosphorus metabolism by increasing the reabsorption of calcium in the renal tubules, decreasing the reabsorption of phosphorus, and mobilizing calcium from bone.

The commonest cause of deficiency of parathyroid hormone is inadvertent surgical removal of the glands in the course of thyroidectomy. Rarely, all parathyroid glands may be destroyed by degenerative disease. When parathyroid hormone is deficient, serum calcium falls, with resultant heightening of neuromuscular excitability. This can lead to tetany, twitching, and seizures. In chronic hypoparathyroidism, calcification may occur about the cerebral arteries, particularly in the basal ganglia. In pseudohypoparathyroidism, a hereditary disorder in which depression of serum calcium is associated with skeletal deformity and short stature, the defect is an inadequate response to parathyroid hormone. Hence therapeutic administration of the hormone is without effect.

An increase of parathyroid hormone may stem from benign or malignant tumors of the parathyroid glands or from diffuse hyperplasia of the glands, either as a primary disorder or in response to chronic hypocalcemia of any cause, including renal failure, rickets, and multiple myeloma. The rise in serum calcium occurs at the expense of bones, which undergo changes characterized as osteitis fibrosa cystica, described in Chapter 26. Hypercalcemia causes muscular weakness, anorexia, increased urinary output, metastatic calcification in blood vessels and kidneys, and urolithiasis.

The usual cause of hypercalcemia is benign adenoma occurring as a solitary nodule in one parathyroid gland and arising from chief cells. The tumor appears as a small brown mass embedded in fat, and may contain zones of hemorrhage and necrosis. The cells are arranged in orderly fashion but appear somewhat larger than normal and may be slightly pleomorphic. In idiopathic hypertrophy of all parathyroids, the glands are seen to contain almost exclusively wasserhelle (water-clear) cells, with small nuclei and very transparent cytoplasm, disposed in sheets, branching cords, and acini.

The Adrenal Glands

The adrenal glands are paired, one being situated atop each kidney. As in the pituitary, each adrenal gland consists of two distinct tissue types that have fused into an anatomically unified structure. The cortex contains cords of cells that produce cortisol for the regulation of carbohydrate and protein metabolism, aldosterone for the control of electrolyte (sodium and potassium) balance, and androgen, which affects the growth of body and facial hair. From outside inward the cortex is divided into three ill-defined zones on the basis of the disposition of its cells: zona glomerulosa (nodules or clusters), zona fasciculata (cords in parallel bundles, radially disposed), and zona reticularis (crisscrossing cords). The cells are cuboidal secretory epithelium containing granules and lipid droplets. The adrenal medulla, which produces epinephrine (adrenalin), consists of clumps and cords of chromaffin cells with variable amounts of granular material in their cytoplasm.

Chronic deficiency of adrenal cortical hormones, resulting from atrophy, tuberculosis, amyloidosis, or metastatic malignancy of both adrenal glands, is called **Addison's disease**. The principal features of this syndrome are weakness, weight loss, increased pigmentation of the skin (especially over the knees, elbows, and knuckles), elevation of serum potassium and nitrogen, and depression of serum sodium and glucose. The heart size decreases and there is a tendency to acute vascular collapse (addisonian crisis). Waterhouse-Friderichsen syndrome is a more acute adrenal cortical deficiency, often fatal, occurring usually in children with meningococcal septicemia (occasionally other coccal infections or *Haemophilus influenzae*) and resulting from bilateral massive hemorrhage of the adrenal glands. In adrenocortical hypofunction due to deficiency of pituitary ACTH, the pigmentation seen in Addison's disease does not occur.

Cushing's syndrome is a constellation of symptoms and signs resulting from excessive levels of adrenal cortical hormones in the circulation. The commonest cause is treatment with adrenocortical steroids. The condition may also result from bilateral adrenocortical hyperplasia affecting the zona fasciculata, or from overstimulation of the adrenals by a basophil adenoma of the pituitary gland (in which case it is called Cushing's disease). The principal features of Cushing's syndrome are obesity, focal edema (moon face, buffalo hump), atrophy and fatty degeneration of muscle, osteoporosis, hypertension, diabetes mellitus, facial hirsutism, and acne.

Conn's syndrome (primary aldosteronism), manifested by retention of sodium and excessive loss of potassium by the kidney, is due to adenoma (occasionally, adenocarcinoma) of the adrenal cortex producing excessive amounts of aldosterone. The symptoms include hypertension, alkalosis, and muscular weakness or paralysis. Secondary aldosteronism, with similar symptoms, occurs in response to certain metabolic imbalances of hydration such as those of nephrotic syndrome, hepatic cirrhosis, and congestive cardiac failure.

Congenital adrenal hyperplasia (adrenogenital syndrome) results from a hereditary inability of the cells of the adrenal cortex to produce cortisol. Pituitary ACTH levels accordingly rise and the overstimulated adrenal glands form excessive amounts of androgen. In female children this androgen produces virilization of the genitalia (clitoral hypertrophy and labial fusion) and often polycystic ovaries. Virilization can result at any age from functioning benign or malignant tumors of the adrenal cortex.

Pheochromocytoma (chromaffinoma) is a tumor of the adrenal medulla that produces excessive amounts of norepinephrine, causing palpitations, tremors, and paroxysmal or sustained hypertension. The tumor is small, lobulated, yellowish-brown, and highly vascular. The cells are large and irregular, with granular cytoplasm. Ten percent are malignant and metastasize to regional lymph nodes, bone, and liver.

The Pineal Gland

The pineal gland or epiphysis cerebri is a cone-shaped body less than 1 cm in greatest dimension, which is attached by a stalk to the roof of the third ventricle of the brain. It has a thin capsule, derived from pia mater, which sends septa into the gland, dividing it incompletely into lobules. These lobules are composed of neuroglia and irregularly shaped epithelioid cells called pinealocytes. The pineal gland undergoes regression after age 7 and contains calcareous concretions (brain sand) after age 15. Its principal secretion, the hormone melatonin, apparently plays a role in sexual maturation and in maintenance of diurnal bodily rhythms.

Asymptomatic cysts of the pineal gland are common and of little significance. Pineal neoplasms occur typically before age 25 and are more frequent in males. They may arise from pinealocytes or neuroglia and occasionally cause ocular or neural symptoms by compression or invasion of adjacent structures. The rare teratoma of the pineal may be associated with precocious sexual development.

Review Questions

1. Why is the pituitary gland sometimes called the master gland?
2. Distinguish *acromegaly* from *gigantism*.
3. Distinguish *myxedema* from *cretinism*.
4. In which sex is thyroid disease more common?
5. What is the most frequent cause for deficiency of parathyroid hormone?
6. Define or explain: *Addison's disease, Cushing's disease, diabetes insipidus.*

26

Bones, Joints, Muscles, and Associated Structures

Gross and Microscopic Anatomy

The microscopic features of bone, cartilage, and skeletal muscle are outlined in Chapter 7. A typical long **bone** is made up of a tubular shaft or diaphysis of compact bone surrounding a marrow cavity and terminating in two expanded epiphyses of cancellous bone. The transition zone between the diaphysis and either epiphysis is known as a metaphysis. A tough membrane of connective tissue, the periosteum, invests all parts of a bone except its joint surfaces. Bones receive a rich blood supply from small vessels entering the haversian canals from the periosteum, as well as from larger vessels entering through nutrient foramina near the epiphyses. Bone growth occurs by expansion of epiphyseal cartilaginous zones called ossification centers (growth centers), which calcify when growth is complete.

The articular surface of a bone is covered by a thin cap of hyaline cartilage, which bears against a similar surface on the other bone forming the joint. Some joints also contain intra-articular plates of fibrocartilage, which provide additional shock absorption while increasing the range of articular movement. Examples are the intervertebral disks and the menisci of the wrist and knee joints. A **ligament** is a flexible but nonextensible band composed of collagenous fibers, attached to both of the bones forming a joint, and so disposed as to allow movement in some directions but not in others. Most joints have several distinct ligaments, each providing stability and limitation of movement in a certain plane. A **joint** is completely surrounded by a capsule or envelope of connective tissue, into which the ligaments blend. This fibrous capsule is lined by a vascular, somewhat redundant synovial membrane of loose connective tissue containing variable amounts of fat and secreting a viscous lubricant, the synovial fluid.

Each **muscle** is surrounded by a sleeve of feltlike connective tissue called deep fascia. The fascial coverings of adjacent muscles blend with one another and with underlying periosteum and overlying subcutaneous fascia. Muscles may be directly connected to the periosteum of the bones on which they act, but more often the attachment is by means of an intervening band or sheet of collagenous fibers. A narrow cable- or straplike connection between a muscle and a bone is called a **tendon**, while a flat, sheetlike connection is an **aponeurosis**. Tendons and aponeuroses are but sparingly supplied with blood vessels. A **bursa** is a small pocket of connective tissue lined with a lubricant-secreting membrane like that found in joint capsules, and so placed as to reduce unwanted friction between moving parts. A **tendon sheath** is a modified bursa of tubular form through which a tendon passes for part of its course.

Pathologic Study of Supporting and Connecting Structures

Bone, joint, and muscle tissue is included in amputated limbs and in surgical specimens removed after severe trauma. Any of these tissues may be sampled by open or closed (needle) biopsy. Specimens of joint tissues for pathologic study may be removed through an arthroscope. Bones and joints are ordinarily not studied at autopsy except in cases of trauma or significant disease affecting these structures, including diseases of the marrow.

Developmental, Inflammatory, and Degenerative Disorders of Bone

Generalized disorders of bone structure, whether congenital or acquired, may affect the connective tissue matrix (osteoid), the deposition of calcium, or both. **Achondroplasia** is a hereditary disorder of cartilage growth and of enchondral bone formation, which results in dwarfism with disproportionately short limbs. The epiphyses of the long bones are bulky, knobby, and irregularly calcified. Microscopic examination shows a chaotic array of osteoblasts in the ossification centers. **Osteogenesis imperfecta** arises from a hereditary defect in the synthesis of connective tissue, including the matrix of bone. Besides excessively fragile bones, affected persons have abnormal dentin and their ocular scleras appear blue because they are so thin that the choroid shows through. The cortices of the bones are thin and porous, the trabeculae slender, and the haversian canals enlarged.

In **Morquio's disease** (osteochondrodystrophia deformans), a hereditary error of mucopolysaccharide metabolism, wedging of vertebrae and other skeletal deformities result from inappropriate synthesis of skeletal matrix, and abnormal accumulations of keratan sulfate are found in cells, particularly macrophages. The hereditary defect in **Albers-Schönberg disease** (osteopetrosis, marble bone disease) is a failure of immature bone to be resorbed, with resulting excessive density of calcification. This leads to skeletal deformities, stunting of growth, and encroachment on marrow cavities with consequent anemia.

The deposition and maintenance of a satisfactory amount of calcium in bone depend on an adequate dietary supply of calcium and vitamin D and a normal level of parathyroid hormone. **Osteomalacia** is any softening of bone due to inadequate calcium content. When severe, it may lead to deformities in the bones of the pelvis, spine, and skull, and susceptibility to fracture after slight trauma. Pathologic examination shows overdevelopment of osteoid with many osteoblasts present but insufficient mineralization and enlargement of marrow spaces. Osteomalacia may result from deficiency of calcium, phosphorus, or vitamin D, or from fluoride intoxication. Failure of calcification resulting from deficiency of vitamin D in childhood, before the ossification centers have closed, is called **rickets**. In rickets there is deformity of bones, particularly in the spine and thorax, with failure of long-bone growth, curving of diaphyses, and hypertrophy of epiphyses. **Hypophosphatasia** is a familial disorder of calcium deposition in osteoid tissue. Skeletal defects include abnormal ossification of growth centers and premature closure of cranial sutures. Hypercalcemia may lead to nephrocalcinosis.

Osteoporosis refers to a reduction in the mass of bone due to both diminished organic matrix and inadequate deposition of calcium. Localized osteoporosis may result from immobilization of a limb after injury (Sudeck's atrophy) or impairment of its blood supply. Causes of generalized osteoporosis include aging, the postmenopausal state, deprivation of calcium and vitamin D, and hyperparathyroidism. Osteoporotic bone has a thin cortex, spindly trabeculae, and increased fatty material in marrow spaces, and shows increased susceptibility to fracture or collapse. Varying degrees of osteomalacia and osteoporosis may occur together.

Hormonal abnormalities can cause either under- or overdevelopment of skeletal structures. Pituitary growth hormone stimulates the normal increase in long-bone length that occurs during growth from infancy to adulthood. Deficiency of growth hormone in infancy or childhood results in pituitary dwarfism, while excess of growth hormone leads to gigantism. In either case, body proportions are normal or nearly so. When the level of growth hormone increases in adulthood, after closure of ossification centers, the result is acromegaly—enlargement and deformity of the bones of the face, thorax, hands, and feet. An excessive level of parathyroid hormone causes a condition called **osteitis fibrosa cystica** (von Recklinghausen's disease of bone). In this disorder, long bones undergo subcortical calcium resorption and show cystic degeneration and fibrous nodules ("brown tumors") along their shafts. Calcium resorption also occurs from the linings of tooth sockets (alveoli). Both organic matrix and calcium deposition are reduced in long bones. Microscopic examination shows excessive osteoclastic activity.

Osteochondrosis is a general term for a group of developmental disorders affecting ossification centers and typically occurring in early adolescence. Clinically these conditions are manifested by local pain and signs of inflammation. The limbs are often affected bilaterally. The pathologic picture varies considerably. Inflammatory changes are generally present. Osteocytes disappear from the affected ossification center and the tissue undergoes a focal degeneration and necrosis with loss of calcium. This is succeeded by a spontaneous regenerative phase, with recalcification. Often some residual deformity persists. Osteochondroses of the more common sites have specific names, as follows.

Freiberg's disease:	head of second metatarsal
Kienböck's disease:	carpal lunate
Koehler's disease:	tarsal navicular
Legg-Calvé-Perthes disease:	head of femur
Osgood-Schlatter's disease:	tibial tubercle
Panner's disease:	capitellum of humerus
Scheuermann's disease:	intervertebral cartilage
osteochondritis dissecans:	knee, elbow

Paget's disease of bone (osteitis deformans) is a disease of middle and later life, of unknown cause, in which repeated periods of bone resorption are followed by excessive attempts at regeneration. Normal bone is replaced by exuberant, inadequately mineralized osteoid. Bones are soft and easily deformed by weightbearing. The bones of the skull show increased mass, and those of the limbs become bowed. This disease is associated with increased risk of osteogenic sarcoma.

Osteomyelitis, or inflammation of bone, is usually due to bacterial infection. Although occasionally the consequence of penetrating injury, it more often results from bacteremia (hematogenous osteomyelitis). Blood-borne infection usually begins in the marrow at the metaphysis of a bone. An acute suppurative process develops and rapidly progresses to focal necrosis, partly because of thrombosis and obliteration of blood vessels. Suppuration may remain confined to a small zone, forming an encapsulated abscess surrounded by dense, sclerotic bone (**Brodie's abscess**). As a rule, however, pus advances through the haversian canals and dissects under the periosteum. Extensive damage to both the cortex and medulla of the bone typically follows, though the epiphyses and joint structures are usually spared. The devitalized portion of the bone, called a **sequestrum**, appears dull gray, rough, and pitted, and is typically immersed in pus. An exuberant granulation tissue called **involucrum** springs up along the margins of the healthy bone and calcifies, producing an irregular nodular contour. Overlying soft tissues show signs of acute and chronic inflammation and may be perforated by draining sinuses.

Tuberculosis of bone is a relentlessly chronic, destructive disease, which shows a greater tendency than pyogenic infections to attack the epiphyses of long bones. Osteoporosis commonly develops, and granulation tissue ossifies but slightly, the net effect being weakening, deformity, and destruction of bone. **Pott's disease**, tuberculous spondylitis, affects the vertebral bodies, particularly in the thoracic and lumbar spine. Growth retardation and spinal deformity typically result, and infection may extend to the intervertebral disks, the spinal dura, and the surrounding soft tissues (cold abscess), sometimes even dissecting beneath the deep fascia of the psoas muscle (psoas abscess).

Focal destructive lesions of bone occur in certain disorders of marrow that are neither infectious nor neoplastic. These include Hand-Schüller-Christian disease (an accumulation of cholesterol in histiocytes of the marrow, ocular orbits, and other tissues), Niemann-Pick disease (accumulation of sphingomyelin in marrow histiocytes), Gaucher's disease (storage of kerasin, a cerebroside, in hyperplastic histiocytes of marrow and lymphoid tissue), and Letterer-Siwe disease (nonlipid histiocytosis, a hyperplasia of histiocytes without lipid storage).

Fractures

Any breaking of a bone by force, from a "hairline" crack in the cortex to wholesale shattering, is called a **fracture**. A comminuted fracture is one in which a bone is broken into more than two pieces. In an impacted fracture the fragments are driven into one another. A break occurring at the site of preexisting disease such as a cyst or tumor of bone is called a pathologic fracture. Most fractures are accompanied by considerable soft-tissue injury. The force causing the fracture may crush or lacerate tissue, and shifting of jagged bone fragments may add further damage. The formation of a hematoma at the fracture site is the first step in fracture repair. Simultaneously, hyperemia, edema, exudation of fibrin-rich fluid, and infiltration of inflammatory cells occur as in any acute injury. The hematoma promptly organizes, the formation of granulation tissue being succeeded by deposition of a hyaline matrix for the formation of new bone. Meanwhile the margins of the fracture undergo necrosis and resorption of calcium. Osteoblastic activity now converts the hyaline matrix to a primitive, nonlamellated, "woven" bone called callus, which welds the fragments together in a rigid union. Finally this callus undergoes a remodeling process whereby its internal architecture approximates that of normal bone tissue, and the original configuration of the broken bone is largely restored.

When a fracture is not immobilized by casting or splinting, excessive movement of the fragments may prevent healing in the manner outlined above. Instead, an excessive cartilaginous matrix may be formed, which calcifies poorly and does not provide a rigid repair. This is called nonunion. Nonunion may also result when the blood supply to one of the fragments is impaired by the injury or by preexisting disease. In this case the ischemic fragment often undergoes avascular necrosis. This outcome is particularly frequent with fractures of the femoral neck and the carpal navicular. Faulty positioning of fracture fragments during and after repair is called malunion.

Cysts and Neoplasms of Bone

Solitary bone cyst is a developmental, perhaps traumatic lesion occurring most often in older children. Focal osteolysis (resorption of calcium) leaves a fluid-filled cyst (occasionally a solid fibrous mass containing giant cells) near an ossification center in a long bone, especially the femur, tibia, or humerus. The lesion is benign but predisposes to pathologic fracture.

Benign solid neoplasms of bone that must be distinguished from malignant ones include osteoid osteoma and osteochondroma. **Osteoid osteoma** forms in the cortex of a long bone, along the diaphysis. It is a small elevated mass consisting of a vascular, cellular connective-tissue center, which forms osteoid trabeculae that do not calcify, and a surrounding shell of dense, sclerotic bone. **Osteochondroma** occurs as a mushroom-like excrescence from the metaphysis of a long bone. It consists of a core of cortical and medullary bone surrounded by a knobby cap of cartilage, attached to the site of origin by a bony stalk. Osteochondromas may be multiple and may become quite large. Those developing later in life sometimes become malignant.

The commonest primary malignancy of bone is **osteogenic sarcoma**, which usually occurs in children and young adults but also affects older persons with Paget's disease or a history of exposure to radiation, as from x-ray therapy or occupational exposure to luminous paint containing radium. The tumor usually begins at the metaphysis of a long bone. The femur and tibia are especially likely sites.

Osteogenic sarcoma arises from osteoblasts, which may retain the ability to form osteoid.

In the usual sclerosing form, the bulk of the tumor consists of an abundant osteoid matrix which calcifies, forming trabeculae that radiate from the central zone. An osteolytic form is also recognized, in which destruction of the original bone is not accompanied by new bone formation. Osteogenic sarcoma is a highly lethal neoplasm that metastasizes most frequently to the lungs and the liver.

A less common malignancy of bone is **Ewing's tumor**, also a disease of children and young adults, which arises from endothelial cells of bone marrow. This is an aggressive malignancy that invades the entire shaft of the bone, elevating the periosteum with several layers of new bone formation and thus creating an "onionskin" appearance on x-rays. Grossly the tumor may contain zones of infarction and necrosis. Histologically it consists of sheets of small round or oval cells with prominent nuclei, scanty cytoplasm, and many mitotic figures. Metastasis to the lungs occurs early.

Giant cell tumor (osteoclastoma) is an uncommon neoplasm that appears as a brittle mass deforming the epiphysis of a long bone, most often the femur or tibia. Expansion can lead to erosion through the bony cortex, invasion of surrounding soft tissues, and involvement of the adjacent joint. The tumor contains zones of infarction, hemorrhage, and fibrosis, and microscopic examination shows spindle cells and giant cells resembling osteoclasts. Though histologically benign, giant cell tumors of bone often recur after excision and occasionally metastasize.

Multiple myeloma, a malignant neoplasm of bone marrow arising from plasma cells, was discussed in Chapter 18. This condition may appear in several bones almost simultaneously. Bone tissue adjacent to a zone of affected marrow undergoes osteolysis, with replacement by a demineralized, gelatinous material that may be responsible for pathologic fractures in the ribs and other bones. The cranial bones are often affected.

Metastatic tumors of bone are commoner than primary malignancies. The spine, pelvis, and femur are the most frequent sites of metastasis. Malignancies are especially likely to spread to the bone from the prostate, breast, kidney, stomach, lung, thyroid, and skin (malignant melanoma). Prostatic malignancies tend to be osteoblastic, the other types osteolytic.

Diseases of Joints

Arthritis is inflammation of some or all of the structures composing a joint. Among the many causes of arthritis may be mentioned trauma, infection, allergy, autoimmunity, degenerative changes, and metabolic disorders. Although any severe or chronic arthritis may involve both the synovial membrane and the articular cartilage, synovitis is the basic response in infectious and antibody-mediated arthritides, while chondritis is more typical of traumatic, degenerative, and metabolic joint disease.

Rheumatoid arthritis, one of the most common of the autoimmune disorders, is typically a disease of early adulthood and middle life. Its course is chronic and it can lead to severe disability and joint deformity. The smaller joints of the extremities (especially the proximal interphalangeal and metacarpophalangeal joints) are most often affected, usually in symmetric fashion. There are edema, hyperemia, and villous hypertrophy of the synovial membrane, with infiltrates of chronic inflammatory cells. Lymphocytes aggregate in typical lymphoid follicles with germinal centers. The joint capsule becomes thickened, and periarticular tissues undergo swelling and other signs of local inflammation, including formation of grossly evident subcutaneous nodules. A rheumatoid nodule is a rubbery gray mass consisting of a necrotic focus surrounded by palisades of proliferating cells. The synovial membrane becomes greatly thickened by a mass of granulation tissue called pannus, which grows across the articular cartilage and may eventually invade and destroy it. Fibrous adhesions may form across the joint, rendering it immobile (fibrous ankylosis), and these may later ossify (bony ankylosis). Osteoporosis and erosion of epiphyseal bone may ensue, with severe deformity. The course of rheumatoid arthritis is unpredictable, and temporary or permanent remissions often occur. The disease is often associated with fever, anemia, weight loss, splenomegaly, and Sjögren's syndrome.

Ankylosing spondylitis (rheumatoid spondylitis, Marie-Strümpell disease) is rheumatoid arthritis of the spine, a progressive disease of young men that affects the intervertebral joints and also the sacroiliac and costovertebral joints. Ankylosis of affected joints eventually renders them rigid. **Juvenile rheumatoid arthritis** (Still's disease), a disease of children, affects growth besides causing ankylosis and deformity of joints. It is regularly accompanied by fever, anemia, splenomegaly, and enlargement of lymph nodes.

Infectious arthritis may be due to a variety of pathogens including staphylococcus, streptococcus, pneumococcus, and gonococcus, which usually arrive in the joint via the blood. Hyperemia and edema of the synovial membrane are accompanied by an increase in the volume of articular fluid, which contains fibrin and leukocytes. The cartilage becomes dull, roughened, and yellowish-gray, and the infection may undermine it, producing zones of necrosis and detaching fragments which cannot heal or regenerate. Ankylosis may follow.

Synovitis is a feature of many systemic conditions, including scleroderma, systemic lupus erythematosus, psoriasis, Reiter's syndrome, and serum sickness.

Degenerative joint disease (osteoarthritis), which affects the articular cartilage of the larger weightbearing joints (knees, hips, and spine), occurs as a result of aging. It is an exceedingly common disorder. In the obese, it begins at an earlier age and progresses more rapidly. Initially the cartilage loses its elasticity and becomes roughened, pitted, scored, and thinned. Progressive erosion exposes the articular surface of the bone, which undergoes a condensation of its mineral content, assuming an ivorylike consistency (eburnation). Simultaneously, new cartilage proliferates about the margins of the articular surface and calcifies to form lip- or beaklike projections (osteophytes, spurs). Lipping of vertebrae often compresses spinal nerve roots, causing peripheral symptoms (pain, paresthesias, hypesthesia). Synovitis may accompany severe degenerative joint disease but pannus formation and ankylosis do not occur.

In **gout**, a metabolic disorder characterized by an abnormally high level of uric acid in the blood, deposits of urate crystals in articular cartilage can lead to extensive destruction of joints. Nodular deposits in other cartilage (e.g., that of the external ear) are called tophi.

A proliferative disorder of certain joints called **hypertrophic** or **pulmonary osteoarthropathy** affects persons with certain pulmonary or cardiac diseases (bronchiectasis, bronchogenic carcinoma, infective endocarditis). The joints of the hands, feet, wrists, and knees are principally affected. Besides thickening and chronic inflammation of synovial membranes, there is bony proliferation at the ends of long bones, producing characteristic deformity (clubbing) of digits. The periosteum and periarticular soft tissues all show inflammatory changes.

Acute or chronic trauma to a joint can cause chondritis, synovitis, or both. Traumatic synovitis is often accompanied by effusion of fibrin-rich fluid into the joint space. Bleeding into a joint is called hemarthrosis; it may occur after very slight trauma in hemorrhagic disorders such as hemophilia and Henoch-Schönlein purpura. A tear in articular cartilage, particularly in a meniscus, heals poorly if at all. A fragment of cartilage or fibrocartilage may become completely separated and interfere with joint mechanics as if it were a foreign body. Joint mice are intra-articular loose bodies formed by separation of fibrotic nodules from chronically inflamed synovial membrane.

Diseases of Muscle and Associated Structures

Albuminoid, hyaline, or waxy degeneration of skeletal muscle may occur in various conditions, including acute febrile illness, toxemia, heavy metal poisoning, and chronic nutritional deficiency. When the causative factors are removed, these disorders tend to resolve. Severe atrophy of muscle due to impairment of blood or nerve supply may be followed by replacement of muscle cells with connective tissue and permanent shortening of the muscle. Volkmann's contracture is such an irreversible change in muscles of the distal part of an extremity due to ischemia, generally following trauma. Several forms of progressive muscular atrophy are recognized, many of them hereditary and some causing symptoms from birth or in early childhood. All are related to degenerative changes in lower motor neurons in the spinal cord.

Progressive muscular dystrophy is a general term for a group of hereditary defects in the metabolism of skeletal muscle cells. In all of these conditions, muscles become atrophic in spite of normal nerve function. Affected muscles appear white or fatty and shrunken. Histologic study shows patchy, random damage to muscle cells, with edema, loss of striations, and necrosis, infiltrates of acute and chronic inflammatory cells, and replacement of damaged muscle tissue by fat and fibrous tissue. Various forms of muscular dystrophy are distinguished on the basis of clinical features. **Duchenne** (pseudohypertrophic) **muscular dystrophy** appears in early childhood and affects chiefly males. Limb muscles first enlarge and then atrophy. **Erb** (scapulohumeral) **muscular dystrophy** occurs in older children and attacks the muscles of the pectoral girdle. In contrast to these severe forms of muscular dystrophy, the **Landouzy-Dejerine** (facioscapulohumeral) **type**, affecting facial and shoulder muscles, and **Gowers** (distal) **type**, affecting muscles of the hands and feet, are milder in expression, beginning in or near adulthood and not appreciably shortening lifespan.

The defect in **myasthenia gravis** is thought to be in the neuromuscular junctions where nerve impulses are transmitted to muscle. More than half of patients with this disorder have hyperplasia or neoplasia of the thymus. Clinically myasthenia gravis is manifested by profound muscle weakness and fatigability. Pathologic changes include thinning of motor end plates and perivascular round-cell infiltrates.

Myositis (inflammation of muscle) results most often from trauma or overuse. **Polymyositis** is an autoimmune disorder coming on usually in middle life and causing atrophy and weakness of the proximal muscles. Microscopic study of affected muscles shows loss of striations, hyaline degeneration and necrosis of muscle cells with fragmentation of fibers, and perivascular round-cell infiltrates. When accompanied by a violet rash of the forehead, neck, and upper trunk, this condition is called dermatomyositis. About one-fifth of persons with polymyositis are found to have visceral malignancies. Severe contusion or tearing of a muscle, particularly in the thigh, may culminate in **myositis ossificans**, in which acute inflammation is succeeded by fibrous repair that goes on to cartilage (osteoid) formation and calcification.

Bursitis, inflammation of a bursa, results commonly from trauma or overuse. Signs of acute inflammation are accompanied by effusion of fibrin-rich and occasionally bloody fluid. Severe or chronic bursitis may proceed to fibrosis and calcification. **Tendinitis** (more accurately tenosynovitis) is inflammation of the synovial lining of a tendon sheath, again usually due to trauma or repetitive wear on the part. Acute inflammatory changes usually resolve spontaneously but may progress to formation of fibrous adhesions about the tendon and calcification. Tenosynovitis of digital tendon sheaths is usually infectious, due to pyogenic organisms introduced by penetrating trauma. A **ganglion** is a thin-walled bland cyst formed as an outpouching of a joint capsule or tendon sheath, and continuous with its synovial lining. Ganglions contain a clear, gelatinous fluid. They usually result from trauma and occasionally accompany a local synovitis.

Review Questions

1. Distinguish *osteomalacia* from *osteoporosis*.
2. Distinguish between *synovitis* and *chondritis* as forms of arthritis.
3. What is the commonest primary malignancy of bone?
4. Define or explain: *involucrum, myositis, sequestrum, tenosynovitis*.

27

The Nervous System and Special Sense Organs

The Nervous System: Gross and Microscopic Anatomy

The nature and organization of nervous tissue and neuroglia are sketched in Chapter 7. The central nervous system (CNS) is that part of the nervous system that is encased by the bones of the skull and the spinal column, i.e., the brain and the spinal cord. The adult **brain** weighs about 1350 g. Although the traditional division of the brain into cerebral hemispheres, diencephalon, midbrain, cerebellum, pons, and medulla oblongata does not accurately represent either the anatomic organization or the functional differentiation of brain tissue, it is useful for purposes of gross description. The right and left cerebral hemispheres are deeply convoluted like the surface of a walnut. The convexities are called gyri and the grooves between them are called sulci. Each hemisphere is divided by deeper grooves or fissures into frontal, parietal, temporal, and occipital lobes. The diencephalon, midbrain, pons, and medulla oblongata, lying in that order from front to back, make up the undersurface of the brain. The latter two structures are called the brain stem and are continuous with the spinal cord. The cerebellum, which looks like a miniature cerebrum, rests on the brain stem.

The central nervous system is protected by three membranes called **meninges**. Of these, the outer dura mater and the inner pia mater are dense and richly vascular sheets of fibrous connective tissue. Between them, and adherent to the pia mater, lies a more delicate meshwork of connective tissue called the arachnoid. The meninges are covered by a layer of simple cuboidal mesenchymal cells called meningothelium. Cerebrospinal fluid (CSF), a filtrate of the blood similar in composition to lymph, circulates through the hollow ventricles within the brain and under the arachnoid membrane of both

252

the brain and the spinal cord, functioning as a shock absorber. The veins of the brain empty into a set of thin-walled venous sinuses formed between folds of the meninges, which in turn carry blood to the internal jugular veins for return to the heart.

Pathologic Study of the Nervous System

Nerve tissue appears incidentally in many biopsy and surgical specimens. Biopsy of the brain may be performed to help in the diagnosis of obscure degenerative disorders. Specimens of cerebrospinal fluid obtained by lumbar or cisternal puncture may be subjected to cytologic study. When the skull is opened at autopsy, the brain and its coverings are examined for evidence of swelling, hemorrhage, suppuration, deformity, atrophy, or tumor. The brain is then severed from its connections and removed for further study. It may be opened at once for internal examination or placed in fixative for several days to harden it and facilitate cutting into thin sections.

Disorders of the Nervous System

The brain and spinal cord are subject to many kinds of developmental anomaly, some of them associated with abnormalities in the skull and spinal column or in other structures. **Cranium bifidum** is a failure of closure of the skull in the posterior midline, and **spina bifida** is a similar malformation of the spinal column. Such a defect may allow protrusion of meninges (meningocele), brain tissue (encephalocele), or spinal cord tissue (myelocele, meningomyelocele). **Hydrocephalus** is an abnormal accumulation of spinal fluid within the skull due to some blockage of its normal flow. When congenital, it leads to enlargement of the skull and expansion of the cerebral ventricles at the expense of brain substance. In the **Arnold-Chiari malformation**, parts of the medulla oblongata and cerebellum protrude from the skull into the cervical portion of the vertebral column. Often there are associated spina bifida and hydrocephalus. **Syringomyelia** is a cavitary dilatation of the central canal of the spinal cord, with loss of nerve tissue. It may be congenital or acquired. A similar condition in the brain stem is termed syringobulbia. **Tuberous sclerosis** (epiloia) includes widespread developmental anomalies, among them hamartomas of glial tissue in the brain and retina.

The response of nervous tissue to irritation, injury, and infection differs somewhat from that of other tissues. Inflammation in the meninges and other supporting structures follows the usual pattern outlined in Chapter 11. In nerve tissue, infiltration of neutrophils and mononuclear cells from the blood occurs only to a limited extent, being found chiefly just outside blood vessels (perivascular cuffing).

Injured, degenerating, or devitalized nerve cells may react by swelling, shrinking (pyknosis), vacuolation, disappearance of Nissl bodies (chromatolysis), deposition of yellow or brown pigment granules in the cytoplasm, or distortion of fibrils within cell processes (fibrillary degeneration). Dead nerve cells disappear either through liquefaction necrosis or by being engulfed by macrophages (neuronophagia).

Neuroglia participates in the response of the central nervous system to inflammation, trauma, circulatory compromise, or toxic or metabolic insult. Glial cells (astrocytes, oligodendroglia) react to these stimuli by swelling, proliferating by mitosis, clustering around damaged nerve cells (satellitosis), and forming meshworks, nodules, or plaques of glial fibrils as a repair material (gliosis). Microglial cells act as macrophages, absorbing degenerating nerve cells and their myelin sheaths.

Disrupted nerve fibers within the central nervous system do not regenerate. Peripheral nerves, however, display marked regenerative potential. **Wallerian degeneration** is a series of changes that take place in a severed peripheral nerve fiber. The portion of the axon distal to the injury swells, becomes granular, and breaks up into irregular fragments, which eventually disappear. The myelin sheath, if one is present, also fragments, forming irregular globules of lipid material before disappearing. The Schwann cells distal to the site of injury enlarge and multiply by mitosis to form a tubular syncytium that will serve as a guide for the regenerating axon. Meanwhile, the proximal end of the severed axon puts forth a bulbous projection, which eventually grows into and along the axon sheath, often dividing into numerous fibrils as it advances. A traumatic neuroma is a nodular growth consisting of an unorganized tangle of hyperplastic nerve fibers and Schwann cells and resulting from aberrant healing of a severed nerve.

Peripheral neuropathy (neuritis) refers broadly to any traumatic, toxic, inflammatory, or degenerative changes in peripheral nerves. The changes may be reversible or may lead to wallerian degeneration, with or without subsequent regeneration. Contusion, compression, or ischemia are the usual reasons for neuropathy of a single peripheral nerve (mononeuritis). Polyneuritis (involvement of several peripheral nerves, often in symmetrical distribution) can result from nutritional deficiency (thiamine, cobalamin), diabetes, bacterial toxins (diphtheria, typhoid fever), or chemical poisons (lead, alcohol, carbon monoxide). Acute idiopathic polyneuritis (Guillain-Barré syndrome) often follows viral respiratory infection.

Cerebral infarction, recognized clinically as a stroke (cerebrovascular accident, CVA), usually results from thrombosis in an arteriosclerotic vessel. Less often it arises from arterial stenosis without thrombosis, or from embolism. The zone of infarction becomes soft, even liquid, and remains so after fixation for pathologic study. Microscopic examination of an early infarct shows edema and neutrophilic infiltrates. Later, nerve cell bodies and axons degenerate, their myelin sheaths liquefying and being engulfed by microglia. During healing, a granulation tissue consisting of capillary loops and proliferating astrocytes forms a fibrous scar. Thrombosis of a venous sinus usually results when infection extends from the eye, ear, face, or jaw. This is a life-threatening condition, causing intense local congestion, meningitis, and encephalitis. Intracranial hemorrhage as a consequence of hypertension combined with vascular disease has a poor prognosis and is often rapidly fatal.

Blunt or penetrating trauma to the head causes various degrees of injury to the brain. **Concussion** implies transitory loss of consciousness without demonstrable injury to the brain or its coverings. In **contusion** of the brain there is mild interstitial hemorrhage without irreversible injury. **Laceration** of the brain involves disruption of nerve tracts and severe hemorrhage. Bleeding within the cranial cavity, usually resulting from head trauma with or without skull fracture, can cause damage or death by compressing soft brain tissue within its unyielding bony case. **Extradural** (epidural) **hemorrhage** most often results from damage to the middle meningeal artery by a blow to the temple, and may prove rapidly lethal. In **subdural hemorrhage**, the bleeding is more often venous. A subdural hematoma may gradually enlarge during days or weeks, producing progressive nervous system symptoms. The adjacent meninges show inflammatory cell infiltrates and fibroplasia. A chronic subdural hematoma often appears encapsulated. Eventually it may be resorbed, with residual hemosiderin staining of the meninges. **Subarachnoid hemorrhage** can result from trauma or rupture of a congenital aneurysm. The prognosis is grave.

When trauma to the spinal cord results in complete disruption of nerve tracts, regeneration does not occur. Compression or contusion of the cord by vertebral fracture, tumor, or herniated nucleus pulposus (slipped intervertebral disk) results initially in edema of nerve tissue, followed by either degeneration or healing, often with gliosis and fibrosis, which may result in meningeal adhesions.

Many varieties of degenerative disease, most of them progressive and of unknown cause, affect the nervous system. Only the most common will be mentioned here. Cerebral atrophy, typically a disorder of middle and later life, assumes various forms. **Alzheimer's disease** is a progressive degeneration diffusely affecting the entire cerebral cortex. Its characteristic lesions are irregular knots or clumps of degenerating fibrils within neurons (neurofibrillary tangles) in the cerebral cortex, particularly in the middle temporal gyrus; neuritic plaques consisting of fragmented axons and dendrites surrounding a central zone of amyloid; and granulovacuolar degeneration and Hirano bodies in the hippocampus. With degeneration of neurons there is progressive reduction in brain volume and weight. In **Pick's disease** the cortical atrophy is more localized, affecting particularly the frontal and temporal lobes. Degenerating neurons contain globular cytoplasmic inclusions (Pick bodies).

The principal pathologic changes of **Parkinson's disease** (parkinsonism, paralysis agitans) are nerve cell degeneration in the basal ganglia and loss of melanin-containing cells from the substantia nigra. Cytoplasmic inclusions called Lewy bodies may appear in neurons of the substantia nigra. Neurofibrillary tangles as in Alzheimer's disease also occur in parkinsonism. **Wilson's disease** (hepatolenticular degeneration), a disorder of copper metabolism, causes degeneration and cavitation of the basal ganglia and putamen. **Huntington's chorea**, a familial disorder first causing symptoms of chorea and mental deterioration in adult life, also affects the basal ganglia. **Kernicterus** results from deposition of unconjugated bilirubin in the basal ganglia of a jaundiced newborn. This condition can lead to lethargy, muscular spasticity and rigidity, and respiratory paralysis.

Amyotrophic lateral sclerosis is a progressive degeneration of motor cells in the brain stem and spinal cord and of the corticospinal tracts. **Friedreich's ataxia** is a familial disorder in which the cerebellum and ascending nerve tracts in the dorsal part of the spinal cord undergo atrophy. In **subacute combined degeneration**, resulting from deficiency of cobalamin (vitamin B_{12}) and hence associated with pernicious anemia, posterior and lateral columns of the spinal cord undergo patchy degeneration with little or no associated inflammatory response.

Multiple sclerosis is by far the most prevalent of the demyelinating diseases, in all of which, for unknown reasons, myelin sheaths of nerve fibers are lost, with deterioration of nerve function. In multiple sclerosis, irregular patches of demyelination occur throughout the white matter of the central nervous system. Destruction of myelin sheaths is followed by gliosis with formation of grossly evident yellowish-gray plaques. In **Devic's disease** (optic neuromyelitis) demyelination occurs in the optic nerve, producing blindness, as well as in the spinal cord. The term **leukoencephalopathy** embraces a group of uncommon childhood diseases resulting from defects in the formation of myelin. These include Schilder's disease (progressive subcortical atrophy), affecting the cerebral hemispheres, and Pelizaeus-Merzbacher's disease, affecting the brain stem, cerebellum, and spinal cord. In Krabbe's disease, demyelination of cerebral white matter with deposits of globoid material results from congenital deficiency of galactosylce-ramidase.

The term **encephalopathy** denotes various acute and chronic dis-turbances of brain function induced by toxic or metabolic abnormali-ties including anoxia, hypoglycemia, lead poisoning, toxemia, severe hypertension, and deficiency of thiamine (Wernicke's encephalopathy). The pathologic changes are various and may be irreversible.

Infections of the central nervous system may be caused by bacte-ria, viruses, or fungi. **Encephalitis**, or inflammation of the brain, is usually viral in origin. The viruses of mumps and herpes simplex, as well as several arthropod-borne viruses, are most often responsible. The brain is edematous, with vascular congestion and focal hemor-rhages. Microscopic examination shows widespread destruction of neurons, perivascular infiltrates of lymphocytes, and glial prolifera-tion. The virus of **rabies**, transmitted in the saliva of infected animals, causes extensive degeneration of ganglion cells in the brain and spinal cord. The brain is edematous, hyperemic, and friable. Histologic sec-tions of brain and spinal cord show degeneration and demyelination of ganglion cells, perivascular cuffing with mononuclear and glial cells, and large eosinophilic inclusions, often containing vacuoles, in the cytoplasm of undegenerated nerve cells (Negri bodies).

Several forms of slowly progressive encephalitis are thought to be due to viral infection (**slow viruses**). Creutzfeldt-Jakob disease causes spongiform degeneration of the gray matter, particularly in the cere-bral cortex. It has been transmitted in corneal transplants. Kuru, also a spongiform encephalopathy, shows a predilection for the cerebellum and occurs almost exclusively in cannibals. Subacute sclerosing panen-cephalitis (SSPE) and progressive multifocal leukoencephalopathy (PML) are rare, progressively demyelinating diseases of the brain believed to be due to slow viruses.

In **poliomyelitis**, due to a virus that enters the body by the gas-trointestinal tract, there is degeneration of gray matter, particularly of the anterior horn (motor) cells of the spinal cord, and to a lesser degree the motor nuclei of the cranial nerves. Punctate hemorrhages occur in affected areas. Microscopic examination shows swelling and chromatolysis of cell bodies with displacement of nuclei, scattered neutrophils, and perivascular infiltrates of lymphocytes. Nerve cells eventually undergo necrosis and are replaced by astroglial scarring.

Brain abscess is caused by pyogenic bacteria, which usually gain access to the cranial cavity from the middle ear or the paranasal sinuses, or via the blood stream in acute systemic infection. A cavity forms in the brain, filled by purulent, necrotic material and surrounded by a capsule found on microscopic study to consist of collagenous fibers, fibroblasts, and macrophages.

Meningitis, inflammation of the meninges, may be viral, bacterial, or fungal in origin. Typically viral (aseptic) meningitis, due to echovirus or coxsackievirus A, is mild and self-limiting. Bacterial meningitis, due to *Neisseria meningitidis, Streptococcus (Diplococcus) pneumoniae,* beta-hemolytic streptococcus, *Haemophilus influenzae,* or staphylococcus, is a life-threatening disease. The spinal fluid appears cloudy, milky, or frankly purulent. The meninges are acutely inflamed, with edema, congestion, and petechial hemorrhages. Microscopic examination shows extensive subarachnoid exudate consisting of neutrophils and tissue debris. Encephalitis (neuronal degeneration) and brain abscess may occur. In *H. influenzae* meningitis, a disease of children, a fibrin-rich exudate with a consistency like putty lies over the brain stem and may cause subdural effusion by impeding the flow of cerebrospinal fluid. **Tuberculous meningitis**, secondary to pulmonary tuberculosis, is a chronic process. A viscous greenish exudate clings to the base of the brain, and miliary tubercles are found in the meninges and often in the brain substance. **Lymphocytic choriomeningitis**, due to an arenavirus transmitted by secretions and excreta of small mammals, may progress to a severe meningoencephalitis, but complete recovery is the rule.

The variety of intracranial neoplasms is very great. Most do not arise from nerve cells. The commonest is the **meningioma**, a noninvasive, histologically benign tumor derived from various cells of the meninges, including meningothelial cells and fibroblasts. **Gliomas** are fairly common malignant tumors derived from neuroglia. Several grades of **astrocytoma** are identified. The higher the grade, the more anaplastic and aggressive the tumor. Grade I (astrocytoma) consists of well-differentiated astrocytes with hyperchromatic nuclei. In Grade II (astroblastoma) the cells are more primitive. Grades III and IV (glioblastoma multiforme) are highly cellular, anaplastic tumors containing many immature glial cells (spongioblasts) and giant cells with bizarre mitotic figures. Astrocytomas of lower grade grow slowly and may undergo cystic degeneration. The higher-grade astrocytomas are the most malignant of all intracranial neoplasms. They often contain focal hemorrhages and zones of necrosis surrounded by glial cells in pseudopalisade formation. These are the only cranial tumors that metastasize outside the cranium. Typically they spread to the lungs and the cervical lymph nodes.

Metastatic tumors frequently invade the brain from the lungs, thyroid gland, gastrointestinal tract, breast, and kidney. They tend to be globular and noninvasive and are frequently multiple.

The Eye: Gross and Microscopic Anatomy

The eyeball consists of three concentric layers or tunics. The outermost tunic, the **sclera**, is a tough shell of collagenous fibers. Anteriorly the sclera is modified to form the transparent **cornea**, through which light rays pass to enter the eye. Most of the cornea is made up of the substantia propria, which consists of many thin layers of collagenous fibers and a few fibroblasts. On the inner surface of the substantia propria lies Descemet's membrane, a thin sheet of elastic fibers, and on its outer surface is Bowman's membrane, a homogeneous layer of noncellular material covered by stratified squamous epithelium.

The second layer of the eyeball is the **choroid** layer or uveal tract, consisting of a rich vascular plexus and many pigment cells. Anteriorly the choroid layer is modified to form two concentric rings containing smooth muscle fibers: the outer **ciliary body**, which supports the lens and changes its shape for focusing, and the **iris**, the colored part of the eye, which forms the margin of the pupil and changes its size in accordance with surrounding illumination. The **lens** is a transparent, elastic structure consisting almost exclusively of layers of fibers with a sheet of simple cuboidal epithelium on its anterior surface.

The innermost coat of the eye is the **retina**, a sheet of light-sensitive nerve cells continuous with the optic nerve (the second cranial nerve) and backed by a pigment layer of hexagonal cells containing the yellowish-brown pigment fuscin. The inner lining of the choroid coat, called Bruch's membrane, is in contact with the retina. Retinal receptor cells are divided on the basis of shape into rods, which contain visual purple or rhodopsin and are concerned with vision at low illumination, and cones, which serve for the perception and discrimination of colors.

The **aqueous humor** is a lymphlike fluid filling the part of the eye anterior to the lens. It is formed by specialized tissue in the ciliary processes adjacent to the ciliary body, and after passing forward through the pupil it is reabsorbed in the canal of Schlemm, a set of endothelial spaces communicating with veins draining the eye. The part of the eye behind the lens contains the **vitreous humor**, a transparent jelly-like medium with a delicate fibrillar structure.

The orbit is a cavity formed by the bones of the skull and lined by a protective layer of fat. The eyelids are composed of connective tissue and covered on their outer surfaces by thin skin. The upper eyelid is reinforced with a tough, curved strip of collagenous fibers, the tarsal plate. Within this plate lie the meibomian glands, composed of cuboidal epithelium, whose secretion, reaching the lid margins by long straight ducts, lubricates them and renders them watertight when the eye is closed. The sebaceous glands of the eyelid, associated with lash follicles, are called the glands of Zeis, and the sweat glands are the glands of Moll.

The inner surfaces of the eyelids are covered by conjunctiva, which also covers the exposed part of the eyeball except for the cornea. Conjunctiva consists of a delicate connective-tissue layer, the substantia propria, covered by stratified squamous or cuboidal epithelium. Small follicles of lymphoid tissue are normally present in the conjunctiva. The lacrimal gland, situated in the upper outer part of the orbit, is a compound tubuloalveolar gland whose serous secretion, the tears, reaches the surface of the eye through several short ducts.

Diseases of the Eye

Congenital malformations of the eye are not uncommon, but many of them impair vision only slightly or not at all. **Coloboma** is the absence of a part of one or more of the layers of the eye as a result of failure of closure during embryonic development. Coloboma iridis, the commonest form, is a pear-shaped defect in the lower portion of the iris. **Keratoconus** is a conical bulging of the cornea, with its apex just below the midline. This malformation is associated with microscopic clefts in Descemet's membrane and deposits of greenish-gray pigment. Congenital cataract (opacity of the lens) occurs as a feature of several hereditary malformations.

Inflammatory conditions of the eye may be traumatic, toxic, allergic, or infectious in origin. **Blepharitis** (inflammation of the eyelid) is often due to chemical irritants or allergens. When caused by bacteria it may progress to ulceration and formation of pustules in lash follicles. A solitary pyogenic infection in one of the glands of Zeis or of Moll is called a **hordeolum** (stye). **Chalazion** is a cystic swelling in a meibomian gland whose duct is obstructed. Microscopic examination shows proliferation of epithelium lining the gland, with lymphocytic infiltrates, hyaline degeneration, Langhans giant cells, and liquefaction of contained debris.

Conjunctivitis (inflammation of the conjunctiva) is a common and usually self-limited disorder. In allergic conjunctivitis there are hyperemia, edema, and a stringy mucous exudate. Vernal conjunctivitis, a particularly severe allergic process, is accompanied by cobblestone granulations of the conjunctiva. Microscopic study shows these to be composed of dense fibrous aggregations with eosinophilic infiltrates. Hyaline degeneration may occur, as well as columnar metaplasia of the epithelium.

In contrast with other kinds of conjunctivitis, trachoma (caused by *Chlamydia trachomatis*) and ophthalmia neonatorum (caused by

Neisseria gonorrhoeae) are capable of causing blindness. **Trachoma** is a severe infection of the conjunctiva that quickly spreads to the cornea. The conjunctiva shows edema, mucopurulent exudate, lymphocytic aggregations, and papillary hypertrophy. Corneal ulceration is followed by a dense fibroplastic process that leaves the cornea opaque. Trachoma is the greatest single cause of blindness in the world. Extraocular infection with *Chlamydia* and other infectious agents causes Reiter's syndrome (conjunctivitis, urethritis, arthritis). **Gonococcal ophthalmia** of the newborn, occurring in a child born to an infected mother, invades all parts of the eye, leading to severe destruction of tissue.

Keratitis (inflammation of the cornea) may be traumatic or infectious. Dendritic keratitis is an acute ulcerative lesion due to the herpes simplex virus. In **interstitial keratitis**, a manifestation of congenital syphilis, there are no ulcers, but the cornea becomes diffusely opaque. **Epidemic keratoconjunctivitis**, due to adenovirus type 8, is characterized by intense edema and hyperemia. Opacities may develop in the cornea during healing, but these commonly resolve after a few months. **Arcus senilis**, a white or gray band around the margin of the cornea, results from cholesterol deposition or hyaline change or both occurring with advancing age. When ulceration or deep abrasion of the cornea removes or destroys all layers down to Descemet's membrane, **descemetocele** (keratocele) may result, with bulging of a sac or bleb of Descemet's membrane through the defect. Bulging of a part of the sclera due to trauma or inflammation, with herniation of the choroid layer, is called **staphyloma**.

Injury or inflammatory disease affecting the anterior chamber (the part of the eye between the cornea and the iris) may culminate in blindness either as a result of opacification of the cornea or by blocking drainage of aqueous humor into the canal of Schlemm and so inducing glaucoma. **Hyphema** is bleeding into the anterior chamber, usually due to trauma. An inflammatory response to such bleeding includes infiltrates of neutrophils and macrophages and may go on to fibrotic scarring of the cornea. **Hypopyon** is a suppurative process in the anterior chamber. Large numbers of neutrophils render the aqueous humor cloudy, and grayish-yellow infiltrates may appear in the cornea. Healing may be accompanied by patches of vascularization and fibrosis in the cornea.

Glaucoma refers to an abnormally high pressure within the eye due to failure of absorption of the aqueous humor. In narrow-angle glaucoma there is an abnormally acute filtration angle. In open-angle (wide-angle) glaucoma the filtration angle is normal, but reabsorption of aqueous humor is diminished all the same. Congenital and post-traumatic forms of glaucoma also occur. All chronic glaucoma lead to progressive visual impairment by causing degenerative changes in the cornea, lens, choroid structures, optic nerve, and retina.

Cataract is a general term for changes in the structure or composition of the lens that impair its transparency. In **senile cataract**, a result of aging which is often aggravated by glaucoma, albuminous deposits form between the layers of the lens, and often crystals of calcium salts, cholesterol, and amino acids are deposited as well. As a result, cloudy gray or amber streaks appear in the lens and by gradually extending and coalescing may render it opaque. Cataracts developing in poorly controlled diabetes begin as fluid-filled vacuoles within the lens and progress to diffuse, cloudy "snowflake" opacities. Cataract can also result from trauma, ionizing radiation, toxic chemicals (naphthalene, dinitrophenol), and prolonged adrenocortical steroid therapy. **Congenital cataract**, as noted earlier, occurs in various inherited malformation syndromes. In **retrolental fibroplasia**, which occurs in premature infants exposed to excessive concentrations of oxygen, a proliferation of fibrous tissue over the posterior surface of the lens renders it opaque.

Uveitis is a general term for any inflammatory condition affecting the choroid structures—iris, ciliary body, and choroid plexus. **Anterior uveitis** may affect the iris alone (iritis) or may also involve the ciliary body (iridocyclitis). These conditions may be traumatic, infectious, or allergic in origin. Iritis occurs in many systemic conditions (rheumatoid arthritis, sarcoidosis) and as a local manifestation of systemic infections (tuberculosis, brucellosis). It may follow inflammatory disease elsewhere in the eye, or injury or disease of the other eye (sympathetic ophthalmia). In Behçet's syndrome it is accompanied by oral and genital ulcers. Iritis occurs in varying degrees and may be acute or chronic. When severe it can lead to extensive destruction of the eye. In **acute iritis** the aqueous humor is clouded by cellular infiltrates, and frank hypopyon or hyphema or both may occur. The cornea assumes a steamy or dewy appearance due to keratic precipitates—grossly visible punctate infiltrates of inflammatory cells in the posterior cornea.

Chronic iritis is usually a granulomatous process, producing a diffuse or nodular fibrotic reaction. Fibrous adhesions may form between the iris and the cornea (anterior synechiae) or between the iris and the lens (posterior synechiae). These can distort the pupil and obstruct the flow of aqueous humor, giving rise to glaucoma. **Choroiditis** (posterior uveitis) has largely the same causes as anterior uveitis, which it usually accompanies. The choroid is subject to various forms of degeneration, most of them due to aging. Drusen are localized thickenings of Bruch's membrane.

The **retina** suffers various inflammatory and degenerative disorders, all of them impairing vision to some degree. **Vascular disease** of the retina associated with arteriosclerosis, hypertension, and diabetes leads to focal and diffuse degenerative changes in ganglion cells and hemorrhages that organize to form fibrotic patches miscalled exudates. Cholesterol and other lipid materials may be found in macrophages in these exudates. Capillary microaneurysms of the retina in diabetes often hemorrhage, the ensuing organization leading to focal fibrotic reaction (retinitis proliferans). **Retinitis pigmentosa** (pigmentary degeneration of the retina) occurs as a hereditary disorder characterized by degeneration of retinal ganglion cells and blotchy clumping of pigment. **Chorioretinitis**, a chronic inflammation of both the retina and the choroid layer, usually results from congenital toxoplasmosis, and causes scattered necrotic and deeply pigmented lesions in the retina. **Macular degeneration**, which affects the central and most important part of the retina (the macula lutea), is a consequence of aging. Retinal degeneration accompanied by infiltrates of foam cells (macrophages stuffed with lipid material) occurs in familial lipodystrophies (Tay-Sachs disease, Niemann-Pick disease). Trauma or degenerative changes may lead to retinal detachment, a separation of the retina from the underlying pigment layer of the choroid coat, to which it is not attached. Trauma or severe intraocular disease causing loss of aqueous and vitreous humor may culminate in phthisis bulbi, a catastrophic condition in which the eye becomes shrunken and lifeless.

Retinoblastoma, the principal intraocular malignancy, occurs primarily in children and is bilateral in one-third of cases. The tumor arises from neural cells of the retina and consists of small, tightly packed round or polygonal cells, which often form rosettes around blood vessels. Cystic degeneration, necrosis, and calcification often occur within the tumor. Invasion of periorbital tissues occurs early.

The Ear: Gross and Microscopic Anatomy

The ear is divided into three parts for anatomic study. The **external ear** is a shallow funnel of elastic (yellow) cartilage, covered and lined by skin, which serves to collect and direct sound waves. The skin of the external auditory meatus (ear canal) is equipped with ceruminous glands, which produce cerumen or ear wax. The sound-transmitting portions of the **middle ear** are the tympanic membrane, a thin, tough sheet of collagenous fibers, and the ossicles (malleus, incus, stapes), three small bones arranged in series between the tympanic membrane and the inner ear. The outer surface of the tympanic membrane is covered by thin skin, the inner surface by a simple squamous mucosa continuous with the lining of the middle ear. The auditory (eustachian) tube, by which the middle ear communicates with the pharynx, has a framework of elastic cartilage and is lined by ciliated columnar epithelium. Adjacent to the middle ear cavity, and communicating with it, are the epithelium-lined mastoid air cells within the mastoid process of the temporal bone.

The **inner ear** or labyrinth consists of a complex conical structure, the cochlea, in which sound waves are converted to nerve impulses, and the semicircular canals, which serve as position sensors for the preservation of balance. Arranged in spiral fashion within the thin bony shell of the cochlea is the organ of Corti, which responds to sound waves as transmitted through the cochlea in its fluid medium, called endolymph. The organ of Corti comprises both neural and epithelial elements. Nonmyelinated axons of nerve cells of the vestibular ganglion terminate beneath the epithelial layer, which is composed of wedge-shaped columnar sustentacular cells resting on a basement membrane and more superficial bottle-shaped hair cells. Each hair cell is equipped with a hairlike process that extends into the gelatinous otolithic membrane and receives sound waves via the endolymph. Both parts of the inner ear—cochlea and semicircular canals—send nerve impulses to the brain by the eighth cranial nerve. The structures of the middle and inner ear are seldom subjected to pathologic study because of the difficulty of gaining access to them without damaging them.

Diseases of the Ear

Congenital malformations of the external ear are common, usually bilateral, and often familial. They occur as part of various congenital syndromes. **Otitis externa**, inflammation of the external ear, is essentially a dermatitis. It may be a feature of a generalized skin disorder such as seborrheic dermatitis or may result from trauma, foreign material, or maceration of the epithelium of the ear canal by water retained after bathing or swimming. Otomycosis is superficial infection of the outer ear by a fungus.

Otitis media, inflammation of the middle ear, usually arises from upper respiratory infection (rhinitis, sinusitis, pharyngitis) by spread of infectious organisms from the pharynx through the auditory tube. Obstruction of the tube by edema at its point of entry into the pharynx is generally an element in the genesis of otitis media. Initially there are hyperemia and edema of the epithelium lining the middle ear, with an effusion of serous fluid and bulging of the tympanic membrane into the ear canal (serous otitis media). When this progresses to frank suppuration (purulent otitis media), there is danger of perforation of the tympanic membrane. Without treatment, otitis media often becomes chronic, with purulent discharge from a perforated tympanic membrane, gradual deterioration of the membrane and of the ossicles of the middle ear, and perhaps invasion of the mastoid air cells (mastoiditis).

An occasional complication of chronic suppurative otitis media with perforation of the tympanic membrane is **cholesteatoma**. This is a nodular growth of squamous epithelium apparently derived from cells in the external ear but developing into the middle ear. Grossly it is a pearly white, shiny, firm, somewhat brittle mass. Microscopic examination shows a cystlike structure consisting of a shell of keratinizing squamous epithelium surrounding a central zone of necrotic cells and debris. Although histologically benign, cholesteatomas may invade or erode surrounding tissues and cause extensive destruction. Occasionally this type of tumor arises elsewhere in the cranial cavity.

Otosclerosis is a dystrophy of the bone forming the otic labyrinth, possibly hereditary. Normal bone is replaced in patches by a spongy, vascular, hyperplastic bone, and fusion (ankylosis) of the stapes to its point of attachment to the inner ear (oval window) results in hearing loss.

Hearing loss may also be caused by degeneration of the neural elements of the middle ear. Aging, toxic substances, certain drugs (streptomycin, kanamycin, furosemide, methotrexate), and acoustic trauma (blast injury, chronic exposure to loud noise) can result in cloudy swelling, degeneration, and atrophy of hair cells in the organ of Corti.

Vestibular schwannoma (acoustic neuroma), a benign neoplasm arising from connective tissue cells in the perineurium of the eighth cranial nerve, accounts for 5–10% of all intracranial tumors. It appears as a slowly enlarging, irregular, encapsulated, nodular or cystic mass, which histologically is composed of slender elongated cells and interlacing fibers. Though it does not invade surrounding tissues it may do extensive damage by expansion and erosion.

Review Questions

1. What is the function of cerebrospinal fluid?
2. Name the three membranes that are collectively called the meninges.
3. Which of the demyelinating diseases is most common?
4. Define or explain: *cataract, cerebral concussion, conjunctiva, encephalitis, glaucoma, gliosis, keratitis, organ of Corti, vitreous humor, wallerian degeneration.*

Part V

Clinical Pathology

28

An Introduction to Clinical Pathology

Clinical pathology, as mentioned in earlier chapters, is the branch of pathology that is concerned with examinations and tests performed on body fluids such as blood and cerebrospinal fluid, wastes such as urine and feces, and abnormal products such as pus and calculi. Most of these examinations yield quantitative data, that is, they count discrete components or measure concentrations, rates, or other features of a specimen that are capable of being expressed numerically. Although many of the procedures proper to anatomic pathology are carried out in laboratories, by convention the expressions *laboratory (lab) test, laboratory (lab) work,* and so on are limited to procedures pertaining to clinical pathology.

Clinical pathology is divided into a number of branches. The names of some of these branches have double meanings, referring both to independent scientific disciplines or to specialties or subspecialties in medicine and to divisions of medical technology. **Hematology** is the study of blood. The term refers both to a subspecialty of internal medicine concerned with abnormalities in the formation and function of blood cells (such as anemia and leukemia) and to a branch of laboratory technology concerned with the performance of quantitative and qualitative assessments of blood cells.

Biochemistry deals with the chemical properties and interactions of all the substances composing the living body. **Clinical chemistry** is the application of biochemistry to diagnostic medicine. In practice, clinical chemistry refers almost exclusively to quantitative chemical analysis of blood specimens. **Urinology** is a branch of medical technology that involves basic microscopic and chemical examination of urine specimens.

Microbiology is concerned with the study of microscopic living things; medical microbiology concentrates on bacteria, fungi, and

269

other microorganisms capable of causing human disease. **Bacteriology, parasitology, mycology** (the study of fungi), and **virology** are divisions of medical microbiology. **Serology** (a branch of immunology) studies antigen-antibody reactions, particularly with respect to the diagnosis of infectious diseases.

The practice of clinical pathology thus comprises an extensive range of physical, chemical, and biological procedures. These include microscopic examination of blood and other fluids for an assessment of the number and type of cells present, both normal and abnormal, and for the identification of pathogenic microorganisms, crystals, and foreign material; qualitative and quantitative chemical analysis of body fluids, particularly blood, for electrolytes, carbohydrates, proteins, lipids, vitamins, enzymes, hormones, waste products, dissolved gases, drugs, and poisons; culture of material for bacterial, fungal, or viral growth; and biological testing for antibodies indicative of previous or current infection or of certain autoimmune disorders or other conditions.

In the following chapters, the most important of these tests will be briefly described or explained and their significance in diagnosis will be outlined. Space does not permit the inclusion of all laboratory tests in current use or the exhaustive discussion of any test.

The purposes for which clinical laboratory tests are performed are essentially the same as for any other diagnostic procedure: to supply data about the patient's condition so as to provide, if not a definitive diagnosis, at least enough information to allow the physician to start treatment on a rational basis. Laboratory procedures can be divided into two broad classes: diagnostic tests and screening tests.

A **diagnostic test** is performed on material from a patient to clarify the nature of his disease. It may be used to help the physician to distinguish among a number of diseases with similar signs or symptoms. Often it is done simply to confirm a diagnosis that has already been made on the basis of history and physical examination. Sometimes it is used to measure the severity of a disease, to assess its response to treatment, or to detect a relapse or recurrence of disease. In each of these cases, a diagnostic test is performed on someone who is sick, or believed to be sick, and there is a strong likelihood that the test will yield an abnormal result. A blood culture in a patient with signs of septicemia would be an example of a diagnostic test.

A **screening test** is one that is performed on a person who is thought to be well or in whom this particular test has a low statistical probability of proving abnormal. Screening tests are done to identify common and potentially serious medical problems before they produce symptoms and perhaps cause irreparable damage. A blood test for phenylketonuria in an apparently healthy newborn would be an example of a screening test.

There can be no sharp distinction between diagnostic tests and screening tests. The difference is largely one of clinical suspicion and statistical probability. A complete blood count done to assess the degree of blood loss in a patient who has had a hemorrhage would be a diagnostic test. The same set of examinations performed on an apparently healthy military recruit would be a screening test.

A third purpose for which laboratory testing may be performed is biomedical research, including research to develop new tests or refine existing ones.

A brief survey of the types of procedures performed in clinical pathology is a necessary preliminary to the discussion of such matters as the concept of normal, reference ranges, and the sensitivity, specificity, and reproducibility of tests.

One basic type of examination is inspection of a specimen by **light microscopy**. The specimen may be examined either in its natural state or after concentration, centrifugation, or treatment with stains or reagents to bring out features that would not otherwise be visible. Microscopic examination can yield various types of information about the material under study. The shape, grouping, and staining characteristics of cells in a fluid such as blood or urine are examples of purely qualitative observations. The size and relative or absolute numbers of various cells present are quantitative measurements. (Often such measurements are made electronically rather than optically.) The microscope is also used to identify pathogenic microorganisms in smears made directly from body fluids or from cultures; to detect and study parasites or their eggs, crystals, and foreign material; and to observe reactions such as agglutination (clumping) or lysis (bursting) of cells in various serologic tests.

Quantitative chemical analysis plays a very large role in modern clinical pathology, and new tests are constantly being developed. Most of these tests are performed on blood or its plasma or serum fractions, but urine, cerebrospinal fluid, saliva, sweat, hair, and other body products and secretions can also be subjected to chemical analysis. Chemical tests are done to measure the levels of normal bodily constituents such as blood sugar or serum calcium, and also to detect and measure substances not normally present in the body, such as waste products of diseased tissue and chemical poisons.

Medical microbiology employs two basic methodologic tools. Besides performing microscopic examinations of fresh or processed smears of pus or other materials, as discussed above, the microbiologist grows pathogenic microorganisms under controlled conditions in cultures. By providing a large number of microorganisms in pure strain, culturing enhances the microbiologist's ability to identify them. In addition, the growth pattern of the organism in the culture medium, which may contain selective nutrients, chemical indicators, or other additives, provides further identifying information. Culturing methods can also be used to test the effectiveness of various antibiotics against a pathogen. Some culturing techniques, such as a colony count of urine, yield quantitative results.

Besides performing direct examinations, measurements, and analyses of specimens, the clinical laboratory technician uses a variety of indirect methods to gather data about a patient's condition. One important type of laboratory determination is **function testing**, in which the capacity of an organ or tissue to perform its normal function is assessed. For example, a measured quantity of a substance may be introduced into the patient's body as a challenge to an organ such as the liver or kidney to incorporate or excrete the substance. The amount of this substance, or of some chemical product or derivative of it, is then measured in the blood, urine, or other fluid, and the functional integrity of the organ under study determined by appropriate calculations.

Several related tests are often performed on one specimen. A group of tests frequently performed together is sometimes called a **panel** (electrolyte panel, liver panel). There are a number of reasons for the practice of performing several tests as a group. The tests composing an electrolyte panel (sodium, potassium, chloride, and bicarbonate) are performed together on the same specimen of blood because the levels of these substances are closely interrelated, are used to calculate other values, and can change from minute to minute. A liver panel includes several tests of liver function, such as direct and total bilirubin, total protein and albumin, AST (formerly SGOT), ALT (formerly SGPT), alkaline phosphatase, LDH, ammonia, and cholesterol. Each of these tests looks at liver function from a different angle. The net result of considering them together is a better balanced and more sharply focused view of the functional status of the liver than could be obtained by doing only one or two of the tests.

Another kind of test panel allows the diagnostician to assess several possibilities simultaneously. For example, an arthritis panel, performed on a patient with acute joint symptoms, might include tests to detect rheumatic fever, rheumatoid arthritis, lupus erythematosus, gout, and metabolic bone disease. Although the patient may have none of these, and certainly does not have all of them, it is more expedient to do the tests simultaneously on a single specimen of blood than to do them one at a time, drawing blood separately for each test and awaiting the result before proceeding to the next test.

Modern laboratory medicine makes use of highly diverse and complex technology, often involving sophisticated and expensive instruments and reagents. Many tests, including frequently performed chemical analyses and counts of blood cells, are done by automatic machinery, which not only performs the requisite tests but prints the results in a standard format.

Frequently a blood specimen is subjected to an automated battery of quantitative analyses for twenty or more substances. A chemistry panel or profile of this type provides a broad range of data from a single specimen, and because it is automated it can be carried out at much lower cost than just two or three of the component tests performed individually by a technician. A chemistry panel is often performed when only one or two of the included tests are relevant to the patient's condition. In this setting, the remaining tests may be considered screening procedures.

Because most clinical laboratory tests yield quantitative results, standardization of units of measure is essential for consistency of reporting and interpretation of tests. Currently efforts are being made to establish an internationally uniform way of reporting laboratory tests. This would not only be based on the metric system but would express all concentrations in fractions whose denominators would be in whole metric units—for example, liters instead of milliliters or cubic millimeters. Widespread acceptance of this plan is far in the future.

At present, counts of blood cells are reported as the number of cells per cubic millimeter of blood. In actual practice, a measured volume of blood is diluted, and the cells in a convenient volume of this fluid are then counted, either optically or electronically. The final figure reported—for example, 4 990 000 RBC/mm^3 (red blood cells per cubic millimeter)—is obtained by calculation.

Results of chemical analysis are usually expressed as concentrations, that is, as a certain weight or volume of the substance in question per unit volume of specimen. Thus, for example, a blood sugar test might be reported as showing 124 mg/dL of glucose. This means that each deciliter (one-tenth of a liter, or 100 mL) of the blood sample was found to contain 124 mg of glucose. In practice, a much smaller volume of blood is actually tested, and the concentration per deciliter is arrived at by calculation.

For some chemical tests, results cannot be reported as weight-per-volume concentrations. For example, in testing for an enzyme in a blood specimen, the clinical chemist does not perform a quantitative analysis, which would be a lengthy and expensive procedure. Instead, the amount of enzyme present is determined indirectly by an assay of its chemical activity. If the enzyme under investigation is an alkaline phosphatase (an enzyme that breaks down phosphate in alkaline medium), then a known volume of the patient's serum is allowed to act on a known quantity of phosphate under controlled conditions. The breakdown of phosphate that occurs during a fixed time interval is then determined, and the amount of enzyme activity is expressed in some arbitrary units.

Units of enzyme activity are often distinguished by the name or names of the persons who developed the test. Thus, a serum alkaline phosphatase test result might be reported as 7.5 King-Armstrong units/dL, 3.0 Bodansky units/dL, or 1.8 Bessey-Lowry units/dL, depending on the test procedure used. Because of inherent differences in the tests, results are not directly convertible from one type of units to another. Currently there is a tendency to adopt one test procedure as a standard and to refer to the units used in that test as international units (IU).

Another type of quantitative test is the serologic titer determined by serial dilutions. Like enzymes, antibodies are identified in a serum specimen not by chemical analysis but by observation of their activity—for example, their ability to clump (agglutinate) cells or particles of latex coated with a specific antigen. In order to form an estimate of the concentration of an antibody in a serum specimen, the technician prepares a series of graded dilutions of the serum. The initial dilution might be 1:7, and each subsequent dilution half of the preceding: 1:14, 1:28, 1:56, 1:112, and so on. The various dilutions are then set out in a row of test tubes and the test material added to each of the tubes. The results of the test are reported as the highest dilution of serum in which antibody activity can still be detected. A report of 1:56 means that antibody activity occurred in all tubes up to and including the one containing the 1:56 dilution of serum, but not at 1:112 or higher dilutions.

The results of two or more tests may be used to calculate rates, ratios, or other derived values. For example, from the three standard measurements of the red blood cell included in the complete blood count—the red blood cell count, the hemoglobin, and the hematocrit—three other values, called red cell indices, are routinely determined: mean corpuscular volume (hematocrit ÷ red blood cell count), mean corpuscular hemoglobin (hemoglobin ÷ red blood cell count), and mean corpuscular hemoglobin concentration (hemoglobin ÷ hematocrit).

The principal proteins of the serum are albumin and globulin. Although these two fractions could be separately measured by chemical analysis, it is technically simpler to determine first the total protein and then the albumin concentration. The globulin concentration is then calculated as the difference between the albumin fraction and total protein.

A crucial factor in the interpretation of any diagnostic test is the concept of **normal**. For most tests, a range of results called a normal range or reference range has been established as being compatible with normal function or absence of disease or impairment. This range is ordinarily based on a statistical analysis of large numbers of results obtained by testing apparently healthy persons. Test results above or below this range are considered abnormal. For some tests, one set of normals is appropriate for women and another for men. Special sets of normal values are applied for the newborn. Most laboratories publish sets of normal ranges based on their own experience and equipment. Normal ranges quoted in the following chapters are average figures based on specific test methods. Normal ranges for some laboratories may vary widely from these figures, particularly when different methods are used. In testing for a substance not normally present in the body, such as lead or arsenic, any amount at all is considered abnormal. The results of a qualitative test—for example, a urine pregnancy test—may be reported as simply positive or negative.

An abnormal test result does not necessarily indicate abnormality in the patient. The result must be interpreted in the light of the patient's history and physical findings and of the results of other tests, or perhaps of the same test performed on different occasions. In some instances, the results of prior tests in a given patient may be the most useful indicator of what later results are to be considered normal for that patient.

Not all laboratory tests are of equal validity or reliability. Numerous factors can prevent the obtaining of a correct result, that is, a result reflecting the subject's true state of health or disease. Among these factors may be mentioned improper securing or preservation of the specimen, contamination of the specimen or of test reagents or materials with extraneous substances or microorganisms, malfunction or improper calibration of equipment, mistakes in reading or recording results, and faulty identification of the source of the specimen.

In practice, all avoidable errors are assumed to have been excluded. It is nonetheless recognized that in any procedure performed by human beings there is a certain margin of error. In addition, because absolute control of test conditions and absolute precision of measurement are never possible, some variance in test results is a built-in feature of the test itself. Hence the reference range for a test allows not only for variations from one healthy subject to another but also for limitations of accuracy inherent in the test.

An abnormal or positive test result in a subject who is healthy or free from the condition tested for is called a **false positive**. A test result that is normal or negative despite the presence in the subject of a disease or condition that would be expected to produce an abnormal or positive test result is called a **false negative**.

Several measures of the reliability or validity of test procedures are applied by statisticians. The **accuracy** of a test is its correctness, that is, its ability to yield a result that truly measures or reflects the condition under investigation. The concept of accuracy implies that there is some independent means of checking on the correctness of the test. Sometimes no such check is possible. In that case, the best indication of the accuracy of a test may be its **reproducibility**. The reproducibility of a test is its ability to yield the same result time after time when performed on the same specimen or material.

The **sensitivity** of a test is its ability to yield abnormal results consistently when performed on abnormal material. Sensitivity is usually expressed as a percent. If the sensitivity of a given test is 90%, that means that when performed on 100 abnormal specimens it would yield 90 abnormal or positive results and 10 false negative results. The **specificity** of a test refers to its ability to reflect only a specific abnormality, and not to be influenced by other factors. If the specificity of a given test is 84%, that means that when performed on 100 normal specimens it would yield 84 normal or negative results and 16 false positive results.

The terms defined in the preceding two paragraphs are often used incorrectly or carelessly interchanged. The term **precision** is somewhat ambiguous in that statisticians consider it synonymous with reproducibility, while physicists, chemists, and engineers use it to refer to the fineness of units (or to the number of significant figures) in a measurement.

The choice of method for performing a given test may be governed by such considerations as cost, speed of performance, availability of special equipment or reagents or of appropriately trained technicians, as well as the comparative sensitivity and specificity of the various methods available. It may be appropriate to accept a method yielding only 90% sensitivity if a more sensitive test costs fifty times as much. Similarly, a test that can be performed by a person having no special training in medical technology may be preferred to a test of higher specificity because of the greater convenience of doing the simpler test at a doctor's office or in the patient's home. Many types of laboratory test equipment are available in kit form for use by untrained personnel outside of a laboratory setting. Such kits may contain premeasured reagents and are often designed to yield unequivocal positive or negative results by means of a color change instead of quantitative results requiring interpretation.

The operation of most clinical laboratories is streamlined and highly efficient, and the performance of most tests quite routine. A few tests are performed only on hospitalized persons, but most tests can also be performed on outpatients, who have blood or other specimens obtained at a physician's office or at the laboratory. Most hospital laboratories perform testing on outpatients as well as inpatients. In addition, there are many free-standing or independent clinical pathology laboratories serving an exclusively outpatient population, generally on referral from physicians' offices.

Securing a specimen for laboratory study may require special techniques and special preparation of the patient. For certain tests (serum cholesterol, fasting blood sugar), the subject must have fasted for several hours before blood is drawn. For others, certain medicines or foods must be withheld for hours or days before testing.

Blood is ordinarily obtained for testing by venipuncture (phlebotomy), that is, by inserting a needle into a vein in the forearm, after antiseptic preparation of the skin, and withdrawing a sufficient volume of blood by means of a syringe or sealed vacuum tube. Other sites of venipuncture may be appropriate in some patients. A specimen for determination of blood gases (oxygen and carbon dioxide) is obtained by arterial puncture. When only a small quantity of blood is needed, an adequate specimen may be obtained by pricking a finger (in infants, a heel). At autopsy, blood can be obtained directly from the heart for diagnostic or forensic studies.

For serologic studies and most blood chemistries, the blood is allowed to clot naturally in the specimen tube. For hematologic testing and some chemical tests, clotting is prevented by the addition of a small amount of anticoagulant. Various anticoagulants are used depending on the tests to be done. Anticoagulants in common use are EDTA (ethylenediaminetetraacetic acid), sodium fluoride, sodium oxalate, sodium citrate, and heparin. All blood specimens and most others, including those for microbiologic study, are collected and stored in sterile containers to prevent deterioration caused by the growth of contaminating microorganisms. In addition, blood and most other specimens are refrigerated as an added precaution against chemical or biological change if some time will elapse between obtaining the specimen and performing the test. For a few tests, however (cold agglutinins, blood culture), refrigeration is not used because it can alter test results.

Specimens of pus, drainage, or secretions for microbiologic study are ordinarily obtained with a sterile cotton swab, which is then transmitted in a sterile tube to the laboratory. The tube may contain a nutrient solution (transport medium) to favor the survival of organisms until they reach the laboratory. Alternatively, the person obtaining the specimen may immediately inoculate a culture plate with the swab. The plate is then transmitted to the laboratory for incubation. Specimens of pleural, peritoneal, and joint fluid are obtained by surgical aspiration of the anatomic region of origin with a sterile syringe and needle.

Regardless of where a specimen is obtained, it must be accompanied by a requisition when it is submitted to a laboratory for study. The requisition is a printed form on which the person obtaining the specimen records the patient's name and other identifying data, the nature of the specimen and the manner of its collection, the test or tests required, the date, the physician requesting the test, the person or place to which the report is to be sent, and perhaps information about billing and insurance. Often the requisition is prepared in triplicate or quadruplicate on variously colored sheets. When the tests are completed, the results are entered in appropriate spaces on the requisition, which then becomes a report form. One copy is retained in the laboratory, another sent to the requesting physician, a third perhaps included in the patient's hospital record, and so forth.

Proper identification of the source of a specimen is of paramount importance in all laboratory work. The specimen container must be labeled with full identifying information, and at every step from the arrival of the specimen at the laboratory to the release of the completed report, procedures are strictly followed to ensure accuracy of identification.

Glossary

The following glossary defines a number of terms and expressions referring to clinical pathology.

aliquot A portion of a specimen that is some known fraction of the entire specimen. Quantitative analyses or other measurements performed on the aliquot can be multiplied by the reciprocal of this fraction to yield figures applicable to the whole specimen.

analyte The substance whose presence is tested for in a qualitative analysis or whose concentration in the specimen is determined in a quantitative analysis.

assay Any quantitative test; applied particularly to measurement of biological activity, as of hormones.

baseline A test performed on an apparently healthy person, or in advance of some other test or procedure, to provide a basis for comparison with results of future tests.

bench test A laboratory test performed manually by a technician, as opposed to one done by automated machinery.

borderline (adjective) Referring to a test result that is close to the border between normal and abnormal.

calibration Adjustment or correction of a testing instrument or method by means of a standard.

control A specimen whose properties are already known, which is subjected to a test or measurement as a means of calibrating an instrument or verifying the accuracy of the procedure.

> **negative control** A specimen that is known to be normal, or that should yield a negative test.
>
> **positive control** A specimen that is known to be abnormal, or that should yield a positive test.

count Any enumeration of discrete objects in a specimen, such as cells of a certain type in blood.

end point The point in an analysis at which the chemical reaction is complete, or at which reading or interpretation of test results is feasible.

high normal A quantitative test result that is near the upper limit of normal, though within the normal range.

in vitro (Latin, 'in glass') Referring to a condition, change, or reaction existing or occurring in a test tube or other laboratory vessel.

in vivo (Latin, 'in the living') Referring to a condition, change, or reaction existing or occurring in the living body.

indicator A chemical substance that changes color in the presence of certain other substances or in response to variations in acidity or alkalinity.

level A numerical (quantitative) test result showing the amount or (more often) concentration of a substance in a specimen.

low normal A quantitative test result that is near the lower limit of normal, though within the normal range.

panic level An abnormal test result level that may indicate a severe or life-threatening condition.

parameter Although this term has a specific meaning in mathematics, in medical jargon it means any variable that can be measured.

QNS Quantity not sufficient; usually indicating that the specimen submitted is inadequate for the performance of the test requested.

rate A laboratory determination involving time; usually a measure of change occurring in a specimen or reagent during a fixed interval of time.

reagent A chemical substance that is made to react with one or more other substances, usually in an analytic procedure.

slide test A test, usually qualitative, performed on a glass, plastic, or cardboard plate, strip, disc, or microscope slide; especially a test designed to be performed simply and rapidly by persons without technical training.

specimen Any material or object that is subjected to scientific examination, measurement, or analysis; generally a sample whose composition is assumed to be representative of the whole from which it is derived.

standard A material of known properties that is used to calibrate an instrument or test system or to verify its correctness.

stat Immediately; refers to medical procedures performed on an urgent basis, including laboratory testing.

substrate The material on which an enzyme acts. The substrate of a phosphatase is phosphate.

titration A measurement or analysis in which an end point is reached after a series of small additions of reagent.

turnaround time The time that elapses between the ordering of a test (or the obtaining of a specimen) and the reporting of the test results by the laboratory.

WNL Within normal limits.

Review Questions

1. Briefly explain the scope of the following branches of clinical pathology: hematology, clinical chemistry, urinology, microbiology, serology.
2. Distinguish between diagnostic and screening tests and give examples of each.
3. List some kinds of information that can be gained by microscopic examination of specimens in the various branches of clinical pathology.
4. List some reasons why several tests are often done together in a group or "panel."
5. Explain the difference between quantitative analysis of serum for a specific enzyme and determination of its activity in serum.
6. Outline the procedure for determining a serologic titer.
7. Give an example of a laboratory value derived by calculation from other laboratory values.
8. How is "normal" defined in practice?
9. What factors govern the physician's choice of a laboratory procedure when several similar methods are available?
10. Define or explain: *accuracy, reproducibility, sensitivity, specificity.*

29

Hematology

The field of hematology embraces the study of the formed elements of the blood (red blood cells, while blood cells, platelets) as well as blood typing and blood coagulation. Procedures performed routinely in the hematology laboratory include counts of blood cells, examination of stained smears of blood, and certain basic chemical tests. Typing and crossmatching of blood for transfusion are ordinarily performed in a separate laboratory associated with the blood bank where blood intended for transfusion is stored.

Most hematologic procedures can be performed on blood obtained by either fingerstick or venipuncture. Some tests, however, require more blood than can be obtained by fingerstick. Unless testing is performed as soon as the blood is removed from the body, the specimen must be treated with anticoagulant.

The basic tool of hematologic diagnosis is a group of tests called the **complete blood count**. The complete blood count comprises enumeration of red blood cells and white blood cells, determination of the hematocrit and the hemoglobin, and examination of a stained smear of the blood for the purpose of making a differential count of white blood cells, estimating the platelet count, and observing all formed elements for abnormalities of appearance. The term **hemogram** is inconsistently applied to the complete blood count or to some of the tests composing it.

As a preliminary to counting red or white blood cells, the technician combines a known volume of the whole blood specimen with a known volume of diluent. Different diluents and different dilutions are used for red blood cells and for white blood cells. The diluted specimen may be either placed in a counting chamber and the count carried out optically with the aid of a microscope, or passed through an electronic counter that rapidly registers each cell in the specimen.

282

Different settings enable the counter to distinguish between white and red blood cells on the basis of their size. Appropriate calculations yield the number of cells per cubic millimeter.

The three basic examinations of the red blood cell, nearly always performed together, are the red blood cell count, the hemoglobin, and the hematocrit. Normal ranges for all three of these tests are 5-10% lower in women than in men.

Basic information about the origin, structure, and function of red blood cells (erythrocytes) is given in Chapter 7. The normal **red blood cell count** is 4 800 000 to 5 600 000/mm³. Elevation of the count (**polycythemia** or erythrocytosis) occurs as part of acclimation to life at high altitude, in compensation for certain forms of pulmonary and cardiovascular disease that impair oxygenation of tissues (pulmonary hypertension, pulmonary emphysema, cardiac valvular lesions), as a feature of some hematologic malignancies, in hypernephroma, and as an idiopathic overproduction of red blood cells (polycythemia vera). Reduction of the red blood cell count (**anemia** or erythrocytopenia) reflects either diminished production of red blood cells (deficiencies of iron, protein, or vitamins; disease or destruction of bone marrow), increased hemolysis (hemolytic anemias, chemical poisoning, transfusion reaction, toxemia, burns, malaria), or acute or chronic hemorrhage.

The **hemoglobin** content of blood (all of it normally within red blood cells) is determined by a quantitative chemical test. The normal hemoglobin level is 12 to 16 g/dL. Broadly speaking, changes in this level are due to changes in the red blood cell count, and occur for the same reasons.

The **hematocrit** is that fraction of whole blood that is composed of cells. A tube of blood is spun at high speed in a centrifuge. This causes the cells to settle rapidly by centrifugal force. The column of cells is then measured as a fraction of the total column of blood in the tube. The normal hematocrit reading is 40 to 48% (or 40 to 48 mL/dL). The hematocrit is sometimes referred to as the volume of packed cells. When the procedure is carried out on a specimen of fingerstick blood in a capillary tube, it is called a microhematocrit. Because the hematocrit measures roughly the same thing as the preceding two tests, changes in hematocrit occur for the same reasons as in those tests.

It is, however, possible to obtain more specific information about abnormalities in red blood cells by determining the **red cell indices**. These values involve no additional testing of blood but are derived by calculation from the three tests just described. Normal ranges for red cell indices are the same for men and women.

The **mean corpuscular volume** (MCV) is found by dividing the hematocrit by the red blood cell count. The normal range is 82 to 92 cubic microns (or 82 to 92 cubic micrometers). Increase in the mean corpuscular volume (**macrocytosis**) means that red blood cells are larger than normal. Because this generally results from defective synthesis of red cells due to lack of vitamin B_{12}, folic acid, or both, macrocytosis is frequently accompanied by reduction in the red blood cell count (macrocytic anemia). Macrocytosis occurs in pernicious anemia and in some anemias associated with pregnancy, alcoholism, hepatic cirrhosis, and malabsorption syndromes. Reduction in mean corpuscular volume (**microcytosis**) occurs in anemias due to deficiency of iron or to chronic blood loss or hemolysis.

The **mean corpuscular hemoglobin** (MCH) is found by dividing the total hemoglobin by the red blood cell count. The normal range is 27 to 31 picograms (or 27 to 31 micromicrograms). This value, representing the average weight of hemoglobin per red blood cell, is of limited significance. A more useful figure is the **mean corpuscular hemoglobin concentration** (MCHC), computed by dividing the hemoglobin by the hematocrit. The mean corpuscular hemoglobin concentration is normally between 32 and 36 g/dL. An increase in this concentration (**hyperchromia**) occurs in hereditary spherocytosis. Reduction of MCHC (**hypochromia**) is characteristic of anemias due to deficiency or malabsorption of iron, certain hereditary anemias, and chronic blood loss.

The origins, structural features, and functions of white blood cells (leukocytes) are discussed in Chapter 7. The normal **white blood cell count** is 5000 to 10 000/mm^3. Elevation of the white blood cell count (**leukocytosis**) occurs in acute or chronic inflammation of any cause and in leukemia and some lymphomas. Depression of the white blood cell count (**leukopenia**) results from suppression of their production by toxic substances, chemotherapy, radiation, or disease of hematopoietic tissue.

The white blood cell count is of limited usefulness in diagnosis. Interpretation of variations in this count depends on the relative numbers of the various white blood cells present. This information is obtained by performing a **differential white blood cell count** (often called simply a differential), a tally of the various types of white cells as identified in a stained smear of blood. The smear is made by spreading two or three large drops of fresh whole blood very thinly across a microscope slide. The smear is air-dried and flooded with a methanol-based polychrome stain such as Wright's (methylene blue and eosin) or Giemsa's (azure II and azure II eosin), which quickly and simultaneously colors nuclear material blue and cytoplasm pink. Usually one hundred white blood cells are counted and the number of each cell type found is expressed as a percent. Differential counting can also be performed electronically, but this method, which distinguishes cells by size, cannot identify abnormalities of cell structure or maturity.

The following table shows normal ranges for the six types of cell encountered in a smear of normal blood. The figures in the middle column are percents obtained by differential counting. Those in the right column are absolute counts of the various cell types, computed by multiplying the percent of each type by the total white blood cell count.

Cell Type	Differential Count	Absolute Count
Neutrophils, segmented	40–70%	2000–6500/mm^3
Neutrophils, bands	4–8%	200–800/mm^3
Eosinophils	2–4%	100–400/mm^3
Basophils	0–1%	40–60/mm^3
Monocytes	4–6%	200–600/mm^3
Lymphocytes	25–40%	1250–4000/mm^3

Variations in the relative numbers of mature (segmented) and immature (band) forms of neutrophils may result from the use of different criteria for segmentation of the nucleus. Some observers consider any constriction in a neutrophil nucleus as evidence of segmentation, while others count all neutrophils as band cells unless their nuclei are separated into at least two lobes with only filamentous connections.

Increase in the absolute number of neutrophils (**neutrophilia**) occurs in acute bacterial infections, toxemia, uremia, acidosis, burns, and myeloproliferative diseases (leukemia, lymphoma). The more acute and intense the neutrophilic response, the greater the number of immature cells (bands) that are likely to be present. An increase in the percent of band cells is called a **shift to the left** or a left shift because at one time cell counts were recorded on a form in which the column for band cells was to the left of the column for mature neutrophils. Relative neutrophilia (increased percent of neutrophils in the differential count without absolute increase) occurs when the absolute number of lymphocytes is reduced.

Reduction in the absolute neutrophil count (**neutropenia**) occurs in toxic states, chemical poisoning (arsenic, antimetabolites, sulfonamides), typhoid fever, some viral infections (measles, influenza), overwhelming bacterial infection, and miliary tuberculosis, and after irradiation. A relative neutropenia without reduction in absolute number of circulating neutrophils appears when there is a marked increase in the absolute number of lymphocytes.

An increase in the number of eosinophils (**eosinophilia**) occurs in various allergic states (asthma, urticaria), parasitism (trichinosis, echinococcosis), polyarteritis nodosa, sarcoidosis, diseases of hematopoietic tissue (Hodgkin's disease, chronic myelogenous leukemia), and after splenectomy. A decrease in the number of eosinophils (**eosinopenia**) occurs after chemotherapy, irradiation, or treatment with adrenocortical steroid.

An increase in the number of basophils (**basophilia**) is seen in chronic myelogenous leukemia, polycythemia, Hodgkin's disease, and after splenectomy. A decrease in the number of basophils (**basopenia**) occurs in hyperthyroidism and after chemotherapy, irradiation, or administration of adrenocortical steroid.

An increase in the absolute number of lymphocytes (**lymphocytosis**) is typical of many viral infections (mumps, infectious hepatitis, infectious mononucleosis), tuberculosis, brucellosis, thyrotoxicosis, and lymphatic leukemia. Relative lymphocytosis accompanies marked neutropenia. Absolute reduction in lymphocytes (**lymphopenia**) is seen in autoimmune disorders, particularly systemic lupus erythematosus, and in some congenital and acquired immune deficiencies. Relative lymphopenia occurs with absolute neutrophilia.

An increase in the number of monocytes (**monocytosis**) occurs in some infections due to bacteria (tuberculosis, infective endocarditis), rickettsiae (typhus, Rocky Mountain spotted fever), or protozoa (malaria, trypanosomiasis), and in some collagen diseases, sarcoidosis, Hodgkin's disease, polycythemia vera, and monocytic leukemia. Reduction in the number of monocytes (**monocytopenia**) is not often recognized but may accompany conditions involving destruction or suppression of bone marrow.

A marked rise in the white blood cell count (over 50 000/mm^3) usually indicates leukemia. Occasionally, however, such a rise reflects a very severe infection or toxemia with intense cellular response. Extreme leukocytosis in the absence of leukemia is called a **leukemoid reaction**. Myelocytic, lymphocytic, and monocytic forms are recognized.

In addition to the six normal types of cell discussed above, several others are occasionally identified in the stained blood smear. **Immature cells** of the myelogenous line not normally found outside the marrow, and immature lymphatic cells not normally found outside lymphoid tissue, may appear in the blood in leukemias or lymphomas or as part of a leukemoid reaction. **Atypical lymphocytes** (also called Downey cells or virocytes) are large lymphocytes with pale or foamy cytoplasm and prominent oval or horseshoe-shaped nuclei resembling those of monocytes. These occur in lymphatic leukemia, brucellosis, viral hepatitis, and various other viral infections. When they exceed 10% of all white blood cells they are virtually diagnostic of infectious mononucleosis. **Plasma cells** appear in peripheral blood in multiple myeloma, plasma cell leukemia, and some viral infections. Coarse basophilic stippling in the cytoplasm of neutrophils, known as **toxic granulation**, usually indicates severe infection or toxemia.

The examination of a stained smear of the blood also enables the hematologist or technician to observe the red blood cells for abnormalities of size, shape, or appearance. Abnormalities of size (macrocytosis, microcytosis) can, however, be more precisely identified by computing the mean corpuscular volume. The degree of variation in red blood cell size can be measured by an electronic counter at the same time as the red blood cell count. The red cell distribution width (RDW) is normally less than 15%, which means that the smallest cell counted varies less than 15% in size from the largest cell counted. Greater variation in red cell size (**anisocytosis**) occurs in many disorders associated with abnormal erythropoiesis, including congenital hemolytic anemias and anemias occurring in deficiency states or chronic disease.

Abnormalities of red cell shape include **spherocytosis** (spherical shape), **ovalocytosis** (oval shape), and **sickling** (sickle shape). Each of these indicates abnormality in the chemical structure of the red blood cell. **Target cells** are erythrocytes with a bull's-eye appearance due to flattening of the cell with a prominent spot of hemoglobin in the center. **Burr cells** have a crinkled profile because of abnormal cytoplasmic architecture. **Nucleated red blood cells** are marrow forms released prematurely into the circulation. Recently formed erythrocytes may contain remnants of nuclear chromatin called **Howell-Jolly bodies**.

In addition to performing a differential count of white blood cells and assessing red blood cell morphology, the technician examining a stained smear of blood estimates the number of platelets present as normal, increased, or decreased. Platelets are discussed further at the end of this chapter under Coagulation.

A large number of hereditary disorders in the synthesis of hemoglobin and the formation of red blood cells have been identified. Information about some of these is presented in Chapter 10. Some of these disorders can be diagnosed on the basis of red cell indices and red cell morphology, but for most of them diagnostic confirmation depends on electrophoretic analysis of hemoglobin. Numerous variants of normal hemoglobin, differing in the amino acid sequences of the globin fraction, occur in the red blood cells of persons with hereditary disorders of hematopoiesis. Often several abnormal hemoglobins are found in the same person. Some hereditary disorders of hemoglobin formation (**hemoglobinopathies**) are without symptoms, but many are associated with diminished production of red blood cells, and most with excessive hemolysis. Hence they are characterized by mild to severe anemia and are often classed as **hereditary** (or **congenital**) **hemolytic anemias**.

Normal adult hemoglobin is designated hemoglobin A. The most commonly encountered abnormal hemoglobin is hemoglobin S, which is characteristic of sickle cell anemia. Hemoglobins C, D, and E are associated with varying degrees of impairment. In some persons, fetal hemoglobin (hemoglobin F) continues to be formed in significant proportions throughout life.

Although persons with some congenital hemolytic anemias may remain asymptomatic, all are at increased risk of certain pathologic changes. Jaundice may appear at times of increased hemolysis. Since most of this hemolysis occurs in the spleen, chronic enlargement of that organ is common. Splenomegaly and hepatomegaly may also indicate extramedullary hematopoiesis. Heightened hemolytic activity raises the bilirubin content of bile and predisposes to cholelithiasis and cholecystitis. Persons with severe hemolytic disease are subject to widespread thrombosis in small vessels and to ischemic ulcers of the legs. Hemolytic crises may be precipitated by reduction in atmospheric oxygen, impairment of pulmonary gas exchange, infection, or other severe physical stress.

The most frequently encountered congenital hemolytic anemia is **sickle cell anemia**, which affects 1 in 600 American blacks. Persons with sickle cell trait (the heterozygous form) produce some red blood cells containing hemoglobin S, and persons with sickle cell disease (the homozygous form) produce more. Red cells containing hemoglobin S tend to assume a sickle shape, particularly under conditions of reduced oxygen tension, and to rupture. Although sickle cell trait is often asymptomatic, sickle cell disease commonly causes developmental abnormalities (cardiomegaly; long, thin extremities), splenomegaly, and recurrent bouts of abdominal and extremity pain. Persons with sickle cell disease are also subject to aseptic necrosis of long bones and to infections with *Salmonella* organisms.

Thalassemia (Mediterranean anemia, Cooley's anemia) is more common in persons of Mediterranean or Far Eastern ancestry. It is associated with abnormal structure of the red blood cell (target cells) and with varying amounts of hemoglobin C, E, and F. Like sickle cell anemia, it occurs in a milder heterozygous form (thalassemia minor) and a more severe homozygous form (thalassemia major). Symptoms and complications are, however, generally milder than in sickle cell anemia. In **hereditary elliptocytosis** (ovalocytosis, Dresbach syndrome), some red blood cells have an oval or cigar shape, and variable amounts of hemoglobin C are present. Because some of the red blood cells in **hereditary spherocytosis** are rounded instead of flattened, they are more readily hemolyzed by changes in osmotic environment. Hereditary **deficiency of glucose-6-phosphate dehydrogenase** (G-6-PD) in red blood cells, also called favism, is a type of hemolytic anemia in which red cells are subject to hemolysis after exposure to certain drugs (primaquine, sulfonamides, nitrofurans), chemicals (methylene blue, toluidine blue), and foods (fava beans). This disorder, which is believed to be the commonest inborn error of metabolism, is frequently asymptomatic.

In addition to electrophoresis to detect aberrations in amino acid structure, hemoglobin can be subjected to chemical testing to identify the presence of abnormal products or compounds resulting from various intoxications. **Methemoglobin** is a form of hemoglobin in which ferrous iron has been oxidized to the ferric state. This form of hemoglobin does not function in oxygen transport. A small amount (less than 3% of total hemoglobin) is normally present. The level is increased in rare hereditary metabolic errors and after absorption of certain oxidizing agents (nitrobenzene, phenylhydrazine, primaquine, nitrates).

The potential gravity of carbon monoxide poisoning is due largely to the fact that hemoglobin shows a greater affinity for carbon monoxide than for oxygen. Measuring the concentration in the blood of **carboxyhemoglobin** (the compound formed by hemoglobin and carbon monoxide) provides evidence of carbon monoxide intoxication and permits assessment of its severity. A level above 5% of total hemoglobin indicates carbon monoxide poisoning. Similarly, hydrogen sulfide poisoning can be detected by determination of **sulfhemoglobin** (sulfmethemoglobin), and cyanide poisoning by determination of **cyanmethemoglobin**.

Other tests performed on red blood cells in the hematology laboratory include the sickle cell preparation, the osmotic fragility test, the reticulocyte count, and the erythrocyte sedimentation rate. In a **sickle cell preparation**, blood is incubated at reduced oxygen tension and the red cells are observed through a microscope for sickling. The **osmotic fragility test** involves incubating specimens of blood in tubes of sterile saline solution of varying osmotic concentration (osmolality), and observing in which tubes hemolysis occurs. Osmotic fragility is increased—that is, hemolysis occurs at osmolalities more nearly normal—in spherocytosis and most other congenital and acquired hemolytic anemias, including those accompanying certain malignancies. Osmotic fragility is reduced—that is, hemolysis occurs at lower osmolalities than with normal red blood cells—in sickle cell anemia, thalassemia, and iron deficiency anemia and some other microcytic anemias.

As mentioned earlier, very young erythrocytes (erythrocytes recently released from the bone marrow into the circulation) may show remnants of nuclear material in their cytoplasm in a stained blood smear. Vital staining (addition of a stain such as methylene blue to whole blood that has been treated with anticoagulant) provides a more distinctive visualization of this material. A smear made of blood after vital staining shows basophilic material forming an irregular network in the cytoplasm of younger red blood cells, which are called reticulocytes. The normal reticulocyte count is 0.5 to 1.5% of all red blood cells. Increase in this count (**reticulocytosis**) suggests heightened erythropoiesis in response to blood loss or hemolysis.

The **erythrocyte sedimentation rate** (ESR, sed rate) is the rate at which red blood cells in a specimen of whole blood, treated with anticoagulant and allowed to stand in a glass column of standard dimensions, settle by gravity to the bottom of the tube. The sedimentation rate (corrected for abnormalities in the hematocrit) is reported as mm/h (millimeters per hour) of settled red blood cells. The normal range depends on the procedure used but is always higher for women than for men. The erythrocyte sedimentation rate is not primarily a reflection of red cell structure or function. It is increased in many acute and chronic inflammatory conditions (viral hepatitis, tuberculosis, acute rheumatic fever, rheumatoid arthritis), acute myocardial infarction, various toxic states, and various malignancies including particularly those accompanied by production of abnormal globulins. Although highly nonspecific, the sedimentation rate is useful in monitoring the course of certain disorders such as rheumatic fever and some malignancies.

Blood Typing

Although all normal blood has approximately the same chemical composition, the antigenic properties of blood vary from person to person. That is, the plasma of some persons contains antibody that will agglutinate (clump) and hemolyze the erythrocytes of some other persons. The classification of blood according to the antigenic properties of the red blood cells is known as blood typing or grouping. The blood type of an individual is genetically determined and remains unchanged throughout life. Blood typing is of paramount importance in blood transfusion and in the diagnosis and treatment of certain conditions associated with pregnancy.

The most important antigen-antibody relationships of the red blood cell are those involved in the ABO system. The essential facts regarding this system are set forth in the following table.

Blood Type	Agglutinogens in Red Cells	Agglutinins in Serum
A	A	anti-B
B	B	anti-A
AB	A and B	none
O	none	anti-A and anti-B

If blood from a type A donor is given to a type B recipient, the anti-A agglutinin in the recipient's serum will agglutinate the donor's red blood cells. To a lesser extent, donor anti-B agglutinin will agglutinate the recipient's red blood cells. A hemolytic reaction due to transfusion of incompatible blood is manifested by fever, chills, shock, and renal failure. The mortality rate is high.

A second kind of erythrocyte antigen is that of the Rh system. About 85% of the population are Rh positive, that is, their red blood cells contain the Rh antigen, which the other 15% lack. Persons who are Rh positive have no antibody to the Rh antigen, and do not form it. Although persons who are Rh negative also lack such antibody at birth, they are capable of forming it after challenge with Rh positive blood. A person who is Rh negative may receive a first transfusion of Rh positive blood with impunity. After forming antibody to the Rh antigen in this blood, however, such a person may not receive further transfusions of Rh positive blood without risk of hemolytic reaction.

Because the Rh positive blood type is transmitted genetically as a dominant trait, an Rh negative woman can conceive and bear an Rh positive child if the father is Rh positive. Although mixing of fetal and maternal whole blood does not normally occur, it may result from minor trauma or during parturition. The mother may then form anti-Rh antibody and continue to do so throughout life. During subsequent pregnancies this antibody, diffusing across the placenta, will hemolyze fetal Rh positive red blood cells, causing the condition known as **hemolytic disease of the newborn** or erythroblastosis fetalis. An Rh positive child born to a previously sensitized Rh negative mother develops jaundice at birth or shortly thereafter because of extensive hemolysis, and nucleated (immature) red blood cells appear in the fetal circulation. Hemolytic disease of the newborn can also result from incompatibility in the ABO system, but this is seldom serious.

Other blood groups that may be of clinical importance are Duffy (Fy), Kell (K), Kidd (Jk), Lewis (Le), and Lutheran (Lu). Testing for these and other minor groups finds its principal application in attempts to disprove paternity. If blood specimens are available from the child, its mother, and the putative father, nonpaternity can be proved in a majority of cases by exhaustive blood grouping.

All blood intended for **transfusion** is typed in the ABO and Rh systems by application of specific agglutinins (anti-A, anti-B, anti-Rh) and observation for clumping of cells. The blood of a prospective transfusion recipient is also typed. Before transfusion, each unit of blood is crossmatched with the blood of the prospective recipient. That is, donor cells are mixed with recipient serum (major crossmatch) and recipient cells are mixed with donor serum (minor crossmatch). Any agglutination or hemolysis in either major or minor crossmatch is evidence of incompatibility and a contraindication to transfusion of that unit of blood to that recipient. In the standard crossmatch procedure, separate major and minor cell-serum mixtures are made in saline, in albumin solution, and in a solution containing antiglobulin to enhance sensitivity.

Blood Coagulation

Blood clots when the soluble plasma protein fibrinogen is converted to insoluble fibrin. Normally this occurs after another plasma protein, prothrombin, is converted to thrombin. Activation of prothrombin can come about through a number of alternative biochemical pathways, variously involving platelets, tissue factors, and plasma proteins other than prothrombin and fibrinogen. All known coagulation mechanisms require the presence of calcium. In addition, Factor V (labile factor), Factor VII (stable factor, proconvertin), Factor VIII (antihemophilic globulin, AHG), Factor IX (Christmas factor), Factor X (Stuart-Prower factor), and Factor XI (plasma thromboplastin antecedent) are all necessary for normal coagulation.

Disorders of coagulation (**coagulopathies**) can be either congenital or acquired. Deficiency or lack of any of the plasma clotting factors, including fibrinogen and prothrombin, can occur as an isolated genetic defect. Classical **hemophilia** (hemophilia A), due to congenital deficiency of Factor VIII, is transmitted as a sex-linked recessive trait, carried by females but expressed only in males. **Hemophilia B**

(Factor IX disease, Christmas disease) shows a similar pattern of inheritance. Acquired deficiency of prothrombin (hypoprothrombinemia) is more frequent than congenital deficiency. It can result from deficiency of vitamin K (an essential chemical building block for prothrombin), hepatic disease (particularly biliary obstruction, which blocks absorption of vitamin K by preventing passage of bile salts into the bowel), or treatment with coumarin anticoagulants. Acquired or congenital deficiency of plasma clotting factors causes a hemorrhagic tendency of variable severity characterized by prolonged bleeding from wounds, hematoma formation, hemarthrosis, and hematuria.

In contrast, congenital or acquired deficiency of platelets (**thrombocytopenia**) is associated with petechiae or purpura. Frank or severe hemorrhage occurs less frequently. **Idiopathic thrombocytopenic purpura** (ITP) is an autoimmune disorder of children, usually benign and self-limited. In **thrombotic thrombocytopenic purpura**, deficiency of platelets may be accompanied by hemolytic anemia, renal impairment, and bizarre neurologic manifestations. The acute form may progress rapidly to a fatal termination. In **Glanzmann's disease** (thrombasthenia), the platelet count is normal but platelet function is impaired.

Hemorrhagic manifestations, usually purpuric, also occur in certain diseases of blood vessels. In hereditary hemorrhagic telangiectasia (Osler-Weber-Rendu disease), recurrent bleeding occurs from telangiectases in the skin and mucous membranes. Von Willebrand's disease is a hereditary hemorrhagic disorder, often mild, characterized by deficiency of Factor VIII, abnormal platelet function, and vascular abnormalities. Examples of acquired vascular disorders accompanied by purpuric bleeding include Henoch-Schoenlein purpura, Cushing's syndrome, and scurvy.

Disseminated intravascular coagulation (DIC), which results from imbalance between the mechanisms of coagulation and of fibrinolysis, can be induced by infection (meningococcal meningitis, Rocky Mountain spotted fever, septicemia), trauma, shock, complications of pregnancy and parturition, and myelocytic leukemia. Clinical manifestations range from widespread bleeding to widespread intravascular thrombosis, and both of these may occur together.

Precise diagnosis of a hemorrhagic disorder depends on the results of several basic tests, which are often performed together as a coagulation panel: bleeding time, clotting time, platelet count, prothrombin time, partial thromboplastin time, and clot retraction. In addition, plasma assay for specific coagulation factors is possible.

Unlike the other procedures mentioned, the **bleeding time** is performed directly on the patient. A small puncture wound is made with a sterile lancet in a convenient place such as an earlobe. The time required for bleeding to stop is called the bleeding time. The normal value when the test is performed by either of the standard methods (Duke or Ivy) is less than four minutes. The bleeding time is prolonged in deficiencies or abnormalities of platelets and in von Willebrand's disease.

The **clotting time** is the time required for a specimen of whole blood, obtained by venipuncture, to coagulate. The normal clotting time by the standard Lee-White method is 6 to 17 minutes. The clotting time is prolonged in deficiency of fibrinogen or of some other plasma clotting factors and after administration of heparin. This test is used to monitor heparin therapy.

The **platelet count** is performed by methods analogous to those for the red and white blood cell counts (optical or electronic). The normal platelet count is 150 000 to 300 000/mm^3 The platelet count may be increased in collagen diseases and some malignancies, particularly those of the bone marrow. The platelet count is decreased in idiopathic thrombocytopenic purpura, thrombotic thrombocytopenic purpura, and disease or toxic states associated with damage to the bone marrow.

The **prothrombin time** (pro time or PT) test is performed by adding a combination of calcium and thromboplastin to a specimen of plasma previously treated with an anticoagulant to bind the calcium that is naturally present. (Thromboplastin is a generic term for substances that convert prothrombin to thrombin.) The prothrombin time is the time required for a clot to form. The results of the prothrombin time test are expressed as both a time (for example, 14 seconds) and a ratio (more correctly, a quotient) obtained by dividing the patient's prothrombin time by a control value for normal serum. Because the potency of thromboplastins varies from one source or batch to another, the precision of the prothrombin time test is enhanced by multiplying the test ratio by a sensitivity index determined for each lot. The resulting International Normalized Ratio has worldwide applicability regardless of the source of the thromboplastin, and makes possible international dialog and accord on diagnostic and therapeutic standards referring to coagulation and its disorders. Prolongation of the prothrombin time, and hence increase of the ratio above 1.0, occurs in deficiency of prothrombin (which may be due to hepatic disease or deficiency of vitamin K), Factor V, Factor VII, Factor IX, or fibrinogen, and after administration of coumarin anticoagulants. This test is used to monitor therapy with coumarin anticoagulants.

The **partial thromboplastin time** (PTT), a modification of the prothrombin time test in which a phospholipid preparation is substituted for thromboplastin, is a more sensitive indicator of deficiency of plasma coagulation factors. The normal PTT is 22 to 37 seconds. Prolongation may be due to deficiency of fibrinogen or of Factor V, Factor VIII, Factor IX, Factor XI, or Factor XII.

One hour or less after a clot forms in whole blood, it begins to retract, that is, to shrink and separate from the portion of the plasma that is still fluid, which is known as serum. Normally this retraction is complete in about six hours, but it may take as long as 24 hours. **Clot retraction** is a function of platelet activity. Prolongation or failure of clot retraction, as measured under standard conditions in the laboratory, indicates either deficiency of platelets or impaired platelet function (thrombasthenia).

Review Questions

1. What examinations make up the complete blood count?
2. List the three basic causes of anemia.
3. How is the hematocrit measured?
4. Distinguish *macrocytosis, microcytosis, hyperchromia,* and *hypochromia* of red blood cells.
5. What routine procedure is used to enhance the diagnostic value of the white blood count?
6. Explain what is meant by saying that lymphocytosis causes a relative neutropenia.
7. What is a leukemoid reaction?
8. What are atypical lymphocytes and what is their clinical significance?
9. What are some symptoms and pathologic features common to most congenital hemolytic anemias?
10. What is the significance of the reticulocyte count?
11. Cite one major difference between agglutinin to type A red blood cells in the ABO system and agglutinin to Rh positive cells in the Rh system.
12. Distinguish *major* and *minor crossmatches.*
13. List some basic tests that are included in a coagulation panel.
14. What is the significance of clot retraction?

30

Chemical Examination of the Blood

Thousands of test procedures are currently available to the clinical laboratory technician to identify and measure hundreds of chemical substances in the blood. Some of these procedures are rarely performed because they are expensive, require special equipment, pertain to rare diseases or conditions, or have been superseded by tests that are cheaper, simpler, faster, more sensitive, or more specific. Others are performed by the tens of thousands every day in laboratories throughout the world. Most of the tests discussed in this chapter are within the standard repertory of virtually all clinical chemistry laboratories.

Although every chemical test of the blood starts with a specimen of whole blood, the initial processing of this specimen varies depending on the type of test to be done. Most chemical tests of the blood seek to determine the concentration of substances in the plasma. Because the concentration of some of these substances (for example, potassium, phosphorus, and some enzymes) is much higher in normal red blood cells than in normal plasma, the cellular elements of the blood must be removed before chemical testing begins.

Although this could be done by allowing the blood to coagulate naturally and waiting for the clot to separate from the serum, this method involves considerable delay and does not yield consistent serum fractions. In practice, the cells are separated from the plasma as soon as possible in a centrifuge, which spins the specimen at high speed so that the cells are caused to sediment rapidly and completely. One type of centrifuge tube, called a separator tube, contains a plug of semisolid material whose specific gravity lies midway between that of cells and that of plasma. The settling cells fall below this plug and the plasma remains above it. Keeping cells and plasma completely segregated in this manner is important; otherwise some red blood cells may leak or burst (hemolyze) and release their contents into the plasma while the specimen is awaiting analysis. Hemolysis in a blood specimen is one of the commonest reasons for false elevations of plasma chemistry levels.

Some tests are done directly on plasma, others on serum (that is, blood with both cells and fibrinogen removed), still others on a protein-free filtrate of plasma. This is prepared by adding to plasma a reagent such as phosphotungstic acid which coagulates all protein so that it can be removed from the specimen by filtration.

Modern clinical chemistry makes use of a wide variety of analytic techniques to identify and measure substances in the blood. Older and more cumbersome gravimetric techniques, requiring precise weighing, and volumetric techniques, requiring drop-by-drop titration, have been replaced by quantitative analytic methods that use electronic equipment. This equipment measures the concentration of various substances indirectly but very precisely by determining various physical properties of a test solution, such as its capacity to transmit light (spectrophotometry) or the wave length of a color change (colorimetry). Other analytic methods include electrophoresis, based on the differing behavior of various solutes in an electrical field; radioimmunoassay, which measures specific proteins by observing their reaction with monoclonal antibodies; and gas, liquid, and thin-layer chromatography.

Automated analytic devices can perform twenty or more tests on blood samples at a rate of one sample or more a minute. Despite their great expense, these analyzers reduce the cost of chemical testing because they are capable of processing a much higher volume of material than a human technician. In addition, they permit better standardization of results and eliminate many potential sources of human error. Automatic analyzers in wide use include the Abbott VP (Abbott Diagnostics), Astra (Beckman Instruments, Inc.), Dade Paramax (American Dade), DuPont ACA (E.I. DuPont), Ektachem (Eastman Kodak Co.), and SMAC (pronounced "smack"; Sequential Multiple Analyzer plus Computer, Technicon Instruments Corporation).

Routine tests performed in all clinical laboratories on venous blood include quantitative analyses for electrolytes, carbohydrates, lipids, proteins (including enzymes), hormones, vitamins, nitrogenous wastes, bile pigments, prescribed drugs, and toxic substances including drugs of abuse. Important examples of each of these classes of test material will be surveyed in the following pages, and their clinicopathologic significance outlined.

The following are representative examples of automated serum chemistry panels (chemistry profiles) comprising six, twelve, and twenty tests (referred to, for example, as SMA-6, SMA-12, SMA-20):

- Six tests: glucose, BUN, creatinine, sodium, potassium, chloride.
- Twelve tests: all of the above plus calcium, phosphorus, uric acid, cholesterol, total protein, bilirubin.
- Twenty tests: all of the above plus alkaline phosphatase, LDH, AST, ALT, direct bilirubin, triglycerides, albumin, iron.

An **electrolyte** is a substance capable of conducting an electrical current when dissolved in water. In chemical parlance, the term *electrolyte* refers to any substance that ionizes in water, that is, that breaks down into ions. An ion is an atom or group of atoms having a positive or negative charge. A cation is an ion that has a positive charge because it has lost one or more electrons, while an anion has a negative charge because it has gained one or more electrons. The principal cations of the plasma are sodium and potassium, and the principal anions are chloride and bicarbonate.

The concentrations and ratios of these substances are held within fairly narrow limits in the normal body, principally by the kidneys, which excrete (or retain) sodium, potassium, chloride, and water, and by the lungs, whose excretion (or retention) of carbon dioxide dissolved in the blood controls the concentration of bicarbonate ion. Disorders of the kidney or of the respiratory system, as well as other conditions causing abnormal loss or retention of body water or dissolved ions, can profoundly alter the levels of serum electrolytes. Determination of **serum electrolytes** (often abbreviated in speech to **lytes**) is a sensitive indicator of a broad range of metabolic disorders, and can also supply valuable indirect information about water balance and acid-base balance.

Sodium, potassium, chloride, and bicarbonate are almost invariably measured together. To facilitate calculations involving these electrolytes, their concentrations are all reported in milliequivalents per liter (mEq/L) or millimoles per liter (mmol/L).

Sodium (Na) is an important constituent of all body fluids, being concerned in maintenance of osmotic pressure, water balance, membrane permeability, and the irritability of nerve cells. The principal source of sodium in the diet is table salt (sodium chloride). Sodium is filtered from the blood by the renal glomeruli, and, under the control of adrenal mineralocorticoids (principally aldosterone), partially reabsorbed in the renal tubules. Most sodium loss occurs through the kidneys, but appreciable losses also occur in sweat and stools.

Sodium is the principal cation of plasma, being present in a concentration of 136 to 145 mEq/L [136–145 mmol/L]. The commonest cause for an increase of sodium concentration (**hypernatremia**) is excessive loss of water due to sweating, vomiting, or diuresis (increased renal excretion of water). Diuresis may be induced by diuretic drugs and also occurs in diabetes mellitus, diabetes insipidus, and various renal disorders. Reduction in serum sodium concentration (**hyponatremia**) may reflect either an increase in serum water content (dilutional hyponatremia), as in congestive heart failure or hepatic or renal disease; or true depletion of sodium, as by vomiting, sweating, or excessive renal excretion of sodium in renal disease, adrenal cortical deficiency (Addison's disease), or as an effect of certain diuretics.

Although present in much higher concentration within cells, **potassium** (K) is an important cation of plasma, with a normal concentration between 3.5 and 5.0 mEq/L [3.5–5.0 mmol/L]. Potassium functions to maintain acid-base balance and osmotic pressure within cells and is essential to normal activity of muscle tissue, especially cardiac muscle. The principal dietary sources of potassium are meats and fruits. It is both filtered from the blood by the glomeruli and secreted (under the influence of mineralocorticoids) by the renal tubules.

Elevation of potassium concentration (**hyperkalemia** or hyperpotassemia) can result from diminished excretion of potassium ions (as in renal disease or adrenal failure) or from additional amounts of potassium in the serum (as from breakdown of muscle tissue or red blood cells). Reduction of serum potassium (**hypokalemia** or hypopotassemia) is most often due to loss of potassium from the body in gastrointestinal secretions (as from vomiting, diarrhea, or prolonged suction drainage from the stomach or intestine). Potassium loss can also occur from the kidney in acute or chronic renal disease, Cushing's syndrome, primary aldosteronism, or (very often) as an effect of diuretic drugs.

Chloride (Cl), the principal anion of intercellular fluid, is also present in significant concentration within cells. Particularly high concentrations are found in cerebrospinal fluid and gastric juice. Chloride helps to maintain acid-base, osmotic, and water balance. A principal dietary source is table salt. Renal excretion of chloride ion tends to parallel that of sodium.

The normal range of serum chloride concentrations is 100 to 106 mEq/L [100–106 mmol/L]. Increase in the concentration of this ion (**hyperchloremia**) may result from dehydration or from reduced excretion of chloride ions in acute renal failure or other renal disease. Decrease of chloride concentration (**hypochloremia**) can be either dilutional (as with excessive fluid retention in congestive heart failure or renal or hepatic disease) or due to depletion by loss from the gastrointestinal tract (particularly by vomiting), from the kidney as a consequence of diuretic therapy or adrenal failure, or from the sweat glands.

The **bicarbonate** (HCO_3^-) ion is measured indirectly, being first converted to carbon dioxide. Hence this electrolyte is often referred to as carbon dioxide (CO_2). The normal serum concentration of bicarbonate is 24 to 30 mEq/L [24–30 mmol/L]. Unlike the other serum electrolytes, whose concentration is determined principally by the kidneys, bicarbonate level depends on excretion or retention of carbon dioxide gas by the lungs. Moreover, this concentration can change very rapidly with shifts in the equilibrium between bicarbonate ion and carbon dioxide.

A principal function of the bicarbonate ion is the regulation of **acid-base balance**. The acidity or alkalinity of a solution depends on its hydrogen ion concentration. This is measured in pH units derived from the logarithm of the hydrogen ion concentration. A pH of 7.0 indicates perfect neutrality. A pH higher than 7.0 indicates alkalinity, and a pH lower than 7.0 indicates acidity. The pH of serum is maintained between 7.35 and 7.45 by a complex set of chemical checks and balances involving renal excretion of hydrogen ions and others, and the buffering effect of cations in the serum. A **buffer** is a substance that resists changes in pH by combining with or releasing hydrogen ions so as to keep their concentration constant in a solution. The principal buffer of the serum is bicarbonate ion. Phosphate ion and the serum proteins (albumin and globulin) also act as buffers, but to a much lesser extent.

A rise in serum pH is called alkalosis and a fall in pH is called acidosis. Either of these conditions can be respiratory in origin, resulting from a disturbance in the excretion of carbon dioxide by the lungs, or metabolic in origin, reflecting abnormalities in the levels of other ions. **Respiratory alkalosis** is due to excessive loss of carbon dioxide via the lungs, as from hyperventilation, while **respiratory acidosis** indicates abnormal retention of carbon dioxide, as from disease of the respiratory or circulatory system that impairs pulmonary gas exchange. The causes of **metabolic alkalosis** include loss of hydrogen ions from the gastrointestinal tract through vomiting and loss of hydrogen ions from the kidneys as a result of diuretic administration, hyperaldosteronism, or Cushing's syndrome.

Metabolic acidosis is divided into two types on the basis of the anion gap of the serum. If the sum of the cation concentrations of serum (sodium plus potassium) is compared to the sum of the anion concentrations (chloride plus bicarbonate), it will be found that the cation concentration is higher. This is because the calculation takes into account only the principal cations and anions, and the anions not included (phosphate, sulfate, protein, and various organic anions) exceed the cations not included (calcium, magnesium, and others).

The difference between cation and anion concentrations when only the four principal ions are included in the calculation is called the **anion gap**, which is normally 12 to 20 mEq/L [12–20 mmol/L].

Metabolic acidosis with a normal anion gap may be due to loss of bicarbonate ion from the bowel through diarrhea, or from the kidney as a result of renal disease (renal tubular acidosis). When metabolic acidosis is accompanied by an increased anion gap, the difference in unmeasured anion is usually due to the presence of excessive anions derived from organic acids. These may be normal anions abnormally retained by a diseased kidney; anions abnormally produced in certain conditions (lactic acidosis, diabetic ketoacidosis); or extraneous substances (salicylate, methanol).

Any shift in serum pH tends to be compensated by whatever mechanism remains unimpaired. Hence, for example, metabolic acidosis leads to increased pulmonary excretion of carbon dioxide, with a resulting tendency towards respiratory alkalosis. Consequently, electrolyte imbalances are frequently complex and difficult to diagnose.

Calcium (Ca) is the principal mineral of bones and teeth and also plays an essential role in nerve and muscle function and blood coagulation. The main dietary sources of calcium are milk and dairy products. The absorption, distribution, and excretion of calcium are controlled by vitamin D, parathyroid hormone, and calcitonin. Most of the excretion of calcium occurs in the stool.

The normal calcium concentration of serum is 8.2–10.2 mg/dL [2–2.5 mmol/L]. This level tends to vary inversely with that of phosphorus. About one-half of the calcium in the serum is bound to protein and the other half is in free (un-ionized) form. Elevation of serum calcium (**hypercalcemia**) occurs in hyperparathyroidism, vitamin D intoxication, sarcoidosis, various malignancies including particularly those of hematopoietic tissue and bone, and any condition favoring bone resorption (such as immobilization).

Serum calcium is reduced (**hypocalcemia**) in hypoparathyroidism, in disorders characterized by low serum albumin (nephrotic syndrome, cachexia), in acute pancreatitis with fat necrosis, and in chronic renal failure with retention of phosphorus.

Phosphorus (P) is widely distributed throughout the cells and fluids of the body, most of it being in chemical combination with calcium in bones and teeth. Phosphorus is abundant in most foods. Its metabolism closely follows that of calcium, and is therefore under the influence of vitamin D, parathyroid hormone, and calcitonin. Phosphate is a minor anion of serum but contributes some buffering effect.

The normal phosphorus concentration of serum is 2.5–4.5 mg/dL [0.8–1.5 mmol/L]. Phosphorus is increased (**hyperphosphatemia**) in hypoparathyroidism, vitamin D intoxication, hematologic malignancies, chronic renal failure, and various disorders of bone (healing fractures, Paget's disease, multiple myeloma, metastatic neoplasm). A reduction of phosphorus level (**hypophosphatemia**) occurs in hyperparathyroidism, renal tubular disorders, osteomalacia, rickets, severe metabolic acidosis, malabsorption syndromes (sprue, celiac disease), and other abnormal nutritional states.

Most of the **magnesium** (Mg) in the body is combined with calcium and phosphorus in bones and teeth. The normal serum level is 1.5–2.3 mg/dL [0.6–1.0 mmol/L]. Increase in this level (hypermagnesemia) occurs in renal failure and in deficiency of thyroid or adrenal cortical hormones. Reduction in magnesium (hypomagnesemia) is seen in malabsorption states, alcoholism, hyperthyroidism, and Cushing's syndrome.

The role of **iron** (Fe) in body chemistry is limited almost entirely to the transport and utilization of oxygen. Iron occurs as a component of hemoglobin, the oxygen-carrying material of red blood cells; myoglobin, a similar compound in muscle; and several substances involved in intracellular metabolism (cytochromes, peroxidase). Under normal conditions, most of the iron in the body is recycled, but intestinal absorption of small amounts from meats and vegetables is needed to offset small losses in urine and stool and to meet needs created by menstruation, normal growth and development, and abnormal blood loss. Acid gastric juice is necessary for proper absorption of dietary iron, most of which occurs in the duodenum. In tissues other than the blood, iron is found in a storage form in combination with the protein ferritin.

The normal serum iron level is 50–160 µg/dL [9.0–28.8 µmol/L] for males and about 10% less for females. Most of the iron in the serum is bound to the protein transferrin. Serum iron is increased (hyperferremia) in hemochromatosis, hemosiderosis due to excessive intake of iron, hemolytic anemia (due to breakdown of red blood cells), and pernicious anemia (due to decreased incorporation of iron in red blood cells). Reduction of serum iron (hypoferremia) is observed in iron deficiency anemia due to malnutrition or to various malabsorptive states (achlorhydria, steatorrhea, surgical absence of stomach or duodenum) as well as after severe hemorrhage.

In order to distinguish among various causes of abnormal serum iron levels it is helpful to determine the **iron-binding capacity** of the blood. The amount of transferrin in normal serum is capable of binding iron to the extent of 250–350 µg/dL [45–63 µmol/L]. Comparison with the normal iron level shows that only 20 to 55% of this binding capacity is normally used (saturated). The iron-binding capacity is increased in anemia due to hemorrhage or dietary deficiency of iron, and decreased in hemochromatosis and in disease states associated with reduction of serum proteins (nephrotic syndrome, chronic infection, hepatic cirrhosis). The saturation of serum iron-binding capacity is increased in hemochromatosis and hemosiderosis and reduced in anemias associated with iron deficiency and chronic disease.

Copper (Cu) is an essential component of enzymes and other proteins concerned in hemoglobin synthesis and bone formation. The normal serum level of copper, most of which is bound to the protein ceruloplasmin, is 0.7–1.5 µg/mL [11–24 mmol/L]. The serum copper level is increased in acute and chronic infections, various anemias, leukemia, collagen diseases, and hemochromatosis, and decreased in Wilson's disease. (The diagnosis of Wilson's disease is established by finding a low level of ceruloplasmin in serum and an increased amount of copper in the urine.)

Glucose is a simple sugar (monosaccharide) that is derived from digestion of dietary carbohydrate (starches and more complex sugars), stored in the liver and muscle tissue as glycogen, and used by body cells as their principal source of energy. The uptake of glucose by cells depends on the hormone insulin. Glucose filtered by the glomeruli from the plasma is normally reabsorbed completely by the renal tubules.

Serum glucose is usually measured in the fasting state to eliminate the variations caused by absorption of dietary carbohydrate. The serum level of glucose in the fasting state (**fasting blood sugar**) is normally between 60–115 mg/dL [3.3–6.4 mmol/L]. (The normal range varies slightly depending on whether glucose is measured by the glucose oxidase, hexokinase, or *o*-toluidine method.) Elevation of serum glucose above the normal range is called **hyperglycemia**. A fasting blood sugar between 115 and 140 mg/dL [6.4–7.7 mmol/L] indicates impaired glucose tolerance and a level above 140 mg/dL [7.7 mmol/L] is diagnostic of diabetes mellitus. Abnormally low serum glucose (**hypoglycemia**) is seen in starvation, insulin reaction, and hyperinsulinism due to tumors of the pancreatic islet cells.

More useful information about glucose metabolism can be obtained by testing the blood glucose at one or several precisely timed intervals after ingestion of a meal or (preferably) after ingestion of exactly 75 mg of carbohydrate. When blood is drawn for testing at several intervals (for example, 30, 60, 90, 120, and 180 minutes), the results can be plotted as a **glucose tolerance curve**. The curve is elevated, with a slow fall towards normal, in diabetes mellitus. A low or flat curve occurs in hyperinsulinism or in decreased digestive absorption of glucose. Variations due to absorption can be avoided by giving the carbohydrate load intravenously.

The most important single value in the glucose tolerance curve is the two-hour postprandial level. Normally this is below 140 mg/dL [7.7 mmol/L]. A two-hour postprandial blood sugar between 140 and 200 mg/dL [7.7 and 11.1 mmol/L] indicates impaired glucose tolerance and a level over 200 mg/dL [11.1 mmol/L] is diagnostic of diabetes mellitus. Several devices are available to enable diabetics to perform frequent checks on blood glucose at home. These devices test fingerstick blood, and despite their simplicity they achieve a high degree of accuracy.

One disadvantage of using the blood sugar level as a means of monitoring diabetes mellitus is that this level fluctuates constantly. A valuable technique for assessing diabetic control over a period of weeks is the measurement of **glycosylated hemoglobin**, a chemical compound of glucose and the A_{1c} fraction of red blood cell hemoglobin. In nondiabetics, glycosylated hemoglobin constitutes less than 6% of total hemoglobin. When diabetic control has been satisfactory during the 8 weeks preceding the test, glycosylated hemoglobin constitutes less than 12% of total hemoglobin.

Cholesterol is a complex organic compound synthesized in the liver and other tissues, widely distributed throughout the body, especially in nerve tissue, and serving as a building block for steroid hormones (cortisol, aldosterone, testosterone, progesterone). Dietary cholesterol from animal fats (including butter fat and egg yolk) is absorbed from the intestine and transported in the serum in combination with lipoproteins. Persons whose diet is high in cholesterol or who have genetic disorders of lipoproteins may show marked elevation of serum cholesterol. Such persons are at increased risk of atherosclerosis, as discussed in Chapter 19.

The normal fasting serum level of cholesterol is below 200 mg/dL [520 mmol/L]. Higher levels (hypercholesterolemia) occur in biliary obstruction, nephrotic syndrome, hypothyroidism, and pancreatic disease as well as in dietary and familial disorders of cholesterol metabolism. In addition, the cholesterol level tends to rise with age. Very low levels (below 50 mg/dL [130 mmol/L]) suggest severe malnutrition or hepatic disease.

Lipoprotein assay provides additional diagnostic information in cases of hypercholesterolemia. The lipoproteins are classified on the basis of their behavior under ultracentrifugation as high density lipoproteins (HDL), low density lipoproteins (LDL), and very low density lipoproteins (VLDL). A relative preponderance of HDL, which carry cholesterol away from tissues, is associated with lower risk of atherosclerosis, while a preponderance of LDL, which deposit cholesterol in tissues, implies increased risk of atherosclerosis.

The term **triglyceride** is a chemical designation for animal fats—compounds of glycerol with fatty acid radicals. The serum triglyceride level has similar implications to those of the cholesterol level. The normal fasting triglyceride level is below 160 mg/dL [1.80 mmol/L]. Elevation of serum triglycerides (hypertriglyceridemia) occurs in hyperlipidemias, liver disease, nephrotic syndrome, hypothyroidism, and diabetes mellitus. Very low levels (below 10 mg/dL [0.12 mmol/L]) suggest severe malnutrition.

The **plasma proteins** vary greatly in structure and molecular weight. The principal plasma proteins are albumin, globulin, and fibrinogen. **Albumin**, which is produced in the liver, has a molecular weight around 69 000 and functions principally in water balance by maintaining the osmotic pressure of the blood. It also acts as a plasma buffer. The normal level of albumin in the serum is 3.5–5.0 g/dL [35–50 g/L]. The level is reduced in liver disease, malnutrition, and chronic infections.

Globulins are a complex mixture of related proteins varying in molecular weight from 150 000 to 1 300 000. On the basis of their stratification in the ultracentrifuge, globulins have been classified as alpha, beta, and gamma globulins. The globulins include the metal-binding proteins transferrin and ceruloplasmin and the lipoproteins, all formed in the liver, which are discussed earlier in this chapter.

The **gamma globulins** or immunoglobulins (Ig), produced by lymphocytes and plasma cells, include all known circulating antibodies. They are divided on the basis of ultracentrifugation and electrophoresis patterns into five classes: IgG (more than 75% of the total globulin fraction), IgA (15%), IgM (10%), IgD (less than 1%), and IgE (less than 0.1%). Study of the electrophoretic pattern of the first three of these can supply clues to a variety of disorders characterized by disturbances in gamma globulin levels (gammopathies), including chronic infection, collagen disease, lymphoma, leukemia, multiple myeloma, immunodeficiency disorders, sarcoidosis, and cystic fibrosis.

The total globulin fraction of serum is normally between 1.5 and 3.0 g/dL [15–30 g/L]. The quotient obtained by dividing albumin level by globulin level is known as the **A/G ratio**. Normally this ratio is between 1.5 and 3.0. In a number of disorders (collagen diseases, nephrotic syndrome, Hodgkin's disease, multiple myeloma, chronic infection, metastatic malignancy), a reduction of serum albumin combined with elevation of one or more globulins causes the A/G ratio to be less than 1.0, a condition loosely referred to as "reversal" or "inversion" of the ratio.

Extensive hemolysis of red blood cells within the circulation releases hemoglobin into the serum. Measurement of the **hemoglobin** level in the serum, of which it is not a normal component, therefore gives information about recent or current hemolysis, as in hemolytic anemia or transfusion reaction. Further information can be obtained by measurement of the level of **haptoglobin** in the serum. Haptoglobins are normal serum proteins that combine with any free hemoglobin resulting from hemolysis. The normal hemoglobin-binding capacity of the serum haptoglobins is 40 to 180 mg/dL [0.4–1.8 g/L]. This level is increased in the presence of acute or chronic inflammation and reduced in hemolysis and liver disease—in the latter case, because of reduced synthesis of haptoglobin.

Fibrinogen, prothrombin, and other serum proteins concerned in blood coagulation are discussed in Chapter 29.

Enzymes are proteins that catalyze biochemical reactions—that is, that accelerate or facilitate these reactions without being permanently altered or consumed in the process. Digestive enzymes in saliva, gastric juice, pancreatic juice, and small intestinal secretions break down carbohydrates, lipids, and proteins to simpler compounds as a preliminary to absorption and utilization. A large number of intracellular enzymes have been identified as being essential to various phases of cell chemistry including energy metabolism and synthesis of cell products such as hormones and other enzymes.

Although only a few enzymes (such as those concerned in blood clotting) perform any function in circulating blood, a number of them can be detected in the serum, at least under certain conditions. Many kinds of cells, when damaged by injury, infarction, or inflammation, leak their cytoplasmic enzymes into the circulation. An elevation of an enzyme level in the serum may therefore indicate disease in its tissue of origin. Because most enzymes are found in a variety of tissues, it is seldom possible to make a specific diagnosis on the basis of a single enzyme level. Typically a group or panel of enzyme tests are done and diagnostic inferences drawn from a consideration of all the information thus gained. As mentioned in Chapter 28, enzyme assays are ordinarily carried out by measuring enzyme activity, which is reported in arbitrarily established units per volume (U/L) rather than by weight per volume.

A group of two or more enzymes having the same action but differing in chemical structure are called **isoenzymes** (or isozymes). Often each isoenzyme can be linked to a specific tissue of origin. Hence, when a rise in the serum level of a certain enzyme is detected, it may be possible to gain more precise information about its source by determining the relative proportions of the various isoenzymes present. Isoenzymes can be separated by electrophoresis, ion exchange chromatography, and other techniques.

An important group of serum enzymes are often found elevated to varying degrees in hepatic disease and in injury or infarction of muscle, particularly cardiac muscle. This group includes creatine phosphokinase, glutamic oxaloacetic transaminase, lactic dehydrogenase, and gamma-glutamyl transpeptidase.

Creatine phosphokinase (CPK) varies from 12 to 80 U/L when incubated at 30°C and from 55 to 170 U/L when incubated at 37°. The level is elevated in degenerative disease or injury of skeletal muscle, cerebral thrombosis with infarction, and in nearly all cases of myocardial infarction. Elevation in myocardial infarction begins in 4 to 8 hours and peaks at 24 hours. Three isoenzymes of CPK have been identified. Of these, the MB isoenzyme rises in myocardial infarction, the MM isoenzyme in cerebral infarction, and the BB isoenzyme (rarely) in uremia, Reye's syndrome, and necrosis of the colon.

Aspartate aminotransferase (AST), also called serum glutamic-oxaloacetic transaminase (SGOT), has a normal level below 35 U/L. The SGOT is elevated in active liver disease, pancreatitis, degenerative disease or extensive trauma of skeletal muscle; also in most cases of myocardial infarction and in some cases of cerebral or pulmonary infarction. In myocardial infarction the elevation begins at 6 to 12 hours and peaks at 24 to 48 hours.

Lactic dehydrogenase (LDH), normally below 110 U/L, is elevated in hepatitis, hemolytic anemia, carcinoma (especially metastatic), pulmonary embolism and infarction, and in nearly all cases of myocardial infarction. The rise in myocardial infarction begins at 12 hours and peaks at 72 hours. Five LDH isoenzymes, designated I through V, have been identified. Elevation of I predominates in myocardial infarction, of II in hemolytic disease and other infarctions, of III and IV in disseminated lupus erythematosus and malignant lymphoma, and of V in hepatic disease.

Serum gamma-glutamyl transpeptidase (or transferase) (SGGT), whose normal level is below 65 U/L, is elevated in biliary obstruction, hepatitis, cirrhosis, pancreatitis, alcoholism, and in 50% of cases of myocardial infarction. Elevation in myocardial infarction begins on the fourth or fifth day and peaks at eight to twelve days.

Alanine aminotransferase (ALT), also called serum glutamic-pyruvate transaminase (SGPT), is elevated in hepatocellular disease and in traumatic and degenerative disorders of skeletal muscle. The normal range is 8–45 U/L.

The alkaline and acid phosphatases are highly useful markers of disease. Serum **alkaline phosphatase**, with a normal level of 20 to

120 U/L, is elevated in hyperparathyroidism, Paget's disease, rickets, biliary obstruction, and hepatic disease, particularly malignant. It is also normally higher in children than in adults. The level of alkaline phosphatase may be depressed in hypothyroidism, malnutrition, and malabsorption. Two other enzymes, serum leucine aminopeptidase (SLAP), normally below 40 U/L, and 5'-nucleotidase, normally below 12.5 U/L, are useful in interpreting elevation of alkaline phosphatase. These typically rise in hepatic disease but not in bone disease. **Acid phosphatase** is found in high concentration in prostatic tissue. The serum level of this enzyme, normally below 0.6 U/L, is usually elevated in carcinoma or infarction of the prostate. It may also be elevated in hepatic disease or metastatic bone disease.

Angiotensin converting enzyme (ACE), produced chiefly by pulmonary endothelial cells, is elevated in sarcoidosis. The test is not sensitive or specific enough for diagnostic use but is helpful in assessing the severity of disease and the response to treatment.

Digestive enzymes may appear in the serum when their tissues of origin are diseased. The serum **amylase** level (normally below 125 U/L) rises in acute pancreatitis, obstruction of the pancreatic duct, and perforation or penetration of a peptic ulcer with pancreatic involvement. It is also elevated in mumps, with or without pancreatic involvement, and in alcoholism. The serum **lipase** (normally below 1.5 U/L) also rises in pancreatic disease but usually remains normal in mumps.

As discussed in earlier chapters, a **hormone** is a chemical messenger or mediator secreted by endocrine tissue and released directly into the blood stream. By definition, then, hormones are normally found in the blood, and their concentrations correlate closely with the condition of their glands or tissues of origin. Depression of a hormone level may indicate disease, atrophy, or absence of its gland of origin, while an elevated level may reflect hyperactivity or a functioning neoplasm. Disease in one endocrine gland can alter the function of another. For example, a reduction in pituitary thyroid-stimulating hormone (TSH) due to disease of the pituitary gland will lead to a decline in the production of thyroxine by the thyroid gland. Conversely, a decline in thyroxine production for any reason other than this will stimulate a rise in the level of TSH.

The blood levels of virtually all known hormones can be determined by radioimmunoassay (RIA). In this technique, a serum specimen is incubated with a known quantity of monoclonal antibody to the hormone under study. By using both radioisotopically tagged and untagged hormone, this method makes possible precise and specific measurement of hormone levels in the serum. Such tests supply invaluable information for the diagnosis of most endocrine disorders. Other analytic methods are also in use for many hormones.

Standard tests are available to measure hormones of the anterior pituitary gland (follicle-stimulating hormone, luteinizing hormone, prolactin, TSH, ACTH, and growth hormone), the posterior pituitary gland (vasopressin), the thyroid gland (thyroxine or T_4, triiodothyronine or T_3, calcitonin), the parathyroid glands (parathormone), the adrenal glands (cortisol, deoxycortisol, aldosterone), the testis (testosterone), the ovary (estradiol, estriol, progesterone), the placenta (chorionic gonadotropin, human placental lactogen), the kidney (renin and the product of its action, angiotensin II), the pancreas (insulin, glucagon), and the stomach (gastrin).

Endocrine disorders are discussed in Chapter 25. Nearly all of the thyroxine (T_4) in the circulation is bound to thyroxine-binding globulin. A calculation based on this value and the T_4 level yields a free thyroxine index (also called T_7), which provides a more accurate measure of thyroid function. In assessing adrenal function it is usual to determine the **plasma cortisol** level at both 8 a.m. (when it is normally high) and at 8 p.m. (when it is normally low). The detection of **chorionic gonadotropin** in the serum is the basis for most serum pregnancy tests in current use.

Measurement of the serum level of some **vitamins** is useful in the diagnosis of certain deficiency states. Quantitative tests are available in most laboratories for vitamins A, B_1, B_{12}, C, and D, carotene, and folic acid. Vitamin deficiencies are discussed in Chapter 10.

Normally the serum level of the amino acid phenylalanine is 2–4 mg/dL [121–242 μmol/L]. More than a tenfold rise may be seen in patients with phenylketonuria, a hereditary disorder of phenylalanine metabolism that causes mental retardation. Testing for this disorder by determining serum phenylalanine is a routine procedure in well-baby care.

The normal daily breakdown of protein in the body produces about 15 g of nitrogen, most of which is excreted by the kidneys. The principal form in which nitrogen is excreted is urea, which is synthesized in the liver. Urea is filtered through the renal glomeruli and neither reabsorbed nor secreted by the renal tubules. Hence the level of urea in the serum, measured as **blood urea nitrogen** (BUN), reflects principally glomerular function. The normal BUN is 5–20 mg/dL [1.8–7.1 μmol/L]. An increase in this level (azotemia) occurs in renal disease, particularly glomerular disease; in conditions causing increased protein breakdown or impairing renal blood flow (prerenal azotemia); and in urinary tract obstruction (postrenal azotemia). The BUN may be reduced in severe liver disease and severe protein deficiency.

Creatinine, also a nitrogenous waste, is a breakdown product formed in muscle tissue from creatine. It is both filtered at the renal glomeruli and actively secreted by the renal tubules. The normal serum level of creatinine is 0.6–1.2 mg/dL [50–100 μmol/L]. Elevation occurs in the same conditions as elevation of BUN, as well as in pituitary gigantism and acromegaly. The ratio of BUN to creatinine is normally about 10:1, but creatinine is considered a more sensitive indicator of renal functional impairment.

Ammonia, yet another nitrogenous waste, is produced in tissues by the normal breakdown of protein, in the intestine by the action of bacteria on dietary protein, and to a lesser extent by the kidneys as part of their regulation of acid-base balance. Ammonia is normally converted by the liver to urea and other products, which are then cleared from the blood by the kidneys. In a healthy person the level of serum ammonia is only 15–45 μg/dL [11–32 μmol/L]. This level rises in hepatic failure of any cause. Ammonia is toxic to the central nervous system, causing tremors, coma, and death.

Uric acid is the ultimate breakdown product of purines (guanine and xanthine), which are components of nucleoproteins in both body cells and food. Uric acid is filtered at the renal glomeruli and both reabsorbed and secreted by the renal tubules. The normal level of uric acid in the serum is 3.4–7 mg/dL [202–416 μmol/L]. An increase in this level (hyperuricemia) occurs in gout, renal disease, and many disorders causing increased breakdown of nucleoproteins, such as hemolytic anemia, hematologic malignancies, and psoriasis. Nonspecific increases occur in many other conditions and in some normal persons, including relatives of persons with gout. Uric acid level is used primarily to diagnose and monitor gout. It is not a sensitive indicator of renal disease.

Approximately 6 g of hemoglobin are turned over each day in the normal breakdown of red blood cells. The heme fraction of this hemoglobin is converted in reticuloendothelial cells to the yellow pigment **bilirubin**, of which about 0.3 g is formed daily. Bilirubin, which is nearly insoluble in plasma, is transported in the blood bound to protein. It is taken up in this form by the liver and conjugated with glucuronic acid, which renders it water-soluble. It is then excreted in the bile. In the intestine, bilirubin is further broken down to urobilinogen. Most of this urobilinogen is eliminated in the stool, but a fraction of it is reabsorbed and re-excreted by the liver.

Both conjugated and unconjugated bilirubin are normally present in the serum. Significant elevation of either or both forms (**hyperbilirubinemia**) results in the temporary yellow staining of the tissues, including the skin, known as jaundice. Conjugated bilirubin is also called direct-reacting bilirubin because it is water-soluble and therefore reacts directly with analytic reagents. The normal level of direct-reacting bilirubin in serum in 0.1 to 0.4 mg/dL [1.7–6.8 μmol/L]. Elevation of this level occurs when bilirubin that has been conjugated by the liver enters the circulation as a result of biliary tract obstruction or disease of the intrahepatic biliary duct system. Because conjugated bilirubin is water-soluble, excessive amounts of it in the blood spill into the urine, where it can be chemically detected and may intensify or alter the color of the urine.

Unconjugated bilirubin is also called indirect-reacting bilirubin because it is insoluble in water and must be treated with methanol before quantitative analysis can be carried out. Unconjugated bilirubin does not appear in the urine. In practice, direct and total bilirubin are determined by quantitative analysis, and the indirect bilirubin is calculated as the difference between them. The normal total bilirubin level is 0.1 to 0.9 mg/dL [1.7–15.3 μmol/L] and the normal indirect-reacting bilirubin level is 0.1 to 0.5 mg/dL [1.7–8.5 μmol/L]. Elevation of indirect-reacting bilirubin occurs in acute or chronic liver disease (viral hepatitis, cirrhosis, hepatic necrosis) and after massive hemolysis. The combination of hemolysis in the neonatal period with immaturity of liver function often produces transient "physiologic" jaundice in newborns.

Monitoring blood levels of certain prescribed medicines is currently standard practice in establishing and maintaining optimum dosage. Analytic methods are available for many common drugs. The **therapeutic range** of a drug is the range of concentrations in serum below which the therapeutic effect is inadequate or absent, and above which toxic effects may occur. Monitoring of drug levels is particularly important with drugs having narrow margins between therapeutic and toxic effects (gentamicin, lithium, theophylline, tobramycin), drugs used to control cardiac arrhythmias (digitoxin, digoxin, procainamide, quinidine), and drugs used to prevent seizures (carbamazepine, phenobarbital, phenytoin, valproic acid).

Quantitative analysis of serum for toxic materials such as drugs of abuse and chemical poisons may provide an explanation for various abnormal conditions, including dementia, coma, and shock. Toxicologic screening by thin-layer chromatography can isolate and identify virtually any extraneous chemical substance, provided that it is present in sufficient concentration in the specimen. Specific quantitative methods are available for alcohol, cannabis, amphetamines, barbiturates, hypnotics, narcotics, salicylate, tranquilizers, and industrial poisons. Testing for quinine may be performed when narcotic abuse is suspected, because street narcotics are nearly always combined with quinine.

Chemical measurement of **arterial blood gases** (oxygen and carbon dioxide) is used to assess the adequacy of pulmonary gas exchange in persons with respiratory or circulatory disease and those receiving oxygen therapy, with or without ventilatory assistance. Ordinarily the pH of the specimen is also determined to identify acidosis or alkalosis and to permit indirect calculation of the bicarbonate ion concentration. The specimen for blood gas determination is drawn from an artery, not a vein. All room air is excluded from the specimen, heparin is added to prevent coagulation, and the specimen is stored in ice until testing is performed. Blood gases are measured in torr (millimeters of mercury).

The normal partial pressure of **oxygen** (P_{O_2}) in arterial blood is 75 to 100 torr. This level normally declines with age. The arterial oxygen may be increased in hyperventilation due to anxiety. Reduction of oxygen tension (hypoxemia) can result from any condition that depresses or inhibits respiratory movements (paralysis, chest injury, pneumothorax, massive obesity, central nervous system depression by drugs, trauma, or disease); any condition that prevents normal oxygen exchange in lung tissue (pneumonia, bronchitis, pulmonary edema, asthma, airway obstruction); or reduction of available oxygen in the atmosphere.

The normal partial pressure of **carbon dioxide** (P_{CO_2}) is 35 to 45 torr. Increase in carbon dioxide tension (hypercapnia) may be caused by most of the same conditions that reduce oxygen (except reduction in available oxygen). Increase in carbon dioxide and bicarbonate ion also occurs in response to metabolic alkalosis. Reduction of carbon dioxide (hypocapnia) occurs in hyperventilation and in response to metabolic acidosis.

Serum pH and bicarbonate ion concentration were discussed at the beginning of this chapter in connection with electrolyte studies on venous blood.

The maintenance of osmotic balance between plasma and intercellular fluid depends on the concentration of solute (electrolytes, proteins, and other substances) in the plasma. The osmotic activity (osmolality) of serum is determined by a physical (nonchemical) measurement. Pure water freezes at 0°C. Adding solute to water lowers its freezing point in proportion to the osmotic activity of the solute. **Serum osmolality**, as determined by the freezing point depression method, is normally 280 to 295 mOsm/kg. Increase of serum osmolality (hyperosmolality) occurs in diabetes mellitus, diabetes insipidus, dehydration, and hypercalcemia. Reduction (hyposmolality) is noted in congestive heart failure, hepatic cirrhosis, Addison's disease, hyponatremia, and inappropriate secretion of antidiuretic hormone.

Review Questions

1. Why is it usually important to separate red blood cells from plasma promptly and completely in a blood specimen intended for chemical testing?
2. What are some advantages of automated chemical testing of blood?
3. What are the principal serum electrolytes?
4. In what units are serum concentrations of these electrolytes reported?
5. Why is the bicarbonate ion sometimes referred to as carbon dioxide (CO_2)?
6. What is meant by saying that metabolic acidosis leads to respiratory alkalosis?
7. In what ways are the glucose tolerance curve and the glycosylated hemoglobin test superior to determination of fasting blood sugar in diagnosing or monitoring diabetes mellitus?
8. What is the point of determining the cholesterol level in an apparently healthy person?
9. What important class of substances is included in the gamma globulin fraction of plasma?
10. What is the principal nitrogenous waste product excreted in urine?
11. List some conditions that both elevate arterial carbon dioxide and depress arterial oxygen.
12. Define or explain: *A/G ratio, anion, buffer, cation, hypercapnia, hypokalemia, isoenzyme, pH.*

31

Laboratory Examination
of Urine and Stool

The history of clinical pathology began with the observation that the urine and stools of sick persons are often abnormal. Pathologic changes in the urine and stool are mentioned frequently in the works of Hippocrates and Galen. Medieval physicians often limited their diagnostic investigations to feeling the patient's pulse and holding a flask of urine up to the light.

In the modern clinical laboratory, microscopic examination and chemical analysis of urine and stool specimens can yield information not only about the excretory and digestive systems but also about other body systems, water and acid-base balance, nutrition, and the presence of toxic substances. A major advantage of urine and stool examinations is that, under ordinary circumstances, both of these materials are readily available, and obtaining specimens calls for no invasive procedures or elaborate equipment.

For most of the tests done in the **urinology** laboratory, the preferred specimen is 60 to 90 mL of freshly voided urine. Although a random specimen is usually suitable, a **first-voided specimen** (the first urine passed after arising in the morning) may be more satisfactory in testing for trace substances because it is usually more concentrated. A **clean-voided specimen** (clean catch) is one obtained after cleansing of the area around the urethral meatus (usually with liquid soap and cotton balls) to prevent contamination of the specimen with material from outside the urinary tract. A **midstream specimen** is one that contains neither the first nor the last portion of urine passed. It is obtained by introducing a specimen container into the urine stream after voiding has begun and removing it before voiding ceases. The purpose of this procedure is to obtain as pure as possible a sample of bladder urine, with minimal admixture of cells or other material from the urethra. A **catheterized specimen** is obtained by urethral catheter (less often by suprapubic needle puncture of the bladder), either because the patient cannot void or to prevent contamination of the specimen. A **24-hour urine specimen** consists of all the urine passed by the patient during a 24-hour period.

A urine specimen is usually collected in a clean, dry bottle or cup of glass, plastic, or waxed or plasticized paper. The container need not be sterile except for bacteriologic work. Examination of urine is carried out as soon as possible after the specimen is obtained because blood cells in urine rupture early and bacterial growth in a standing specimen may alter its chemical composition. When a delay is expected, the specimen is refrigerated. A one- or two-gallon jug is used to collect a 24-hour urine specimen. The jug may be kept on ice during the collection period, and one of several preservatives may be placed in the jug before collection begins.

The principal diagnostic procedure in urinology is the **urinalysis**, a set of routine physical and chemical examinations. In most laboratories, the urinalysis includes direct observation of the specimen for color, turbidity, and other obvious characteristics; determination of specific gravity; microscopic examination of sediment for cells, crystals, and other formed elements; determination of pH; and chemical testing for glucose, protein, occult blood, and perhaps bilirubin and acetone.

Variations in color and clarity of urine usually reflect variations in concentration of solutes, including pigment. Because the daily solute load is fairly constant, changes in concentration are nearly always due to changes in volume of water excreted. Turbidity (cloudiness) may be due to the presence of phosphates, which are insoluble in alkaline urine. A smoky brown color ("Coca-Cola urine") often indicates the presence of hemolyzed blood. Color changes may be due to abnormal waste products (bilirubin, porphyrins), drugs (methylene blue, phenazopyridine), or pigments from foods (beets, blackberries). Mucus shreds, fragments of tissue, or calcareous material may be grossly evident in the specimen.

The **specific gravity** of urine is determined by noting the depth to which a hydrometer sinks in the specimen. The normal specific gravity is 1.005 to 1.030. The specific gravity varies in direct proportion to the concentration of dissolved materials. The specific gravity is increased in dehydration (with normal renal function), toxemia, congestive heart failure, acute glomerulonephritis, and diabetes mellitus with glycosuria. The specific gravity is decreased (hyposthenuria) after ingestion or infusion of fluid (with normal renal function), in diabetes insipidus, and in renal failure with loss of concentrating ability.

Microscopic examination of the urine is usually preceded by centrifugation of the specimen to concentrate any cells or other formed elements present. A polychrome stain such as the Sternheimer-Malbin stain (crystal violet and safranin in ethanol) may be added to the sediment to enhance the distinctive features of various cells, but is not essential. Microscopic examination is carried out on a small volume of fluid urine placed on a slide and covered with a cover slip. Dried smears of urine are not ordinarily suitable for examination.

Formed elements frequently found in urine are red blood cells, white blood cells, casts, crystals, bacteria, epithelial cells, and amorphous sediment. Cell counts are recorded as cells per high-power field, obtained as an average after examination and counting of several fields. A small number of red and white blood cells are present in normal urine. A finding of more than 1 or 2 **red blood cells** per high-power field (RBC/hpf), called microscopic hematuria, indicates either bleeding in some part of the excretory system or contamination of the specimen with blood, possibly menstrual. Hematuria occurs in acute glomerulonephritis, urolithiasis, hemorrhagic diseases, infarction of the kidney, tuberculosis of the kidney, benign or malignant tumors of any part of the urinary tract, and many cases of simple cystitis. The presence of more than 1 or 2 **white blood cells** per high-power field (WBC/hpf), known as pyuria, usually indicates infection in some part of the urinary tract.

Casts are microscopic cylindrical bodies that have been formed by concretion of cells or insoluble material within renal tubules and subsequently excreted in the urine. Casts are always abnormal. They are reported as the number counted per low-power field. Hyaline and waxy casts are homogeneous casts varying in refractility. They consist of coagulated protein and are found in conditions associated with leakage of protein through glomeruli: nephritis, nephrotic syndrome (including lupus nephrosis and Kimmelstiel-Wilson disease), toxemia, and congestive heart failure. Granular casts are formed by aggregation of red or white blood cells or both in renal tubules and occur in many of the same conditions as hyaline and waxy casts.

A variety of **crystals** may be found on microscopic examination of the urine. Their chemical composition can usually be deduced from their shape. Crystals of uric acid, cystine, calcium oxalate, and triple phosphate may appear in the urine of persons who excrete abnormal quantities of these materials and are subject to stone formation. **Bacteria** in significant numbers in a freshly voided specimen (bacteriuria, bacilluria) suggest urinary tract infection. Some squamous **epithelial cells** (squames) are often found in urine and have little significance. **Amorphous sediment** is a general term for ill-defined solid material seen on microscopic examination of urine. It consists of chemical and cellular debris and is of no diagnostic importance.

Routine chemical testing of urine is usually performed with a "dipstick," a commercially produced strip of plastic or paper bearing a series of dots or squares of reagent, each designed to assess a specific chemical property of urine. The dipstick is immersed briefly in the urine and the test squares are observed for color changes. These tests are semiquantitative and are read by comparing the degree of color change in each square with an appropriate color chart. Results of dipstick tests other than pH are reported as either positive on a scale of 1 to 4 (1+, 2+, 3+, 4+) or negative.

The **pH** of urine (traditionally called the "reaction") is normally about 5.5. The urine may be alkaline (pH 8) in vegetarians and in persons with urinary tract infection due to urease-producing organisms such as *Proteus,* which split urinary urea to ammonia in the bladder.

The presence of **protein** in the urine (proteinuria) is usually due to leakage of albumin from the glomeruli. Hence it is often termed albuminuria, even though routine tests for protein in urine do not distinguish which proteins are present. Protein loss from the kidney occurs in glomerulonephritis, nephrotic syndrome, renal infarction, fever, and toxemia. In addition, most chemical tests for protein are positive in the presence of hematuria or pyuria.

Normally all of the plasma glucose that appears in glomerular filtrate is reabsorbed in the renal tubules. The detection of **glucose** in the urine (glycosuria) generally indicates an abnormal elevation of plasma glucose. The renal threshold for glucose is about 180 mg/dL [10 mmol/L]. That means that at plasma levels above 180 mg/dL, more glucose appears in glomerular filtrate than can be reabsorbed by the tubules. Glycosuria is a cardinal finding in diabetes mellitus. It also occurs after rapid absorption of dietary glucose (alimentary glycosuria) and in some persons with abnormally low renal thresholds for glucose (renal glycosuria).

Occult blood refers to blood present in insufficient quantity to alter the color of the urine. A positive test for occult blood has generally the same significance as the finding of red blood cells in urine. **Acetone** and other ketones appear in the urine in diabetes mellitus with acidosis, in starvation, thyrotoxicosis, and high fever. As noted in the preceding chapter, only bilirubin that has been conjugated with glucuronic acid is soluble in water. Hence the appearance of **bilirubin** in the urine (bilirubinuria, choluria) is noted in obstructive jaundice, in which conjugated bilirubin enters the blood stream from bile, but not in jaundice due to hemolysis or liver disease, in which only unconjugated bilirubin is elevated in the plasma.

Qualitative testing for **hemoglobin** (not normally present in urine) is positive in disorders causing release of hemoglobin into the plasma (hemolytic anemias, burns, malaria) and in hematuria of any cause with extensive hemolysis of red blood cells in the urine. A qualitative test for **myoglobin** in urine is positive in some diseases of muscle, in crush syndrome, myocardial infarction, and various toxic states (carbon monoxide poisoning, alcoholism, diabetic acidosis).

Precise quantitative determinations of several substances in the urine are important in the diagnosis of certain conditions. Because of wide variations in urine volume and concentration due to variations in water intake and in nonrenal water losses (sweating, vomiting, diarrhea), analysis of a 24-hour urine specimen and computation of 24-hour excretion of the analyte provide much more useful information than analysis of a random specimen.

Quantitative determinations of **electrolytes** (sodium, potassium, chloride) in urine may help to clarify renal, adrenal, or metabolic disease in which serum electrolytes are abnormal because of inappropriate renal loss or retention. Measurement of **calcium** and **phosphorus** excretion supplies information about parathyroid function and the security of the body calcium pool. **Amino acid** screening of the urine can identify renal tubular defects associated with failure to reabsorb certain amino acids. Urinary **urobilinogen** excretion (normally below 4 mg/24h [6.8 mol/d]) is increased in hemolytic anemias, large hematomas, pulmonary infarction, and hepatic disease (viral hepatitis, cirrhosis), and reduced in biliary obstruction and starvation. Urinary excretion of **coproporphyrin** (a product of hemoglobin breakdown) is normally below 180 μg/24h [276 nmol/d]. Increases occur in porphyria, lead poisoning, and hepatic disease (viral hepatitis, cirrhosis). Excretion of **delta-aminolevulinic acid** (normally below 7 mg/24h [53 μmol/d]) is also increased in lead poisoning.

Identification of various products of neoplastic tissue in urine is sometimes more expedient than diagnostic studies of the blood. Excretion of both **catecholamines** and **vanillylmandelic acid** (VMA) is increased in pheochromocytoma and neuroblastoma. In carcinoid tumor with carcinoid syndrome, urinary excretion of **5-hydroxyindoleacetic acid** (5-HIAA) is increased. Adrenal cortical hyperplasia or neoplasia, or increased production of cortical steroids due to excessive secretion of ACTH by the pituitary gland, is reflected in an increase of urinary **17-ketosteroid** excretion. **Bence Jones protein** in urine (as detected by electrophoresis or immunoelectrophoresis) suggests multiple myeloma but may also be found in some collagen diseases and lymphomas. Urine **estrogen** or **androgen** levels may be increased by functioning gonadal neoplasms.

Urine pregnancy tests depend on identification of chorionic gonadotropin in urine. Measurement of urinary **urea** or **creatinine** is essential for determination of glomerular filtration rate as a function of urea or creatinine clearance, as mentioned in Chapter 30. One means of testing for intestinal malabsorption is to administer a test meal of **D-xylose** and measure urinary excretion. The **Schilling test** is a radioisotope study designed to identify persons with pernicious anemia. Oral administration of vitamin B_{12} tagged with radioactive cobalt (^{57}Co or ^{60}Co) is followed by collection of a 24-hour urine specimen. Recovery of less than 3% of administered radioisotope in the urine indicates impairment of vitamin B_{12} absorption. Repetition of the test with administration of intrinsic factor shows normal absorption of vitamin B_{12} in pernicious anemia but not in intestinal malabsorption.

Analysis of urine for toxic chemicals and drugs of abuse is a routine screening procedure in many occupational settings and in competitive athletics.

Urine **osmolality** (osmotic activity of total solute content) can be measured by the freezing point depression method, as described for serum osmolality in the previous chapter. The normal range of urine osmolality is 500 to 1200 mOsm/kg. Abnormally low urine osmolality despite restriction of water intake indicates renal disease with impairment of concentrating ability. In severe renal tubular disease the osmolality of urine approximates that of plasma (isosthenuria).

For urine culture, with or without colony count and sensitivity testing, the specimen is obtained under sterile conditions in a sterile container. Culture is performed in the microbiology laboratory.

Laboratory examinations of **stool** specimens are performed less frequently than examinations of urine. This is partly because procuring a stool specimen is esthetically objectionable to patients, but more importantly because only limited information can be gained by examining the stool. Tests that are routinely performed on stool specimens are qualitative analysis for occult blood and fat; quantitative determination of urobilinogen; smears for leukocytes, parasites, and parasite ova; Gram stain for pathogenic organisms; and culture in infectious diarrheas.

The **occult blood** test is useful in identifying gastrointestinal hemorrhage at any level, and is widely used in screening for malignant disease of the colon. For maximum specificity of the test, the patient should be on a meat-free diet for three days before collection of the specimen. A more sophisticated test for gastrointestinal bleeding involves determination of radioactivity in the stool after tagging of some of the patient's red blood cells with radioactive chromium (^{51}Cr). A finding of excessive **fat** in the stool by testing with Sudan III suggests steatorrhea (malabsorption of fat). Quantitative testing for fat normally shows less than 7 g/24h. Testing for steatorrhea is more sensitive if the patient consumes at least 60 g of fat daily for three days before collection of the specimen. Stool **urobilinogen** (normally 40 to 280 mg/24h [68–473 μmol/d]) is increased in hemolytic anemias and reduced in severe intrinsic liver disease and biliary obstruction.

Microscopic examination of stool normally shows undigested vegetable and muscle (meat) fibers, some fat, epithelial cells, and bacteria. A few white blood cells are also seen. Increase in white blood cells suggests inflammatory disease of the bowel. Bacteriologic smear and culture of the stool are performed in the microbiology laboratory. For the detection of intestinal parasites (protozoa, helminths, cysts, ova), a stool specimen is subjected to repeated concentrations (washing and centrifugation). Serologic studies may be more reliable for diagnosis of parasitism than isolation and identification of organisms from the stool.

Review Questions

1. What procedures can be used to limit contamination of a urine specimen by cells or secretions from outside the urinary tract?
2. What examinations make up the standard urinalysis?
3. What formed elements may be found on microscopic examination of a centrifuged specimen of urine?
4. What is the origin of casts in the urine?
5. What conditions other than diabetes mellitus may account for the appearance of glucose in the urine?
6. List some constituents of urine for which analysis requires collection of a 24-hour specimen.
7. What constituent of the stool is likely to be increased in malabsorption syndromes?
8. Define or explain: *choluria, clean catch, glycosuria, occult blood, pyuria, reaction of urine, specific gravity.*

32

Laboratory Examination of Other Body Fluids and Materials

Although blood and urine are the principal objects of scrutiny in the clinical laboratory, any other body fluid or product, normal or abnormal, can be subjected to microscopic inspection, chemical analysis, and bacteriologic culture. For some fluids (cerebrospinal fluid, amniotic fluid, semen), certain examinations are routine. For others (sputum, gastric aspirate), the diagnostic focus determines what examinations are done.

This chapter reviews only the more common and useful laboratory examinations of specimens other than blood, urine, and stool. Procedures for cytologic study of transudates, exudates, and aspirates for malignant cells are discussed in Chapter 4, and microbiologic examinations are discussed in Chapter 33. Most of the other tests performed on body fluids consist of either microscopic examination of stained or unstained smears or quantitative chemical analysis for substances increased or decreased in certain diseases or conditions.

Cerebrospinal fluid is obtained by lumbar puncture ("spinal tap") (less often by cisternal puncture) in cases where central nervous system infection (meningitis, encephalitis), neoplasm, or hemorrhage is suspected, and in various other conditions. Separate specimens are routinely obtained for cell count, chemical testing, and culture. The normal **cell count** is less than 10 cells/mm³, and normally all cells found are mononuclear. A rise in mononuclear cells occurs in viral encephalitis and meningitis and in tuberculous meningitis. Appearance of polymorphonuclear leukocytes indicates pyogenic (bacterial) meningitis or encephalitis or brain abscess.

The total **protein** concentration of spinal fluid (about 90% of it albumin) is normally 15 to 45 mg/dL [0.15–0.45 g/L]. Protein is increased in encephalitis, meningitis, poliomyelitis, neoplasm of the brain or spinal cord, and cerebral or subarachnoid hemorrhage. A rise in protein without a rise in cell count (albuminocytologic dissociation) is characteristic of Guillain-Barré syndrome. The **glucose** level of spinal fluid is normally about 20 mg/dL [0.2 g/L] less than that of the blood. Hence for proper interpretation the blood level must be tested at the same time as the spinal fluid level. Spinal fluid glucose is increased in diabetic coma and reduced in bacterial meningitis.

Pleural, pericardial, and peritoneal fluid obtained by needle aspiration can be tested for specific gravity and protein concentration in order to distinguish between a transudate (specific gravity less than 1.016 and protein less than 3.0 g/dL [0.03 g/L]) and an exudate (specific gravity 1.016 or more and protein 3.0 g/dL or more). A finding of polymorphonuclear leukocytes in a stained smear indicates pyogenic infection.

Synovial fluid obtained by needle aspiration from a joint in acute or chronic arthritis with effusion is subjected to cell count and examination by compensated polarized light microscopy for crystals. A white blood cell count over 200/mm^3 suggests inflammation and over 2000/mm^3 suggests infection. Very high counts (to 100 000/mm^3) are seen in septic arthritis. Uric acid crystals are found in gout, calcium pyrophosphate crystals in pseudogout.

Gastric analysis (testing of the acid content of gastric juice obtained by nasogastric tube) is carried out both in the basal state and after stimulation with histamine. The normal basal production of acid is 2 to 5 mEq/h, and one hour after stimulation with histamine this may rise to 20 mEq/h. Gastric acid secretion is increased in duodenal ulcer and greatly increased in Zollinger-Ellison syndrome. It is decreased or absent in gastric carcinoma, achlorhydria, and pernicious anemia.

A smear of **nasal secretions** stained by the Wright or Giemsa method shows eosinophils in allergic rhinitis.

Sweat electrolytes (concentrations of sodium and chloride in sweat) are increased in cystic fibrosis.

On **semen analysis**, more than 50 000 000 spermatozoa/mL should be found. More than 60% of these should be motile and fewer than 50% should show morphologic abnormalities.

Chemical analysis of **urinary calculi** helps to identify disorders that cause renal excretion of abnormal substances or of normal substances in abnormal amounts.

Amniotic fluid, obtained by needle aspiration from the amniotic sac at or after the fourteenth week of gestation, supplies fetal cells for karyotyping, described below, and can also be tested chemically. Elevation of alpha-fetoprotein (AFP) occurs in neural tube defects (anencephaly, spina bifida). The lecithin/sphingomyelin ratio, determined by thin-layer chromatography, is less than 1.0 before fetal lungs mature, more than 1.0 when lung maturity has been attained.

Cytogenetics, the study of the chromosomal structure of cells, can be used to verify the genetic sex of an individual, to identify chromosomal abnormalities such as Down's syndrome (mongolism), Turner's syndrome, and Klinefelter's syndrome, and to diagnose various inborn errors of metabolism before birth.

Sex chromatin analysis is relatively simple and can be performed on a stained smear of any body cells. A smear from the buccal mucosa is most often used. For prenatal sex determination, chromatin analysis is performed on cells from amniotic fluid obtained by amniocentesis. The Barr body, a solitary, very small, solid mass lying just within the cell membrane and visible by light microscopy, is present in about half of all the body cells of a genetic female. The Barr body is absent from all cells of a genetic male. Y bodies, which indicate maleness, can be detected by more elaborate procedures.

For **chromosomal analysis** or karyotyping, blood cells or tissue cells obtained by biopsy are first grown in tissue culture. Slides of these cells are then prepared and specially stained to show chromosome banding. Chromosome counts are performed on a number of cells and the results collated. Fetal chromosome analysis is performed on cells from amniotic fluid or from biopsy of chorionic villi. Fetal cells can also be subjected to DNA analysis for prenatal identification of certain genetic diseases such as cystic fibrosis and muscular dystrophy. Cytogenetic study of tissue specimens for the presence of **oncogenes** (mutant genes responsible for converting normal cells to malignant tumor cells) and for the absence of tumor suppressor genes is used to diagnose and stage various neoplasms. More than 150 cytogenetic abnormalities have been associated with specific neoplasms. Examples are the Philadelphia chromosome, found in marrow cells in chronic myelogenous leukemia; *ras* oncogenes, characteristic of carcinomas of the colon and rectum; and absence of the tumor suppressor gene *p53*, which occurs in more than 75% of colorectal carcinomas.

Review Questions

1. What routine examinations are performed on cerebrospinal fluid?
2. What is meant by albuminocytologic dissociation in the spinal fluid?
3. In what conditions are abnormalities of gastric acid secretion noted?
4. What diagnostic procedures can be performed on amniotic fluid?
5. List some clinical applications of cytogenetics.

33

Microbiology and Serology

Virtually all of the procedures performed in a microbiology laboratory pertain to infectious disease—confirming the presence of infection, identifying the causative organisms, selecting antibiotics effective against them, and verifying microbiologic cure after treatment. Infectious diseases are discussed in Chapter 11. In medical microbiology, diagnostic focus is of paramount importance. No laboratory procedure or group of procedures can isolate or identify all possible pathogens. The source of a specimen provides some clues as to which pathogens are likely to be found and hence some direction as to the choice of culture techniques. Ideally, however, the patient's medical history and physical findings, the results of other laboratory tests, the response to treatment, and the clinician's tentative diagnosis are all taken into account in processing a microbiologic specimen.

Most of the routine work is in **bacteriology**, whose two principal diagnostic methods are the microscopic examination of stained smears and the culture of microorganisms. A **smear** is a translucent layer of fluid or semisolid material thinly spread over a microscope slide. A smear can be prepared from any natural body fluid, waste product, or abnormal secretion. Standard procedures are in use for making smears from throat, nasopharyngeal, vaginal, and anal swabs and from sputum, stool, wound drainage, and pus. Clear fluids such as spinal fluid, urine, and serous exudates may be centrifuged or filtered, as described in Chapter 4 under cytologic techniques, to improve the yield of bacteria.

Bacteriologic smears are routinely stained by Gram's method, as discussed in Chapter 11. The technician examining the smear notes whether one or several kinds of organism are present and, by considering their size, shape, grouping, and Gram-staining characteristics, forms a judgment as to whether the smear contains only normal flora (nonpathogenic organisms normally found in the source material or bodily region in question) or whether infection is present, and if so what kind. Specimens of sputum or other material can also be stained by the acid-fast method (described in Chapter 11) when infection with *Mycobacteria* is suspected. Special stains designed to identify specific organisms are occasionally used.

Besides being treated with chemical stains, bacteriologic smears can also be examined by a **fluorescent antibody** technique. In this method, the smear is treated with a combination of monoclonal antibody to a suspected organism and a fluorescent dye such as rhodamine. If the anticipated antigen-antibody reaction occurs, sites of fixation of the fluorescent antibody can be observed by microscopic examination of the smear with fluorescent lighting. This method is valuable in identifying intracellular organisms, such as *Chlamydia,* which stain poorly if at all by standard staining techniques.

A **culture** is a growth of microorganisms under controlled artificial conditions in the laboratory. Culturing offers several advantages over the simple smear for diagnostic purposes. When only a few organisms are present in a specimen, they may be missed in a smear. Theoretically every viable organism in the specimen will generate a separate, pure colony in a culture. Hence culturing permits isolation of various organisms from a mixture for individual study. Observation of the growth characteristics of organisms in a culture supplies additional identifying data, and pure colonies from the culture can be studied in stained smears. Smears or suspensions made from pure cultures are also more suitable for study with serologic reagents such as agglutinins applied to detect the presence of specific organisms.

By the addition of nutrients and inhibitors to a culture medium, certain types of organisms can be favored while others are suppressed. Reagents and indicators added to the culture medium allow prompt detection of distinctive products of bacterial growth. For more precise identification, organisms from a culture can be subcultured in one or more special media. For **antibiotic sensitivity testing**, disks impregnated with known concentrations of various antibiotics are incorporated in the culture medium. Zones of inhibition of bacterial growth around certain disks indicate sensitivity of the organism to those antibiotics.

Several kinds of bacteriologic media are in regular use, each with its specific purpose. Fluid media, usually called broths, are placed in sterile glass test tubes stoppered with cotton wool, which allows entry and exit of gases but prevents contamination of the culture by bacteria and molds from the air. Many media contain a vegetable gum called agar which gives them a stiff gel-like consistency below 45°C. Organisms grown on agar present more distinctive cultural characteristics than those grown in broth, and individual colonies can be observed and sampled. In addition, the use of sensitivity disks requires a solid medium. When an agar medium is placed in tubes, the tubes are usually allowed to cool in a slanted position so as to provide a larger surface area ("agar slants"). More often, agar media are placed in shallow transparent glass or plastic plates called Petri dishes. Each Petri dish has a loosely fitting cover which allows entry of oxygen and escape of gases but prevents contamination of the medium.

Introduction of infectious material into a culture medium is called **inoculation**. A minute amount (inoculum) of the specimen may be picked up with a sterile wire or wire loop and immersed in broth or streaked across the surface of an agar plate or slant. Streaking can also be done with a cotton swab, as in the case of a throat culture. Blood cultures are inoculated by adding freshly drawn whole blood to a nutrient broth in a culture flask.

After inoculation, cultures are ordinarily **incubated** at human body temperature (37°C) for 48 to 72 hours and observed periodically for growth. Growth of certain microorganisms is favored by incubation in an atmosphere with little or no oxygen or with increased carbon dioxide. Organisms that grow best at very low oxygen tension are called anaerobes. Cultures for acid-fast organisms (*Mycobacteria*) require six to eight weeks of incubation.

Throat cultures are performed on **blood agar**, a medium containing whole blood of animal origin, to facilitate identification of streptococci. Alpha-hemolytic streptococci and some other organisms cause greenish discoloration of the medium due to partial hemolysis. Beta-hemolytic streptococci and some other organisms cause the medium to become perfectly transparent around each colony by more complete chemical breakdown of blood. A disk impregnated with bacitracin may be included in the medium to distinguish Group A beta-hemolytic streptococci, whose growth is inhibited by bacitracin, from other beta-hemolytic organisms, which are resistant to bacitracin. **Chocolate agar**, so called because of its color, contains blood that has been chemically altered by heating. Chocolate agar is a preferred medium for certain organisms, such as *Neisseria* and *Haemophilus*. Thayer-Martin medium is chocolate agar containing various antibiotics to inhibit the growth of organisms other than *Neisseria*. Differentiation among similar colon bacilli is achieved by simultaneous incubation in media containing various sugars (glucose, maltose, lactose, sucrose) ("differential sugars") and observation of growth patterns. Identification of organisms in a culture may depend on chemical detection of biochemical products such as hydrogen sulfide, indole, or nitrites from nitrates.

Quantitative techniques have been developed for culturing some specimens, notably urine. The standard urine **colony count**, requiring precise dilution of the specimen before inoculation, is reported in colonies per cubic millimeter of urine. A colony count over 100 000/mm^3 is regarded as evidence of urinary tract infection, but lower counts may also be significant for some organisms or in some patients.

Medical **mycology**, the study of pathogenic fungi, employs techniques similar to those of bacteriology. However, most fungi cannot be stained by Gram's method or others routinely used in bacteriologic work. On the other hand, fungal material is more resistant than human cells to digestion by potassium hydroxide (KOH) solution, and treatment of material such as sputum or wound drainage with this alkali often leaves fungal hyphae or spores clearly visible on microscopic examination. Special culture media are required for fungi. Sabouraud's agar, containing peptone and dextrose, is the most widely used. Incubation, usually at room temperature, must be continued for several weeks.

In contrast, diagnostic **virology** generally does not make use of direct techniques like those of bacteriology. Viral particles cannot be seen by light microscopy, and cannot be cultured in artificial media. Although electron microscopy and cell culture techniques are available for the study of viruses, in practice the laboratory diagnosis of most viral infections can be made more promptly and less expensively by serologic testing, usually by demonstrating specific antibody to the virus in the patient's serum.

The methods of diagnostic **parasitology** are also different, in that, while staining and culture of parasites are often not feasible, many kinds of parasite are visible to the naked eye or are so distinctive in smears or tissue sections as to leave no doubt as to their identity. Standard procedures are in use for examination of stool, urine, and sputum for protozoan parasites, worms, cysts, and ova. Malarial parasites, trypanosomes, and leishmaniae are detectable in appropriately stained blood smears. Pinworm infestation (enterobiasis) can sometimes be diagnosed by finding ova on a Scotch tape swab taken from the perianal region in the morning upon arising. Vaginal trichomoniasis can be diagnosed by finding motile trichomonads in a wet mount or hanging drop preparation of vaginal secretions.

Serology, broadly speaking, embraces all those diagnostic technologies and strategies based on antigen-antibody reactions, including a number of procedures that do not involve testing of serum. Antibody formation in response to infecting organisms and allergens is discussed in Chapter 11. Currently of major importance in the diagnosis of viral infections, serologic methods are also used to identify infections due to bacteria, fungi, and parasites. In addition, serologic testing has been applied to the diagnosis of some noninfectious diseases, particularly neoplasms.

Serologic testing is often easier, less expensive, faster, and more specific than routine procedures for isolation and identification of infecting organisms. The basic laboratory procedure in serology is the identification of an antibody or an antigen by bringing about an antigen-antibody reaction under controlled conditions. Antibodies are sought in serum by challenge with specific or nonspecific antigens. A specific antigen is chemically or biologically identical to the one that elicited antibody formation—for example, an extract of *Salmonella* organisms used in a serologic test for antibody stimulated by *Salmonella* infection. A nonspecific antigen reacts with one or more antibodies even though it is biologically different from the antigen that elicited antibody production—for example, sheep or horse red blood cells that react with heterophile antibodies in infectious mononucleosis.

The reaction between antigen and antibody can take many forms in the laboratory. The antigen and antibody, separately suspended in solution or gel form, can be combined in a plate or tube in such a fashion that a turbid, opaque, or insoluble complex is formed between them. Such a reaction is called **precipitation**. When the precipitate appears to consist of irregular fleecy masses it may be called **flocculation**. The reaction between antigen and antibody can be accelerated by passing an electric current through the system, which promotes migration of proteins towards the cathode (**immunoelectrophoresis**). In an **agglutination** test, suspended particles of antigenic material are caused to clump by exposure to antibody. These particles may be killed microorganisms, red blood cells, or inert material such as latex coated with antigen. Sometimes antibody is more readily detected by an indirect method. In **inhibition** reactions, competition between two antibodies prevents precipitation or agglutination that would otherwise have occurred. In **complement fixation** (CF) tests, a reaction between antibody and antigen is shown to have taken place by the absorption of complement, a serum protein essential to such reactions.

Precipitation tests are generally qualitative, but most of the other tests mentioned can be made quantitative. The use of serial dilutions to establish the **titer** of an antibody is described in Chapter 28. In the serologic diagnosis of an acute infection it is customary to draw blood as soon as possible after the onset of illness and again approximately two weeks later. Simultaneous testing of the two specimens should show at least a fourfold rise in the titer of antibody to the infecting organism from the "acute serum" to the "convalescent serum." A past history of certain infections (or of active immunization against them), and presumed protection against reinfection, is shown by finding a protective titer of antibody to the infecting organisms.

Some serologic methods involve application of antibody to detect antigen. Fluorescent antibody (FA) testing has been mentioned already as a means of identifying certain bacteria in smears under the fluorescence microscope. This is an example of **direct immunofluorescence**. In **indirect immunofluorescence**, the antibody that reacts with the antigen in the specimen is not fluorescently tagged. After this initial reaction, a fluorescent antibody to the first antibody is applied. In **radioimmunoassay** (RIA) procedures, the antigen or antibody is radioactively tagged. In an **enzyme-linked immunosorbent assay** (ELISA), the antigen or antibody is tagged with an enzyme, whose activity, measured after addition of a suitable substrate, gives a measure of the antigen or antibody bound in the reaction.

Antibody testing using specific antigens is employed routinely in the serologic diagnosis of acute infection, or in establishing prior history of infection, with measles, rubella, mumps, herpes simplex, varicella-zoster, human immunodeficiency virus, cytomegalovirus, and various fungal and parasitic diseases, including toxoplasmosis. The **antistreptolysin O** (ASO) titer is a standard means of detecting recent streptococcal infection. A level of 500 to 5000 Todd units is seen in active rheumatic fever and acute glomerulonephritis. Slide tests for rapid diagnosis of streptococcal pharyngitis (**strep screen**) employ agglutination or ELISA methods and are performed directly on material from throat swabs. The Widal agglutination test for typhoid fever determines antibody to two antigens (0 and H) derived from *Salmonella* organisms. The *Treponema pallidum* **immobilization** (TPI) test is a specific antibody test for syphilis, as is the **fluorescent treponemal antibody** (FTA) test, which uses indirect immunofluorescence.

Several routine tests for the diagnosis of infectious disease use nonspecific antigens. In the **heterophile agglutination** test, sheep or horse erythrocytes are agglutinated by the serum of a patient with acute or recent infectious mononucleosis. The serum is first treated with an extract of guinea pig kidney to adsorb nonrelevant antibodies. A titer of 1:112 or higher is typical of acute disease. Several qualitative slide tests based on this reaction are available. The **VDRL** (Venereal Disease Research Laboratories) test for syphilis, and its modification, the **RPR** (rapid plasma reagin), use beef heart cardiolipin as an antigen. Sometimes the term **serology** is used in the narrow sense of "serologic test for syphilis," which may also be abbreviated STS. In the Weil-Felix test, antigens from various strains of *Proteus vulgaris* are used to identify antibody to various rickettsiae such as those causing typhus and Rocky Mountain spotted fever. Patients with mycoplasmal pneumonia form antibodies called **cold agglutinins**, which agglutinate type O human erythrocytes at 4°C but not at 20° or 37°.

A panel of tests for various **febrile agglutinins** is sometimes performed in cases of fever of unknown origin. A typical panel includes agglutination titers for typhoid (Widal O and H), paratyphoid, brucellosis, tularemia, and rickettsiae (Weil-Felix).

Methods are available to detect viral and other antigens in serum with monoclonal antibody. Testing for three antigenic fractions of the hepatitis B virus (hepatitis B core antigen or HB_cAg, surface antigen or HB_sAg, and e antigen or HB_eAg) in serum provides information about the stage of the disease.

A number of newer molecular biology techniques allow identification of very small concentrations of antigen or antibody in specimens. In the **Western blot** (immunoblot) procedure, known antigens are separated electrophoretically into bands and then blotted (transferred by direct contact) to a nitrocellulose membrane, where they retain their relative positions. Antibodies present in specimen material bind to corresponding antigens when exposed to the membrane. **Dot-blot hybridization** detects specific DNA (deoxyribonucleic acid) sequences in a small spot of specimen material that has been blotted to a membrane. A **polymerase chain reaction** (PCR) can raise the concentration of DNA in a specimen to a level at which it can be detected by molecular biology techniques. In this process, specimen DNA is made to combine with specially designed primers and then enzymatically induced to replicate many times.

Blood typing (grouping), discussed in Chapter 29, makes use of type-specific antisera. In addition, serologic testing is used to identify acquired hemolytic anemias including those arising from Rh incompatibility. In the **direct Coombs** test, the patient's red blood cells are tested with antiserum to determine whether they have become coated with an antiglobulin. This test is positive in a newborn with erythroblastosis fetalis and in persons with acquired hemolytic disease due to production of abnormal globulins, as in leukemia, lymphoma, and collagen diseases. In the **indirect Coombs** test, the patient's serum is tested for antiglobulin by incubation with erythrocytes. The indirect Coombs test is positive in the mother of an infant with erythroblastosis fetalis and in any person with anti-Rh antiglobulins or other acquired hemolyzing antibodies, as in hematopoietic malignancies and collagen diseases. Both direct and indirect Coombs tests are negative in hereditary hemoglobinopathies.

Serologic testing also finds application in the diagnosis of allergy, autoimmune disease, and certain neoplasms. The **radioallergosorbent test** (RAST), a modification of radioimmunoassay, uses isotopically tagged allergens to detect IgE antibodies to these allergens in the serum of allergic persons. Several laboratory tests have been found useful in identifying abnormal globulin activity in persons with autoimmune disease. The **lupus erythematosus cell test** (LE cell prep) is performed by incubating the patient's blood under controlled conditions and then observing a stained smear for LE cells. The LE cell is a neutrophil with a very large cytoplasmic inclusion produced by the action of the patient's abnormal antibodies on the cell nucleus. The test is positive in disseminated lupus erythematosus and in some cases of scleroderma, dermatomyositis, and rheumatoid arthritis. More sensitive but not more specific tests for **antinuclear antibody** (ANA) can be performed by complement fixation or immunofluorescence techniques. The **anticytoplasmic antibody** (ACPA) test, which detects autoantibodies to components of neutrophilic cytoplasm by immunofluorescence, is useful in diagnosing Wegener's granulomatosis and gauging its extent and severity.

Rheumatoid factor is an IgM antibody that is directed against the patient's own IgG. It can be detected by various tests, including a latex agglutination test in which the patient's serum is incubated with latex particles coated with human IgG. These tests are positive in about two-thirds of patients with rheumatoid arthritis and in some persons with other autoimmune disorders. **Human lymphocytic antigens** (HLA), which occur in some autoimmune disorders, can be defined and typed by serologic methods. HLA-B27 is found in patients with ankylosing spondylitis, Reiter's syndrome, Graves' disease, myasthenia gravis, multiple sclerosis, and several other systemic diseases.

Certain glycoproteins detectable by radioimmunoassay appear in the serum of some patients with certain malignant neoplasms. Tests to detect these tumor markers are used to screen populations at risk for certain malignancies, to stage malignancies after diagnosis, and to detect recurrences after treatment. **Carcinoembryonic antigen** (CEA) is present in many cases of carcinoma, particularly of the lung, digestive tract, and pancreas. Because it is also elevated in other malignancies and in nonmalignant inflammatory diseases of the bowel, as well as in many heavy smokers, it is not of much use in screening or diagnosis. It is valuable, however, in testing treated cancer patients for recurrence or metastases. **Prostate specific antigen** (PSA), a protease produced by prostatic epithelium, is found elevated in primary and metastatic adenocarcinoma of the prostate as well as in some cases of prostatitis and benign prostatic hyperplasia. **Alpha-fetoprotein** (AFP) is a globulin produced by the liver and other tissues of the fetus and newborn. Its level normally declines after one year of age. Elevation of alpha-fetoprotein occurs in hepatocellular carcinoma, viral hepatitis, hepatic cirrhosis, and various teratocarcinomas and embryonal carcinomas of gonadal origin. As mentioned in the preceding chapter, an elevated level of AFP found in amniotic fluid suggests the presence of a neural tube defect in the fetus.

Review Questions

1. What are the two basic laboratory procedures in bacteriology?
2. In what ways can culturing a pathogenic microorganism contribute to its identification?
3. What is the standard medium for throat cultures?
4. What basic type of reaction is studied in a serologic test?
5. What are some reasons for preferring serologic testing to culture of pathogenic microorganisms?
6. Give an example of a diagnostic antibody test that uses a nonspecific antigen.
7. List some serologic tests that are used to diagnose diseases or conditions that are not infections.
8. Define or explain: *agar, convalescent serum, febrile agglutinins, normal flora, sensitivity test, STS.*

Glossary

Note: A glossary of clinical pathology terms and expressions is found on pp. 279–280. Those entries are not duplicated here.

ABC Aspiration biopsy cytology.

acellular Without cells.

adhesion An abnormal fibrous connection between two structures or surfaces.

adipocere A waxy material formed by the decomposition of fatty materials in a dead body, especially one submerged in water or buried in damp ground.

aerobic Living, growing, or taking place in the presence of oxygen.

afferent Conducting towards a structure.

agminated Clustered, aggregated.

agonal Referring to the last moments of life.

amastigote An immature form of *Leishmania*, lacking a flagellum.

amniocentesis Removal of a quantity of amniotic fluid from the pregnant uterus for diagnostic purposes.

amorphous Without form or shape.

amphophilic Attracting stains of both acidic and basic reaction.

anaerobic Living, growing, or taking place in the absence of oxygen.

anencephaly Congenital absence of the cranium and of most or all of the cerebrum.

anisonucleosis Abnormal variation in the sizes of cell nuclei.

anlage The earliest discernible rudiment of a structure during embryonic development; primordium.

anorexia Loss of appetite.

anoxia Deficiency of oxygen.

antimesenteric Referring to the side of the bowel opposite the attachment of the mesentery.

apatite A calcium phosphate salt found in bones and teeth.

apoptosis Fragmentation of a cell into particles, each of which is surrounded by a membrane.

arthralgia Pain in one or more joints, with or without evidence of inflammation.

asplenia Absence of the spleen.

atresia Congenital absence or closure of an orifice or passage.

atypia Irregularity, departure from expected appearance.

azurophilic Showing an affinity for blue aniline stains.

bacteremia The presence of bacteria in the blood circulation.

BAL Bronchoalveolar lavage.

Bard-Parker blade Proprietary name for disposable scalpel blades available in a variety of shapes and used in surgery and in performing autopsies.

beefy Having the appearance or texture of raw lean meat.

Betz cell A pyramidal ganglion cell of the cerebral cortex.

bifurcation Division of a vessel or other structure into two branches.

bioptome A cutting instrument for obtaining biopsies.

bland Without evidence of inflammation.

boss A rounded prominence or knob.

bosselated Marked or covered by bosses.

burrow A linear cutaneous lesion created by the migration of a parasite beneath the skin surface.

calcinosis Deposition of calcium salts in tissue.

calvarium The top of the skull.

cancerization Malignant degeneration.

carneous degeneration Tissue change producing a fleshy texture.

carnification Same as the preceding.

cast An elongated mass formed by inspissation of semisolid material in a tubular structure.

Caves-Schutz-Stanford bioptome An instrument for obtaining a biopsy of the myocardium via a transvenous catheter.

chancre The primary lesion of syphilis, a painless indurated ulcer.

Chiba needle An aspiration biopsy needle.

chilblain Local cutaneous inflammation caused by exposure to cold and damp.

choristoma A mass of heterotopic tissue.

chylous Containing or resembling chyle, the milky fluid containing absorbed nutrients passing from the digestive tract to the circulatory system via the thoracic duct.

circumscribed Surrounded, clearly demarcated from adjacent structures.

coagulopathy Any disorder of blood coagulation.

colic A sharp, intermittent pain in the trunk of the body, generally due to smooth muscle spasm or obstruction of a tubular structure.

concretion A gritty or sandy material, usually formed by deposition of mineral salts.

congenital Present from birth.

Cook needle An aspiration biopsy needle.

coryza The common cold, or any similar condition with nasal congestion and discharge.

Councilman chisel An autopsy instrument used for splitting bone.

crenated Having a shriveled or pitted surface.

crepitation, crepitus Crackling.

cribriform Perforated like a sieve.

cutis anserina Gooseflesh; erection of the hairs in response to cold or fear.

cyanotic Showing an abnormal bluish discoloration.

cyst Any fluid-filled abnormal structure.

debris Amorphous material resulting from injury, degeneration, or necrosis of tissue.

denuded Uncovered, deprived of a normal surface.

depth The deepest portion of a surgically excised specimen, as in "The margins and depths of the specimen are free of malignant cells."

dilated Enlarged.

DIC Disseminated intravascular coagulation, a condition in which widespread clotting of blood in vessels consumes clotting factors and leads to hemorrhage.

ectasia Expansion or dilatation of a duct or vessel.

ectopia Abnormal location of a tissue or structure.

efferent Conducting away from a structure.

effusion An oozing or outpouring of fluid.

emphysema Abnormal presence of air within tissues.

endosteum The connective-tissue lining of the marrow cavity of a bone.

enterotome An autopsy instrument used for opening the intestine.

eosinophilia 1. Affinity for eosin and other acidic stains. 2. An abnormal increase of eosinophils in the circulating blood or in tissue.

epistaxis Nosebleed.

erythema Abnormal redness.

erythema nodosum A hypersensitivity reaction to various abnormal conditions, characterized by formation of tender red nodules beneath the skin, especially over the shins.

erythroderma Redness of the skin.

eschar A crust or scab of exudate or devitalized tissue forming at the site of a burn or other injury.

etiology The study of the causes of disease; often used in the sense of "cause."

excrescence An abnormal nodule or mass growing away from a surface.

exophytic Growing away from a surface.

extravasate To leak or ooze from vessels.

fascicle A small bundle.

fibrofatty Consisting of fibrous and fatty connective tissue.

fibrovascular Consisting of fibrous connective tissue and blood vessels.

filiform Threadlike.

flaccid Limp, not spastic or rigid.

flagellum A whiplike process characteristic of certain protozoans.

florid Fully developed, as in "florid cirrhosis."

focal Confined to one or several distinct sites or foci.

frank Fully developed, obvious, unequivocal, as in "frank pus."

Franseen needle A needle used for aspiration biopsy as well as for removal of a solid core of tissue.

friable Crumbly, readily broken up.

fungating Growing rapidly and irregularly, like a fungus, usually said of a neoplasm.

fusiform Spindle-shaped; an elongated structure that is thicker in the middle than at either end.

gemistocyte A swollen astrocyte with an eccentric nucleus.

Gluck rib shears An autopsy instrument used to cut through the costosternal joints.

granular Speckled or grainy in appearance or texture.

Greene needle A biopsy needle used for aspiration and also for removal of solid tissue specimens.

grumous Lumpy; said of a liquid or semisolid material with small, denser masses or bodies suspended in it.

gumma A rubbery nodule of inflammation and necrosis, characteristic of tertiary syphilis.

hematemesis Vomiting blood.

hemoglobinuria The presence of hemoglobin, as distinct from whole blood, in the urine.

hemoptysis Coughing up blood from the respiratory tract.

hepatomegaly Enlargement of the liver.

hepatosplenomegaly Enlargement of the liver and spleen.

hereditary Inherited; affecting the genetic makeup of an organism.

host The person or animal in whom an infection or infestation occurs.

Howship's lacuna A pit or cavity resulting from resorption of calcium from bone.

Hutchinson's teeth Notched incisor teeth in congenital syphilis.

hypercapnia Excess of carbon dioxide in the blood.

hypoxia Deficiency of oxygen.

iatrogenic Referring to a condition, abnormality, disease, or injury that results from medical or surgical treatment or from a diagnostic procedure.

idiopathic Arising as if spontaneously; said of a disease or abnormality whose cause is unknown.

in situ In its original or normal position; said of a malignancy that has not begun to extend or invade beyond its tissue of origin.

induration Abnormal hardening of tissue.

injection Hyperemia; dilatation of blood vessels causing redness of a surface or tissue.

inoculation Introduction of infectious material into a living host or culture medium.

inspissated Dried out, thickened; said of fluid or semisolid materials.

Jamshidi needle A biopsy needle.

karyorrhexis Fragmentation of cell nuclei.

keratoacanthoma A benign epidermal tumor resembling squamous cell carcinoma.

koilocytosis A hollow appearance of cells.

lamellated Layered.

laminated Layered.

Lee needle A cutting biopsy needle.

lesion Any local, objectively perceptible abnormality in tissues resulting from injury or disease.

leukocytosis Abnormal increase in circulating leukocytes.

leukoderma Abnormal whiteness of skin.

leukopenia Abnormal decrease in circulating leukocytes.

ligneous Woody.

lipidosis Any abnormal condition characterized by an increased amount of lipid.

lipophage A macrophage that has ingested lipid material.

macrometastasis A grossly evident metastasis.

Madayag needle A biopsy needle used for aspiration and also for removal of solid tissue specimens.

malar Pertaining to the cheeks.

marantic Pertaining to cachexia or wasting.

marasmus Wasting, cachexia, particularly when due to protein and caloric deficiency in children.

meaty Having the appearance or texture of raw meat.

mediastinum That part of the thoracic cavity lying between the lungs.

melena Tarry black stools, generally due to bleeding within the digestive tract.

mesangial Pertaining to the mesangium, a membrane that supports the capillary loops of a glomerulus.

metabolism A general term referring to the sum of biochemical processes taking place in a living organism, or to specific groups of such processes, as in "carbohydrate metabolism."

microfilaria The prelarval stage of various tissue worms.

micrometastasis A microscopic metastasis.

mongolism Down's syndrome, a chromosomal disorder characterized by skeletal abnormalities and mental retardation.

mononucleosis Excessive numbers of mononuclear cells in circulating blood.

morphology The study of the shape or appearance of structures; often used as a synonym for "shape" or "appearance."

mottled Irregularly covered with darker or lighter spots.

mucopus A mixture of mucus and pus.

mummification Necrosis of tissue (as in gangrene) or of a dead body accompanied by extreme drying and shriveling, with only slight evidence of putrefaction.

myalgia Muscular pain.

mycosis Any fungal infection.

mycotic aneurysm An aneurysm due to local infection with a fungus. Although this is the literal meaning of the term, in practice it usually refers to local infection caused by bacteria carried in the circulation from another site.

nephrocalcinosis Deposition of calcium salts in the tissue of the kidney.

normocephalic Having a normal head.

nosocomial Pertaining to a hospital, and particularly to an infection contracted by a hospitalized person.

nuclear dust Fragments of a nucleus that has undergone karyorrhexis.

obliteration Complete removal of a structure, or complete filling of a cavity or passage.

oliguria Abnormal reduction in the volume of urine.

opportunistic Said of microorganisms that seldom invade healthy persons but often cause infections in persons with diminished immunity or in tissues already damaged by injury or disease.

organogenesis Formation of organs during embryonic development.

orthochromatic Showing normal or expected staining properties.

osteoblastic Referring to development or overdevelopment of bone tissue.

osteolytic Referring to absorption or destruction of bone tissue.

ostium A small orifice.

palisade A configuration created by structures lined up like the palings of a fence.

palpation Feeling a structure or tissue for diagnostic purposes.

papillary Showing nipplelike projections.

paracentesis Removal of fluid from a cavity, especially the abdominal cavity, with a hollow needle.

patchy Occurring in irregularly shaped and irregularly distributed areas.

patent Open, unobstructed.

pedunculated Attached to a surface by a stalk.

percutaneous Through the skin.

perforation Creation of an abnormal opening, usually in a hollow structure.

perfusion The flow of fluid through the vessels of a structure, generally referring to blood circulation.

perichondrium The connective-tissue covering of cartilage.

peristalsis The coordinated wave of muscular contractions in a tubular organ such as the intestine by which its contents are propelled forward.

phlebolith A calcified thrombus inside a vein.

phlegmon An indurated zone of inflammation and necrosis caused by pyogenic bacteria.

plantar Pertaining to the sole of the foot.

plasmacytic Pertaining to plasma cells.

pleocytosis An increase in the number of cells, particularly in the cerebrospinal fluid.

pleomorphic Occurring in various forms.

polarity Orientation of elongated structures, particularly with respect to an axis.

polygonal Many-sided.

polyhedral Many-sided.

porencephaly The presence of cysts or cavities in the cerebral cortex.

prenatal Before birth.

primary Said of a disease or condition not known to result from some other disease or abnormal condition; cf. *secondary.*

primordium The earliest discernible rudiment of a structure during embryonic development; anlage.

probe patent Allowing the passage of a probe; said of an orifice or hollow or tubular structure.

proliferation Reproduction, growth through increase in number of components.

protuberant Bulging, protruding.

proudflesh Granulation tissue of skin or mucous membrane.

pruritus Itching.

psammoma body A small, concentrically laminated mass of calcareous material found in certain neoplasms.

pseudomembrane A film of exudate or tissue debris resembling a membrane.

punctate Forming or resembling a spot or dot.

pyriform Pear-shaped.

refractile Transmitting light rays in the manner of glass or water, with deviation of rays as they pass into the surrounding air.

Rein rib-cutting knife Autopsy instrument for severing the costosternal joints.

rest 1. A mass of surviving embryonic cells. 2. A mass of cells misplaced during embryonic development (e.g., adrenal tissue in the kidney).

retroperitoneal Behind the peritoneal cavity.

rosette A ring-shaped cluster.

Rotex needle A cutting biopsy needle.

rouleau A roll of erythrocytes like a stack of coins.

saddle embolus An embolus consisting of a thrombus that comes to rest at the bifurcation of an artery, blocking both branches.

sand, brain Gritty material found in the pineal body, the choroid plexus, and other structures within the brain.

saponification Formation of soap or soaplike material.

sarcoplasm The cytoplasm of striated muscle fibers.

satellite A cell, structure, or lesion found in association with a larger one.

scaphoid Boatlike; said of an abdomen that appears concave when the subject is supine.

sclerosis Hardening.

secondary Due to some other condition or disease; as in "secondary hypertension" and "ischemia secondary to vascular occlusion." Cf. *primary.*

siderophage A macrophage that has ingested hemosiderin, a product of broken-down erythrocytes.

skin slip Abnormal mobility of the skin over subcutaneous structures due to early putrefactive changes in a dead body.

slough Complete separation of inflamed or devitalized tissue.

spondylitis Inflammation of one or more vertebrae.

stable Firm, displaying no abnormal mobility or looseness.

stellate Star-shaped.

stenosis Abnormal narrowing of an orifice or tubular structure.

stippling Speckling with fine dots.

storage disease A metabolic disorder that causes excessive accumulation of a substance such as glycogen in cells or tissues.

suture, cranial A joint between two of the bones of the cranial vault.

syndrome A combination of symptoms or abnormal signs having a common cause.

teratology The study of congenital and developmental abnormalities.

thermocoagulation Coagulation of tissue by excessive heat.

thora(co)centesis Removal of fluid from the thoracic cavity.

tortuous Twisted, winding.

toxicology The study of poisons and their effects on living organisms.

traction artifact Abnormal appearances created in tissue by suction or stretching during the obtaining of a biopsy specimen.

transect To cut across.

transudate A fluid low in fibrin and cells that has passed through a membrane.

trocar A sharp pointed instrument used to puncture a cavity.

Trucut needle A cutting biopsy needle.

Turner needle A biopsy needle for aspiration and cutting of solid tissue specimens.

umbilicated Having a central pit or dimple.

unattended death Death of a person not under medical care.

unremarkable Displaying no abnormal or unusual features.

urticaria Hives; a transitory eruption of itchy white papules (wheals) usually due to allergy.

vasoconstriction Constriction of blood vessels, principally arterioles.

vasodilatation Dilatation of blood vessels, principally arterioles.

vesicular Resembling a bladder; said of a cell nucleus whose chromatin has been displaced to the margin of the nucleus, creating a hollow or open appearance.

Virchow chisel An autopsy instrument used for splitting bone.

viremia The presence of a virus in the blood.

Westcott needle A cutting biopsy needle.

whorl A circular swirl or vortex.

xeroderma Abnormal dryness of the skin.

zymogen granules Secretory granules in the cytoplasm of glandular epithelium, representing precursors of enzymes.

Index

About the Author

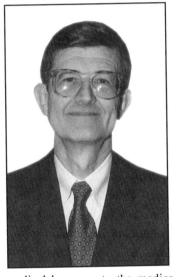

John H. Dirckx, M.D., has been director of the student health center at the University of Dayton in Dayton, Ohio, since 1968. His longstanding interest in classical and modern languages has led to the writing of several books and numerous articles on the language, literature, and history of medicine.

He is author of *The Language of Medicine: Its Evolution, Structure, and Dynamics,* 2nd ed. (New York: Praeger Publishers, 1983), *H & P: A Nonphysician's Guide to the Medical History and Physical Examination* (Modesto, Ca.: Health Professions Institute, 1987), and *Roundsmanship: An Introductory Manual* (Modesto: Health Professions Institute, 1987). He is a frequent contributor of articles on medical language to the medical transcription periodicals, *Perspectives on the Medical Transcription Profession* and *Journal of the American Association for Medical Transcription,* and is medical consultant for The SUM Program for Medical Transcription Training developed by Health Professions Institute.

He has acted as an editor, editorial consultant, or translator for various medical journals. His essay on the history and etymology of medical English appeared in the first edition of *Webster's Medical Desk Dictionary* (1986).

His hobbies include book-collecting and music. He is married, the father of five daughters, and has seven grandchildren.